CONTEMPORARY TOPICS IN IMMUNOBIOLOGY
VOLUME 4

CONTEMPORARY TOPICS IN IMMUNOBIOLOGY

A Continuation Order Plan is available for this series. A continuation order will bring delivery of each new volume immediately upon publication. Volumes are billed only upon actual shipment. For further information please contact the publisher.

CONTEMPORARY TOPICS IN IMMUNOBIOLOGY

VOLUME 4

INVERTEBRATE IMMUNOLOGY

EDITED BY
E. L. COOPER

Department of Anatomy
School of Medicine
University of California
Los Angeles, California

PLENUM PRESS • NEW YORK AND LONDON

Library of Congress Cataloging in Publication Data

Cooper, Edwin Lowell, 1936-
  Invertebrate immunology.

  (Contemporary topics in immunobiology, v. 4)
  Includes bibliographies.
  1. Immunology. 2. Invertebrates—Physiology. I. Title. II. Series. [DNLM: 1. Inver-
tebrates—Immunology. W1CO77 v. 4 1974 / QL362 I64 1974]
QR180.C632 vol. 4 [QR181] 574.2'9'08s
ISBN 0-306-37804-3   [592'.02'9]   74-6092

© 1974 Plenum Press, New York
A Division of Plenum Publishing Corporation
227 West 17th Street, New York, N.Y. 10011

United Kingdom edition published by Plenum Press, London
A Division of Plenum Publishing Company, Ltd.
4a Lower John Street, London W1R 3PD, England

Contributors to This Volume

R. T. Acton   *MRC Immunochemistry Unit, Department of Biochemistry, University of Oxford, South Parks Road, Oxford, QX13 QU, England*

R. S. Anderson   *Pathology Research Laboratories, Variety Club Heart Hospital, University of Minnesota, Minneapolis, Minnesota 55455, U.S.A.*

D. G. Baskin   *Department of Zoology, Seaver Laboratory, Pomona College, Claremont, California 91711, U.S.A.*

C. J. Bayne   *Department of Zoology, Oregon State University, Corvallis, Oregon 97331, U.S.A.*

Z. Brahmi   *Institut Pasteur d'Algerie, Alger, Algerie.*

W. J. Burdette   *The University of Texas (Houston), M. D. Anderson Hospital and Tumor Institute, Houston, Texas, U.S.A.*

F. M. Burnet   *School of Microbiology, University of Melbourne, Parkville, Victoria 3052, Australia*

Ann Cali   *Institute for Pathobiology, Lehigh University, Bethlehem, Pennsylvania 18015, U.S.A.*

T. C. Cheng   *Institute for Pathobiology, Lehigh University, Bethlehem, Pennsylvania 18015, U.S.A.*

J. D. Collins   *School of Biological Sciences, James Cook University of North Queensland, Townsville 4810, Australia*

E. L. Cooper   *Department of Anatomy, School of Medicine, University of California (Los Angeles), Los Angeles, California 90024, U.S.A.*

R. R. Cowden   *Department of Anatomy, Albany Medical College, Albany, New York 12208, U.S.A.*

Sherrill K. Curtis   *Department of Anatomy, Albany Medical College, Albany, New York 12208, U.S.A.*

T. G. Dix   *School of Biological Sciences, James Cook University of North Queensland, Townsville, 4810, Australia*

S. Y. Feng   *Marine Research Laboratory and Biological Sciences Group, University of Connecticut, Noank, Connecticut 06340, U.S.A.*

W. H. Hildemann   *School of Biological Sciences, James Cook University of North Queensland, Townsville, 4810, Australia*

H. R. Hilgard   *Division of Natural Sciences, University of California (Santa Cruz), Santa Cruz, California 95064, U.S.A.*

W. E. Hinds   *Division of Natural Sciences, University of California (Santa Cruz), Santa Cruz, California 95064, U.S.A.*

R. K. Hostetter   *Department of Antomy, School of Medicine, University of California (Los Angeles), Los Angeles, California 90024, U.S.A.*

C. R. Jenkin   *Department of Microbiology, University of Adelaide, Adelaide, South Australia*

C. A. Lemmi   *Department of Antomy, School of Medicine, University of California (Los Angeles), Los Angeles, California 90024, U.S.A. and Transplantation Laboratory, Department of Surgery, Harbor General Hospital, Torrance, California 90502, U.S.A.*

D. McKay   *Department of Microbiology, University of Adelaide, Adelaide, South Australia*

T. C. Moore — *Transplantation Laboratory, Department of Surgery, Harbor General Hospital, Torrance, California 90502, U.S.A.*

A. J. Nappi — *Biological Sciences, State University of New York (Oswego), Oswego, New York, U.S.A.*

L. Nyhlén — *Institute of Physiological Botany, University of Uppsala, Uppsala, Sweden*

G. B. Pauley — *Eastern Fish Disease Laboratory, Leetown, Route 1, Box 17, Kearneysville, West Virginia 25430, U.S.A.*

G. O. Poinar, Jr. — *Division of Entomology and Parasitology, Agricultural Experiment Station, College of Agricultural Sciences, University of California (Berkeley), Berkeley, California 94720, U.S.A.*

W. Schwemmler — *Institut Für Biologie II, Lehrstuhl Für Mikrobiologie, Universitat Freiburg, D-7800 Freiburg i. Br., B.D.R.*

S. Shostak — *Department of Biology, University of Pittsburgh, Pittsburgh, Pennsylvania 15260, U.S.A.*

Christiane Stang-Voss — *Anatomical Institute, University of Freiburg, 78 Freiburg i. Br., B.D.R.*

J. E. Stewart — *Fisheries Research Board of Canada, Halifax Laboratory, P.O. Box 429, Halifax, Nova Scotia, Canada*

M. R. Tripp — *Department of Biology, University of Delaware, Newark, Delaware, U.S.A.*

C. J. Tyson — *Department of Microbiology, University of Adelaide, Adelaide, South Australia*

T. Unestam — *Institute of Physiological Botany, University of Uppsala, Uppsala, Sweden*

P. Valembois — *Laboratoire de Zoologie de l'Université de Bordeaux I, Institut de Biologie Animale, Avenue des Facultés, 33405 Talence, France*

R. H. Wander   *Division of Natural Sciences, University of California (Santa Cruz), Santa Cruz, California 95064, U.S.A.*

P. F. Weinheimer   *Department of Medicine, Division of Clinical Immunology and Rheumatology, University of Alabama (Birmingham), Birmingham, Alabama 35294, U.S.A.*

B. M. Zwicker   *Fisheries Research Board of Canada, Halifax Laboratory, P.O. Box 429, Halifax, Nova Scotia, Canada*

Foreword

This fourth volume of *Contemporary Topics In Immunobiology* treats invertebrate immunity. Specifically, the results represent several approaches to humoral and cellular immunity. It is evident that invertebrates do have functioning immune systems. For example, cellular immunity is characterized by both specificity and memory, but it is still problematical whether vertebrate immune capacity evolved directly from invertebrates.

Most of the manuscripts were formally presented at the International Symposium on Invertebrate Pathology, University of Minnesota, August 1972, held in connection with the 25th anniversary celebration of the American Institute of Biological Sciences.

I wish to express my appreciation to the contributors and to beg their indulgence in what may have been overzealous editing. This was done, though, in the interest of clarity and to seek uniformity. Because of earlier problems, time limitations did not permit consultations between submission of manuscripts and final editing.

For assistance, I extend a special note of gratitude to Mrs. Lois Gehringer who unselfishly retyped many of the manuscripts.

The preparation of this volume was aided partially by NSF Grant GB17767, two grants from The California Institute for Cancer Research, and a grant from The Brown-Hazen Corporation.

E.L.C.

Contents

Chapter 23. **Hemagglutinins: Primitive Receptor Molecules**
      Operative in Invertebrate Defense Mechanisms
      Ronald T. Acton and Peter F. Weinheimer

Chapter 24. **Tumors in *Drosophila* and Antibacterial Immunity**
      Walter J. Burdette

Chapter 25. **A Final Comment on Invertebrate Immunity**

Introduction

"One only understands the things that one tames, said the fox."

The Little Prince (p. 67)
Antoine De Saint-Exupéry

One significant milestone in the history of immunology was the discovery of phagocytosis by Metchnikoff. A Russian zoologist, Metchnikoff arrived at the Pasteur Institute during the latter half of the 19th century. Prior to his arrival in France, he had observed that starfish larvae (Phylum Echinodermata) are transparent, a condition which allowed easy viewing of their mobile amoeboid cells. After sticking thorns into these larvae, he discovered on the next day, that the thorns had been surrounded by amoeboid cells. Later, he studied this same phenomenon in *Daphnia* (Phylum Arthropoda), this time using the destruction of the yeast *Monospora bicuspidata,* a pathogen for the water flea. These discoveries culminated in his theory of phagocytosis, which has persisted as an antecedent of modern cellular immunology. Furthermore, of equal importance, much of invertebrate immunology today, reviewed in this volume, traces its history from these observations.

As you will understand after reading the first chapter by Sir MacFarlane Burnet, immunology should be again indebted to him, this time for alerting us to the relevance of invertebrate immunology. Since the proposal of the clonal selection theory, a more recent concern is immunologic surveillance. Burnet seeks to define how cells recognize the difference between *self* and *not-self* — a fascinating question of general interest to immunobiologists — but, more importantly, a question whose answer may illuminate how neoplastic cells are recog-

1

nized and disposed of. He offers several examples of recognition among sponges (Phylum Porifera) and colonial ascidians (Subphylum Urochordata) and then addresses himself briefly to self-incompatibility in plants, probably a pseudoimmunological response. Finally, he sets the stage for what we may derive from an understanding of the relationship among hemagglutinins, opsonins, and his hypothetical immunocyte ancestors, the primitive invertebrate mobile cells. The complex hemagglutinins could have acted as recognition units, bound to cell surfaces, ready for discriminating between self and pathogenic not-self. According to Burnet:

> From the point of view of comparative immunology, the most interesting future development could be a demonstration that invertebrate hemocytes (or some subgroup of these cells) were capable of differentiation into forms analogous to immunocytes, i.e., multiple clones of cells each with a distinctive pattern or range of patterns of steric reactivity. There are phenomena which hint at specific adaptive immune responses in coelomate invertebrates, but until immunocytes with specific receptors are defined, one must remain skeptical.

For those actively studying invertebrate cellular and humoral immunity, there is both cautious praise and criticism. Although Burnet recognizes the existence of immune responses in invertebrates with resemblances to vertebrate immune responses, he warns against searching for precise equivalence of invertebrate and vertebrate reactions. With concurrence, the following may still be offered in response to this cogent observation. Most invertebrate immunologists are usually first biologists, aware of the animals and their particular habits. Secondly, they are immunologists, often groping for definitions, criteria, and parameters which many times only come from those established by vertebrate studies. A way out of the dilemma is continued, but more imaginative, research and mutual tolerance between invertebrate and vertebrate immunologists.

It is appropriate that a symposium devoted to *Invertebrate Immunology* consider some detailed events in phagocytosis, which is exceedingly important to invertebrates and vertebrates. Resistance and recovery from pathogenic infections is impossible without this ubiquitous capacity, even in the unicellular protozoans. Although protozoans combine food-getting and defense in the single act of phagocytosis, the two reactions become separate in multicellular animals with cell·specialization. Three chapters deal with phagocytosis, beginning with the fate of bacteria injected into the land snail, observations of oyster granulocytes by electron microscopy, and the metabolism of cockroach hemocytes.

The work of Bayne is concerned with the clearance of massive doses of *Serratia marcesens* from the hemolymph of snails. He arrives at astronomical calculations based on clearance rates, suggesting almost impossible feats. To account for this, Bayne stresses that phagocytosis is apparently not the sole mechanism for clearing small particles and implies that substantial elimination occurs in certain tissues and organs. That the response could be specific remains to be determined.

In the descriptions of Cheng and Cali, bacteria phagocytosed by oyster granulocytes can be found later within cytoplasmic vacuoles situated between vesicles. In the light microscope, vesicles are cytoplasmic granules that appear to be membrane-bound. By means of transmission and scanning electron microscopes, they derive a terminology describing granule structure, composed of a membrane, cortex, and core. The core, devoid of inclusions, is the site of active degradation of foreign material and glycogen synthesis. Once inside the cytoplasm, bacteria are digested within cytoplasmic vacuoles. Presumably after complete or partially complete degradation, the material is passed on to the vesicles, and this is followed by glycogen synthesis. Although oyster granulocytes are a part of a complex multicellular animal, they still retain the capacity for defense by phagocytosis; nutrition is a by-product of the process as well.

Anderson's chapter is unique in comparing the activities of an invertebrate hemocyte with an analogous mammalian cell. Glycolysis is stimulated in cockroach hemocytes and mammalian leukocytes by the process of ingestion. Despite this one similarity, there is one major difference, i.e., the myeloperoxidase-halide-hydrogen peroxide antibacterial system of mammalian leukocytes is apparently nonfunctional in cockroach hemocytes. Anderson's studies point out that defects in leukocyte metabolism from patients with chronic granulomatous disease result in failure to kill certain microorganisms permitting expression of the disease.

Baskin's beautiful electron micrographs provide glimpses of the structural complexity of nereid coelomocytes. His observations are important for those delving into cellular immunity in general but earthworms in particular. Nereids are polychaete or marine annelids, and earthworms are oligochaete or terrestrial annelids. Baskin acknowledges the confusion that prevails when one views blood cells, and I would add that similar cloudiness prevails whether one studies blood cells derived from marine worms, manure worms, or mice. For example, the important phagocytic eleocyte is often referred to as phagocyte, amoebocyte, or leukocyte. He cautions that combined morphologic and developmental studies must precede a final adequate understanding of coelomocytes in worm defense reactions. Nevertheless, they, like other invertebrate blood or coelomic cells, conform to Burnet's hypothetical wandering cell, which recognizes and reacts to antigen. We are left with choosing the appropriate cells and determining, by rigorous analyses, how they are sensitive to (recognize) and how they react to (affect) antigens.

The electron micrographs of Stang-Voss provide oligochaete cells complementary to Baskin's polychaete coelomocytes, but she has added two additional cell types, the coagulation cell and the erythrocytelike cell of molluscs and arthropods. The electron micrographs are exquisite and, aside from the wealth of scientific information relevant to immunity, they provide an esthetic respite from the usual tables, curves, and histograms. One suspects that the central aim is to understand blood cell differentiation from the comparative viewpoint; thus this skill could be extended to several invertebrate groups. She makes the somewhat startling revelation that the hemoglobin-containing hemolymph of *Eisenia foetida* possesses two types of cells: eleocytes derived from chlorogogen tissue and phagocytic amoebocytes which differentiate from cells of the septal and parietal peritoneum. According to her observations, the eleocytes of *Eisenia* act as erythrocytelike cells containing hemoglobin crystals and deposits of ferritin. The presence of effete eleocytes suggests that pigment is released into the hemolymph. She does not mention coelomocytes from the coelomic cavity. We have worked with the marine annelid *Glycera* which contains numerous hemoglobin-bearing erythrocytes. Unlike the blood of *Eisenia*, which appears clear to us without formed elements, the blood of *Glycera* contains, in addition to the erythrocytes, leukocytes, which for most earthworms are lodged separately from the blood, in the coelomic cavity. We now know something of the cytologic complexity of invertebrate immune cells.

The electron micrographs of Cowden and Curtis are valuable not so much because of their clarity, but because they represent, for the first time, descriptions of leukocytes derived from a discrete invertebrate organ. As a result, the octopus *white body,* long known to be a leukocyte source, can now join ranks with the vertebrate thymus and lymph nodes. We could witness mass migrations to the Zoological Station at Naples where octopi are readily available in the shadow of Vesuvius. Is there demonstrable specific activity *in vivo* in cells of the white body? Can these cells be grown in *in vitro*? How do they respond to antigens? For the future, let us deemphasize straight morphology in favor of more physiologic experiments. These three papers by Baskin, Stang-Voss, and Cowden and Curtis, taken together, indicate a hitherto unknown complex structure of invertebrate immune cells, both at the free-cell and organ-confined levels.

Three laboratories (Cooper, Duprat, Valembois) have worked independently since the early 1960's on graft rejection in earthworms. Two of the groups, however, are represented in this volume by three relevant contributions. Earthworms clearly do recognize the difference between self and not-self. Their mechanisms for handling tissue antigens, according to the present information, is characterized as highly specific and accompanied by an anamnestic component. Coelomocytes mediate graft rejection, a contention based on ordinary histology, adoptive transfer experiments, electron microscopy, and quantitative comparisons of coelomocyte reactions to autografts, xenografts, and wounds.

The paper of Hostetter and Cooper is informative, particularly because of the excellent hypothetical schemes accounting for immunity in earthworms. These have never been published and represent entirely independent observations by Hostetter. Our most recent observations show that coelomocytes can reveal specific memory responses only to xenografts, not autografts nor wounds. Lemmi is aware of current trends in mammalian cellular immunology con-

ceptually, and he uses them to approach earthworm coelomocyte characteristics. His hypotheses are not entirely fanciful and should serve as exciting
stimuli for future work. Valembois's account is both necessary and informative, for it reviews current experimentation on earthworm graft immunity in
France. His ideas are important since they account, for the first time, for
immunity in coelomate *vs.* acoelomate invertebrates. According to his scheme,
coelomate animals (e.g., earthworms) possess a system of cells, the coelomocytes, capable of reacting specifically to various foreign insults. Only recognition
occurs in more primitive phyla.

Shotak's transplantations in hydra are intriguing. Cnidarians have reached
a level of organismic complexity so that transplantation techniques can be used
advantageously for analyzing such developmental problems as growth and form.
Of more pertinence to us, incompatibilities occur after grafting that clearly
resemble graft destruction in advanced invertebrates. Shostak supports the
compromise position between those interested in "the [ambiguous] biological
roots of recognition, sensitivity, specificity, and anamnesis," and those [with
predetermined views] searching for [the] "characteristics of the immune
systems found in primitive organisms." Thus, he pursues such questions as "what
does a primitive organism do in response to a challenge a vertebrate would
respond to with its immune system?"

With skill, patience, and a genuine concern for the well being of their sub-
jects, Hildemann, Dix, and Collins have provided us with a unique account of
transplantation among diverse marine invertebrates such as: corals (*Acropora*),
pearl oysters (*Pinctada margaritifera*), and certain echinoderms, e.g., the sea
cucumber (*Cucumaria tricolor*) and the horned sea star (*Protoreaster nodosus*).
Hildemann's links with vertebrate immunology often provide us with the needed
bridge, term, or concept, since essentially all our information comes from vertebrate research. Furthermore, his biologic predilection reminds the cautious, but
forces the inexperienced, to beware of the pitfalls of animal husbandry and
technique when dealing with exotic animals. Finally, his beginning analyses of
transplantation reactions in these newer species introduce other invertebrates
where characteristics of cell-mediated immunity can be analyzed.

One of the first contributions to invertebrate immunology which made a
strong case for the existence of cellular receptors was the clever approach used
by Hilgard, Wander, and Hinds. Hilgard ackowledges the increasing evidence that
cellular immune memory does occur in several invertebrates (e.g., annelids) but
assumes that invertebrates lack memory. According to his idea of an invertebrate immune system which lacks memory, there are several criteria: immunocompetent cells bear specific surface receptor molecules. When such a cell meets
an antigen, if it has the complementary receptor, a receptor—antigen complex is
formed that signals the synthesis of new receptor molecules to replace those
already complexed with antigen. In the presence of free antigen to combine with

receptors, new receptors are synthesized rapidly. However, when all the antigen is complexed, the system returns to its original state, i.e. a "background" number of cells producing receptors at the same rate as before encounter with antigen. This system accounts for recognition of nonself, with specificity, but no immune memory and therefore no accelerated clearance of antigen. Aside from those receptors needed to complex with antigen, there are no antibodies or overproduction of receptors. Hilgard's kind of analyses, if extended to other invertebrates, should be appropriate to elevate invertebrate coelomocytes from the mire of mere phagocytes to receptor and effector cells.

More to the heart of the problem of recognition of foreignness in invertebrates is a situation that creates a direct confrontation between invertebrate immune cells and antigen. Tyson, McKay, and Jenkin in their careful studies observed the interaction between crayfish hemocytes and erythrocytes and bacteria. Since crayfish are easily obtained and maintained in the laboratory and provide from $2-5 \times 10^6$ hemocytes/ml, they are ideal animals for cellular recognition studies. Their results suggest that the hemagglutinin in crayfish hemolymph is equivalent to the opsonin since erythrocytes must be pretreated with hemolymph to ensure phagocytosis. Adsorption of hemolymph from one type of erythrocyte removes the hemagglutinin and opsonin for that erythrocyte, and both opsonic and hemagglutinating activity are always found in the same fraction. With their work, we are somewhat closer to pinpointing the executors of nonself recognition.

Not all investigations dealing with immunity are concerned with cell-mediated responses to cells, particulate antigens, or microbes. A substantial amount of work has treated invertebrate immune reactions to parasites, especially nematodes. Poinar presents a review of the several known insect defense reactions including simple encapsulation, usually by hemocytes that isolate parasites within capsules. He warns against confusing encapsulation, phagocytosis, and encystment. Encystment is effected by a parasite itself, resulting in the formation of a membrane or cyst around itself. In the case of melanotic encapsulation, surrounding hemocytes produce a dark pigment, melanin, around the body of a parasite. Humoral melanization can occur within one hour after a parasite enters the host by means of homogeneous deposits of pigment granules. These enlarge and coalesce to form layers of melanin around the deposit. Finally, tissue reactions represent a fourth type of immune response to parasitic nematodes. In this reaction, once parasitized, surrounding cells form syncytial giant cells.

As threats to the lives of invertebrates, fungi are active against crustacean arthropods. Indeed, Unestam and Nyhlin inform us that unlike vertebrates, fungi "compete" successfully with bacteria in insects. In fact, with regard to diseases of invertebrates other than insects, fungal infections outnumber those caused by bacteria. In the case of arthropods, the first reaction is growth of hyphae penetrating the outer tough chitin. With regard to the crayfish plague fungus, hemocytes first encapsulate *Aphanoncyces astaci* and other phycomycetes which penetrate the European crayfish, *Astacus astacus,* or the American, *Pacifastacus leniusculus.* Reactions in internal organs rarely occur since hyphae never seem to penetrate further than the outer integument. Like the insect response to parasites, crustaceans synthesize melanin in the cuticle, constituting the most concentrated known host response to fungal attack.

The account of Nappi is all encompassing since he details several interlocking areas, namely, mechanisms of recognition of foreignness by insect hemocytes, and controls of the process — the endocrine system. He draws largely from his own work and from that of the pioneer investigator Salt. Nappi stresses that we are unable to answer fundamental questions about hemocyte kinetics and interactions owing to a lack of comparative and quantitative studies of hemocyte activities during infection. He recognizes further that there is little information on blood cell differentiation. For future experimentation, he suggests that hormonal imbalances cause hemocytic changes resulting in encapsulation and melanization of parasites. Such results could naturally lead to a genetic analysis of tumor development, which in turn could lead to studies of hemocyte reactions to tumors.

Schwemmler provides an interesting model of symbiosis involving the small leafhopper, *Euscelsis plebejus* F., whose existence depends on intracellular symbionts. At least two symbionts exists (*a* and *t*), and they are placed as "protoplastoids" between viruses and mycoplasma. The model involves several processes which should be of interest to students of differentiation and those concerned with recognition mechanisms. The model is clearly outlined and involves hemolymph and factors such as lysozyme and hormones.

Lysozyme is a universal macromolecule found in plants and animals. According to Feng's review, it can occur in animals other than invertebrates, in body fluids, in tears, mucus, or milk. It was found in oyster hemolymph and mantle mucus first by McDade and Tripp. Feng has extended these observations considerably by linking oyster lysozyme to humoral immunity. Lysozymes in numerous invertebrates are lytic since they (1) reduce the turbidity of a suspension of isolated cell walls of *Micrococcus lysodeikticus,* (2) release reducing groups, (3) liberate acetylamino sugar complex of glucosamino and the acidic hexosamine. By physicochemical analyses, Feng showed that oyster lysozyme is not related to egg white lysozyme. It contains two anodal bands and is a basic protein, unlike egg white lysozyme, which is cathodal and acidic in electrophoresis. From these comparisons, he concludes that the lysozymelike activity found in oyster hemolymph might represent a case of functional convergence during the course of biochemical evolution.

According to Stewart and Zwicker, the American lobster, like other animals, is vulnerable to a fatal infection, a microorganism, *Gaffkya homari,* causing gaffkemia. Apparently the disease appears when the lobster's phagocytic, bactericidal, and agglutinating capacities are incapable of reducing its severity. Lobster hemagglutinin agglutinates a wide variety of microorganisms but none of the four strains of *G. homari*. Even after phagocytosis *in vivo*, *G. homari* remains in the host, causing massive decline in circulating hemocyte numbers prior to death. Stewart and Zwicker's only successful attempts to induce resistance to the disease were injections of lobsters with vaccines prepared from avirulent strains of *G. homari* which gave a degree of resistance to virulent strains. These studies are of obvious practical importance. Here we recognize a known disease and can apply the techniques of invertebrate immunology to an immediate mission.

The arthropods, particularly the crustaceans, have been essential to understanding hemagglutinin structure and function. Pauley's account is important because, for the first time, we have information on the blue crab, *Callinectes sapidus*. It appears universal that all advanced invertebrates possess naturally occurring agglutinins. Pauley provides us with a firsthand account of the approaches used by invertebrate "hemagglutinologists." Furthermore, he reviews and compares the sea hare *Aplysia californica* agglutinins with those of the crayfish, *Procambarus clarkii*, both experimental animals from his laboratory. Pauley believes that the blue crab agglutinin, like other agglutinins, is equivalent to an opsonin.

The chapter by Brahmi and Cooper is a straightforward approach to a rather "new" animal, the scorpion, and an old problem, hemolymph agglutinins. It is noteworthy that these studies represent satellite observations peripheral to the special task of preparing antiserum against scorpion venom, a potent threat to the people of Algeria. Secondly, a more detailed study should lead to independent confirmations of what Marchalonis and Edelman found in the horseshoe crab. One additional advantage of the scorpion, like the octopus, is the presence of a discrete organ from which the hemocytes are derived. Invertebrates with such organs provide easily approached cellular systems whereby cells can be analyzed from several viewpoints *in vitro*: their labeling qualities, responses to various antigens, reconstitutive abilities. For those with "thick skin," scorpions are quite easy to maintain, husband, and handle.

Acton and Weinheimer's review of hemagglutinins is crucial for several reasons. Because of their intense work in this aspect of invertebrate immunity and their ties with vertebrate immunologists, they are able to view relationships (where they exist) between invertebrate humoral components, such as agglutinins, hemolysins, lysins, *etc.*, and vertebrate immunoglobulins. They are versed in both camps and have given, therefore, complete reviews and stimulating hypotheses. For example, they draw from their own physicochemical analyses and the investigations of other workers (notably Marchalonis and Edelman, Hammerström and Kabat, Jenkin and Rowley, Fuller and Doolittle, and Tripp) to offer the following hypothesis: hemagglutinins and other components, such as opsonins, are the primitive receptor molecules of invertebrates. A primordial gene coded for a molecule of approximately 20,000 molecular weight. By various alterations certain genes evolved coding for hemagglutinin molecules of about 69,000, as in the spiny lobster. By other considerable further mutations, molecules with diverse functions were produced. A final suggestion is based on the work of Marchalonis and Edelman on the lamprey. The lamprey (primitive vertebrate) hemagglutinin molecule, which differs from the lamprey immunoglobulin, deserves intense investigation; it could be a linking remnant between invertebrates and vertebrates.

Cancer is of international interest because it is a dreaded human disease. Its riddance is poorly understood and still more dismaying, its *raison d' etre*. That the immune system may be involved in preventing spread of cancer may not be readily obvious. However, Burnet's concept of immunologic surveillance indicates that the immune system evolved not only to prevent extinction by disease and parasites, but to guard against the possibility of unchecked cancerous growth resulting from mutant cells. This is accomplished by immunocytes recognizing not-self cells which must somehow be sequestered prior to destruction of a host organism. Since Burnet's concept is rooted partially in evolution of immune mechanism, we are in the advantageous positon of reporting on primitive immune mechanisms in some animals which do develop recognizable neoplasms.

Looking at antibacterial immunity and tumors in *Drosophila*, Burdette offers us a glimpse into another area of deep concern — comparative oncogenesis. Fruit fly tumors are melanotic, gradually dissolve as larvae approach metamorphosis, are benign, and apparently are controlled by multiple genes. Nitrogen mustard, 20-methylcholanthrene, irradiation, and other agents increase tumor incidence in certain populations. Similar results are obtained when oncogenic RNA and DNA viruses are introduced by feeding and inoculating flies. As also mentioned by Nappi, insect tumors, *Drosophila* no exception, respond to the stimulus of molting and juvenile hormones. To unite tumor formation and bacterial immunity, Burdette found that humoral immunity was impaired in the tumor strain with a high incidence of spontaneous melanotic tumors. Because the tumors may result from altered hemocyte behavior, a link is suggested between immunity and tumorogenesis.

It was not our intention to include techniques in this series of papers, yet some few details of methods remain. This volume should be of sufficient general interest to a wide audience, not only immunologists, zoologists, and pathologists, but also to another important group — ecologists and environmentalists. Thus, some minutia stays, if for no other reason than to stimulate thought and criticism relative to our approaches. Finally, for the forgetful or the newcomer, a taxonomic scheme is provided. In it can be seen examples of those familiar creatures that we either eat, swat, despise, use for bait, or exterminate. Regardless of the niche they occupy in the order of one's esthetic preferences, they are exciting and valuable tools for immunology. In these austere days of antiscience, less expensive animals for immunologic research, with alluring habitats, are welcome.

A NOTE ON TAXONOMY

The following classification scheme is modified from many sources. It is included to acquaint you with those animals not commonly used in immunology research. It would do us well to recognize their importance, since according to Hickman (1967), "at present, about 1,200,000 different species of animals have been named, and about 10,000 new species are added to the list each year. More than 90% of these species belong to the invertebrates." Of that total, at least 75% of all species belong to the phylum arthropoda.

A CLASSIFICATION OF ANIMALS

Phylum Protozoa	Acellular animals, usually unicellular
Phylum Porifera	The sponges
*Phylum Coelenterata or Cnidaria	Aquatic, mostly marine, tissue grade organisms; jelly fishes, sea anemones, hydra
Phylum Platyhelminthes	Flatworms
Phylum Aschelminthes	Rotifers, round worms, arrow worms, horsehair worms, gastrotrichs
Phylum Acanthocephala	Spiny headed worms
*Phylum Annelida	Segmented worms, terrestrial (earthworms); marine (*Nereis*)
*Phylum Mollusca	Slugs, oysters, clams, snails, octopuses, squids
*Phylum Arthropoda	Insects, crayfish, lobsters, crabs, spiders, scorpions
*Phylum Echinodermata	Starfish, sea urchins
Phylum Chordata	Chordate animals: notochord, pharyngeal gill slits
Subphylum Hemichordata	Acorn worms
Subphylum Cephalochordata	Lancelets
Subphylum Tunicata (Urochordata)	Ascidians

*Indicates phyla actually represented in this volume.

Subphylum Vertebrata
    Superclass Pisces   Aquatic vertebrates (fishes)
    Superclass Tetrapoda   Terrestrial vertebrates (tetrapods)
      Classes
        Amphibia, Reptilia,
        Aves, Mammalia

E.L.C

REFERENCE

Hickman, C. P., 1967, *Biology of the Invertebrates,* C. V. Mosby Company, St. Louis.

Chapter 1

Invertebrate Precursors to Immune Responses

F. M. Burnet

School of Microbiology
University of Melbourne
Parkville, Victoria, Australia

INTRODUCTION

As long as there are useful invertebrates like earthworms, oysters, or honey bees to be protected, and others like tapeworms, slugs, and mosquitoes to be destroyed, there will be a utilitarian justification for studying invertebrate pathology and whatever is equivalent in them to what we study in vertebrates as immunology. Nevertheless, I fancy that most contributors to this symposium are interested mainly in what, if any, light such studies of invertebrates can throw on the evolution of the processes of inflammation and immunity as we see them in man and the experimental mammals of the laboratory. Since Darwin, much of the "fun" of biological research has been to interpret what directly interests one in evolutionary terms. This introduction is stimulated almost wholly by my interest in the phylogeny of the immune responses and will touch only on findings that appear to be relevant to that theme.

SELF AND NOT-SELF

Current hypotheses suggest that chloroplasts and mitochondria are, in a fairly literal sense, the descendants of prokaryotes, approximately equivalent to blue-green algae and bacteria, respectively, which developed as symbionts in some early organisms on the borderline between prokaryotic and eukaryotic character. At that stage there must often have been situations in which there was no clear *individuality* of organism in these tentative cooperations between primitive forms. However, once well defined eukaryotes, animal or plant, emerged, each organism, and to some extent each cell, had its own definable existence as an individual.

13

In this paper I am concerned primarily with animal forms, although it is already clear that in flowering plants the need to avoid self-fertilization has resulted in the evolution of what might be called a para-immunological approach to its prevention. I have included a brief note about these phenomena, which perhaps are not as well known to immunologists as they should be.

If we accept an amoeba or any typical protozoon as a prototype animal, the relationship of self and not-self becomes immediately important when digestion of food particles, often living microorganisms, within the cytoplasm becomes the standard form of nutrition. In some way, the food particle, with its proteins of much the same character as those of the ingestor, must be disintegrated without more than minimal harm to the cytoplasm. The same requirement, progressively refined, holds equally for phagocytic cells in all metazoan forms, and the more the substance of the cell or cell fragments taken in as food resembles the substance of the ingesting cell, the more refined will have to be the differentiation between self and not-self.

With the development of multicellular animals, from the sponges upward, a new necessity arose to prevent "intrusion" of any other type of living system into cells of the organism. By the time this stage had been reached, every organism was the product of some millions of years of independent evolution during which each line had developed its own elaborations and modifications of the basic biochemical mechanisms. In every functioning organism, hundreds of simultaneously active functions must be coordinated, and it is clearly intolerable that a different set of reactions should intrude into a region where they must distort the normal pattern. An equally important requirement for evolutionary survival that had to develop is the capacity to repair a traumatized region of the body. In broad terms, a cell must present a surface which delimits it and offers some resistance (appropriate to its situation) to intrusion of microorganisms or larger cells but which is also capable of "recognizing" and interacting physiologically with cells that are appropriately in contact with it, i.e., those which are genetically identical and are there either as established structural cells or as part of a repair process. On general grounds, the most effective counter to a damaging mechanical, chemical, or biological intrusion into a cell is to segregate the damaged cell from adjacent undamaged tissue, reject it, and repair the gap. That statement is made in *a priori* form but does, of course, also outline the general quality of responses in higher forms. In any case, it provides a suitable framework in which to discuss some of the types of not-self recognition that are seen in invertebrate situations.

"SELF-RECOGNITION" IN COLONIAL MARINE FORMS

Sponges

The classical example of self/not-self differentiation in invertebrates was described by Wilson in 1907, using marine sponges. He found that when living sponge tissue was dissociated into single cells in sea water, the cells soon formed small aggregates which eventually developed into sponges typical of the species. When cells from two sponges of different colors were mixed, they sorted themselves out to form aggregates, each composed of one species of cell and giving rise to typically distinct sponges. Moscona (1968) has carried out much recent work with this system, using the sponges *Haliciona* and *Microciona*. In both species, auto- or isografts, even with individuals from distant localities, were readily accepted, but grafts from the foreign type were rapidly rejected. When Wilson's experiment is done using sea water lacking divalent cations, reaggregation does not occur. Moscona considers that specific reaggregation is due to the presence of a surface glycoprotein which in the presence of Ca^{++} and Mg^{++} acts as a specific ligand. Curtis (1972) considers the evidence quite inadequate to establish this view. Adhesion between cell surfaces is extraordinarily complex physically, and very critical experiments would be needed to establish the molecular mechanism of a specific example of adhesion. He believes, however, that when cells from two distinct races (α and δ) of the fresh-water sponge *Ephydatia fluviatilis* are mixed and allowed to reaggregate, they form units specific for race. Analysis of the process led to the conclusion that the strains produce soluble substances which act on cells of heterologous strains to diminish their adhesion while increasing the adhesion of cells of the homologous strain (Curtis and Van de Vyver, 1971). In Curtis' view the specificity resides in the control of the strength of adhesion and not in the mechanism of the adhesion itself. His approach, therefore, is a purely negative one which has no bearing on the question of the genetic control and molecular nature of the specificity. It does, however, make it necessary to realize the extreme complexity of biological systems. Whenever the existence of a recognition process is postulated, its nature must eventually be defined by isolation and characterization of the interacting molecules if the hypothesis is to be accepted. This need not, however, inhibit analysis at the genetic and para-immunological level of specific interactions in the search for evolutionary analogies.

Colonial Ascidians

Probably the best studied example of self-recognition by lower invertebrates concerns colonial ascidians of the genus *Botryllus*. These have been studied in Japan by Oka and his associates and by Sabbadin in Italy. These organisms multiply both by budding and sexually, and conditions in nature are such as to virtually enforce heterozygosity. They are hermaphroditic, but self-fertilization is prevented in the European form by an asynchrony between ripening of the oocytes and liberation of the sperm (Sabbadin, 1971). Self-fertilization is possible in the laboratory but is significantly less effective in producing viable offspring. There is, however, no evidence of self-incompatibility as almost equally high percentages of eggs are fertilized in suitably timed self-fertilizations as in

Table I. Rules of Fusion in *Botryllus*[a]

Genotype of colony	Fusion occurs with		None with	
AC	AB, AC, AD, BC	AB-AC	BD	
AD	AB, AC, AD, BD	AB-AC	BC	
AC-AD	AB, AC, AD	AB-AC	BD, BC	AC-BC

[a] After Oka (1970) and Mukai (1967).

natural cross-fertilizations. The Japanese form, *B. primigenus*, is said by Oka (1970) to be incapable of self-fertilization, and in a footnote he comments that the situation appears to be analogous to self-incompatibility in plants.

All authors agree that any two colonies found in their natural environment can be accepted as heterozygous in regard to the fusion qualities that concern the present topic, and can be given the designations AB and CD, representing the alleles responsible. The F_1 generation will include AC, AD, BC, and BD forms, which can be sorted out by a series of fusion experiments. When separated portions of two natural colonies, AB and CD, are placed together with cut edges in apposition, early interaction between the vascular tubes results in a zone of necrosis and failure to fuse. Two pieces of colony AB, placed similarly in apposition, fuse, and their vascular tubes rapidly establish continuity. Results with F_1 and F_2 colonies are consistent with the rule that fusion occurs when either one or two alleles are common to the interacting pieces. AC will fuse with AC, AB, AD, BC, and CD, but not with BD. When a semihomologous fusion occurs (e.g., AC with AB), there is interchange of soluble and cellular components, and, according to Mukai (1967), if the pieces are separated again after four days, each has become equivalent to the other and can be represented AB—AC. The general rule seems to be that whenever there is a heterologous pair (e.g., AC, BD) involved, directly or indirectly, fusion fails to occur; the existence of a homologous component in such complex pairs does not prevent failure of fusion. This adds a complication which will require much careful experimentation on the cellular and molecular conditions in the semihomologous chimeras in order to elucidate an explanation. In a fairly simple-minded approach, one can at least assume that some form of mutual recognition — steric complementarity — is concerned in mediating the differences in responses. When we are dealing with a biological situation where specificity is determined by multiple (in this case very numerous) alleles, we can eliminate with reasonable certainty any suggestion that the small, primitive organism has a battery of receptors, each tuned to any one of a hundred or more foreign patterns. The recognition must be a positive one between two of its own constituents, the damaging effect being a nonspecific process that can be inhibited by the occurrence of the specific recognition. In a previous paper (Burnet, 1971) I suggested that in an AC animal each cell is likely to have *A, a,* and *C, c* surface proteins in which *A* and *a* have a specific steric relationship, as do *C* and *c.* As long as an adequate number of *Cc, aA, aC,* or *Aa* contacts are made, the relationship is stable. If none, or an inadequate number, can be made, damaging interaction occurs. This is very much an *ad hoc* hypothesis which leaves the whole nature of the necrotic effect unexplained. Many more facts are needed, in particular a clear molecular demonstration that complementary pairs such as *A* and *a* do actually exist. Even if their presence is accepted, it does not necessarily follow that interaction produces anything resembling an antigen—antibody union. All that may be necessary is that highly reversible specific contact should initiate an effective signal to one or both cells concerned. This might take place without experimental demonstration of specific cell adhesion.

General Aspects

There may well be a common genetic requirement for colonial invertebrates to be able to distinguish their own colony from another, though it does not follow that the same method of doing so is always used. Findings somewhat similar to those in *Botryllus* have been reported by Theodor (1966, 1970) for the Gorgonians (Anthozoa), *Eunicella* and *Lephogorgia. Eunicella,* the form used in most experiments, is found in the form of branching colonies, each branch having a firm scleroprotein axis which supports a fused mass of living tissue made up of many individual zooids. Theodor used a simple technique of taking branch segments 25–30 mm long and denuding a central 2–3 mm. The denuded areas of two segments were then brought together to form the meeting point of a right-angled cross. When such preparation are maintained in a suitable environment, regrowth occurs at the denuded region. If both segments are from the same colony, all four growing surfaces fuse without any sign of discontinuity. When one segment is from colony A and the other from colony B of the same species, the two races do not fuse and a clear line of demarcation is visible. If pieces from two different genera are similarly tested, there is both failure of fusion and evidence of damaging interaction in the form of "blistery tissue" where contact occurs.

In view of the existence of rather similar recognition phenomena in sponges, coelenterates, and ascidians, it is likely that equivalent capacities are present in all metazoa. One can probably generalize that cells of similar genetic origin, when brought into experimental contact, find it easy to establish a working relationship, but that beyond a certain genetic distance, effective fusion becomes impossible and there is some degree of mutual damage and rejection. From our point of view, the question to be answered is how the recognition of foreignness is mediated, particularly when the genetic evidence points to the existence of very large numbers of alleles or pseudoalleles. Any discussion must, in the present state of knowledge, make no pretension to interpret the phenomena at molecular or physical levels. Only genetic and what one can call para-immunological concepts are admissible. It may be legitimate to generalize from what has been said earlier about *Botryllus* and say that the most likely basic hypothesis is that in all animal cells the cell membrane carries discrete structures or molecules whose specificity can be represented as *A* and *a*. Contacts *Aa* and *aA* between adjacent cell membranes are essential for functional association between the cells. This does not eliminate the possibility that there are many other mutual requirements, but it allows us to localize a situation which could form a basis for the evolution of a wide range of allelic specificities. The genetic requirement is that when *A* changes as a result of mutation to *B*, *a* must change either simultaneously or eventually by mutation to *b*, if the organism is to remain fully functional. As Oka has pointed out, the situation in *Botryllus* is formally analogous to self-incompatibility in flowering plants. This is a topic which has interested botanists for many years without, as yet, any interpretation at the molecular level having been established. In view of its potential interest to immunologists, a brief note on incompatibility in plants may be relevant.

A NOTE ON SELF-INCOMPATIBILITY IN PLANTS

There seems to be a widespread advantage for survival among species of flowering plants if self-fertilization can be avoided. The subject was opened up by Darwin, who showed that at least three methods had been evolved to effect this: There may be two alternate flower structures on the same plant (heterostyly), the pollen grains and ovaries may mature at different times, or pollen may be incapable of developing an effective pollen tube in its own race but is competent to fertilize any other race.

In this, as in the previous discussion (Burnet, 1971), I am concerned only with incompatibility resulting from failure of pollen tube development. Detailed study of cross-pollinations may show as many as fifty or more groups, which are defined by showing mutual incompatibility only within the group. The accepted interpretation is that the differences correspond to the presence of multiple alleles at a single locus. The mechanism has not been analyzed at a molecular level but is regarded by most workers concerned as representing a pseudo-immunological recognition between molecules on the pollen (or liberated from it) and another recognition factor in the style (Lewis, 1952; Linskens, 1961; Knox and Heslop-Harrison, 1971; Townsend, 1971). It is assumed that union of the two factors triggers a reaction (remotely equivalent to the liberation of lymphokines by antigen from a sensitized lymphocyte in mammals) by which the normal association of pollen tube and stylar tissue is prevented from developing.

The point of chief interest in the present context is that if each self-incompatibility group is defined by a single allele, it is extremely difficult to picture a complementary and specific interaction between two examples of the same gene product. If detailed study can confirm preliminary indications that there is such a specific complementary relationship, some difficult problems in genetics will have to be faced. It seems impossible to conceive that a single "gene" can simultaneously produce two complementary protein patterns. The alternative is to assume that two closely linked genes are concerned and that mutation in one will result in relatively inefficient descendants until eventually a mutation in the other can again produce a complementary pattern. Any more detailed genetic interpretation will have to await isolation and analysis of the relevant gene products.

COELOMATE INVERTEBRATES

There is no doubt that a similar capacity to recognize the difference between genetically identical and foreign cells or tissues is present in earthworms and, presumably, many or all coelomate invertebrates. I am not, however, convinced that an effective case has yet been made for the existence in any invertebrate of responses which have more than an incomplete and perhaps superficial resemblance to the classical cellular and humoral immune responses of warm-blooded vertebrates.

As there are a number of papers on this theme in the present volume, I shall not attempt to discuss responses in annelids in any detail. Instead, I shall try to foreshadow the directions of research on coelomate invertebrates (annelids, molluscs, arthropods, and echinoderms) which might be expected to throw light on the origin of the characteristic immune responses of vertebrates. My chief quarrel with much current work is the effort to force results obtained in invertebrates into the pattern of vertebrate immunology without regard to the extreme differences in physiology.

When one looks at mammalian immunology from first principles it involves:

1. The genetic and somatic genetic development of a very wide diversity of immune patterns which can become available for immunocyte receptor or antibody.
2. A process of phenotypic restriction by which an immunocyte can express only one such pattern. This determines the specificity both of its surface receptors and of any antibody it liberates.
3. Immunocytes reactive with antigenic determinants present and accessible in the body are either destroyed or rendered nonfunctional.

The elimination of such cells and antibodies makes available a means of recognizing self from not-self.

4.   Antigenic stimulation of an immunocyte can cause it to proliferate, producing descendant immunocytes of similar specificity.

5.   Some immunocytes develop capacity to synthesize and liberate excessive amounts of receptors (B-cells, antibody), others remain as effector cells and memory cells.

6.   Effector cells and antibody can deal in biologically effective fashion with foreign cells and microorganisms appearing in the body.

From the point of view of evolutionary discussion, everything else is virtually irrelevant. As has already been indicated, some forms of recognition of the difference between self and not-self are evident in invertebrates. From the point of view of comparative immunology the most interesting future development could be a demonstration that invertebrate hemocytes (or some subgroup of these cells) are capable of differentiation into forms analogous to immunocytes, i.e., multiple clones of cells each with a distinctive pattern or range of patterns of steric reactivity. There are phenomena which hint at specific adaptive immune responses in coelomate invertebrates, but until immunocytes with specific receptors are defined, one must remain skeptical.

HEMAGGLUTININS AND OPSONINS

However, recent work (much of it recorded in this volume) is already approaching ways of demonstrating specificity more reproducibly than is possible in allograft and xenograft experiments. More and more attention is being concentrated on the natural hemagglutinins of body fluids and on the cells (hemocytes) that are always present in coelomic fluids. Both components have been considered by McKay *et al.* (1969) in work on an Australian fresh-water crayfish. Their tentative conclusion is that the hemagglutinin can serve as an opsonin, facilitating phagocytosis of sheep red cells by crayfish hemocytes. They and other groups have also provided evidence, by cross-absorption experiments, that the hemagglutinin comprises more than one molecular species. Despite all the current interest in agglutinins for mammalian red cells and red-cell rosette formation around hemocytes, this is clearly only a convenient laboratory reagent. It is inconceivable that mammalian erythrocytes have ever played a part in the evolution of arthropods or molluscs. Whatever their biological significance, these hemagglutinins are widely distributed among coelomate invertebrates of several phyla, and a similar substance is even reported to be present in the sea lamprey (Pollara *et al.,* 1968). It is, of course, possible that there is no uniformity of chemical structure among invertebrate hemagglutinins, but at least some general resemblance seems likely, and that of the king crab, *Limulus,* may be taken as a prototype. The chemical study by Marchalonis and Edelman (1968) shows that the substance(s) has no resemblance to mammalian immunoglobulins. It is a protein of molecular weight around 400,000, which is apparently built up from 22,500 MW units. The macromolecule is an aggregate of six subunits, each of which is made up of 3 of the 22,500 MW monomers.

All who have studied invertebrate hemagglutinins agree that they are quite unrelated to vertebrate immunoglobulins. Nevertheless, it is an attractive hypothesis, implicit in several discussions, that evolutionary needs have produced a certain diversity of pattern among molecules of soluble protein that is crudely parallel to later vetebrate developments.

HEMOCYTES

A broadly similar viewpoint can be adopted toward hemocyte function. It is clear enough that throughout the whole course of animal evolution phagocytic cells have played a major role, first in nutrition, when this was predominantly microorganismal in origin, and subsequently in defense against microbial infection. One can reasonably assume that genetic instructions for the differentiation of phagocytic cells have persisted in the genome through some route from invertebrate to the early chordates and thence to true vertebrates. At each stage further differentiation of primitive phagocytic cells to special functions appropriate to the organism must have taken place. Hemocytes have been extensively studied in a variety of arthropods, and Salt's review (1970) of work in insects can be taken as a basis for discussion. Experimental work with a variety of species has shown that when foreign particles are introduced — a larval parasite, a bacterial vaccine, or a little carbon black — there is a standard type of response. The foreign particle sticks to the hemocyte or, if the particle is larger, the hemocyte sticks to it. Small particles are phagocytosed. With a larger intruder, a larval parasite, for example, the attached cells flatten against it. Further cells become attached and eventually the parasite is encapsuled within several layers of cells, and if it is of a species not specifically adapted to parasitize the caterpillar in question, it will be killed. Parasites in their "usual" host have means of discouraging hemocyte response (Salt, 1965).

ANALOGIES WITH VERTEBRATE IMMUNE RESPONSES

Even with our present limited knowledge, an outline of what happens in the invertebrate coelom is beginning to take form. Circulating hemocytes must *ipso facto* not adhere to or be damaged by contact with any cells they may encounter in the normal organism. In some way, they must be able to differentiate between the normal surfaces and, if not "anything else," at least a wide range of foreign materials. What is perhaps most needed at the experimental level is work on the fate of hemocytes from one species transferred to the body cavity of another species, particularly if such studies could cover a representative range of species chosen for graded genetic distance from the donor form. The other major need, already referred to, is to determine whether or not hemocytes comprise a number of different clones, each with distinctive receptors and a corresponding range of reactivity. Tyson *et al.* (personal communication) have recently concluded that, in the Australian fresh-water crayfish, recognition of foreignness is a function of both the soluble hemagglutinins and similar factors associated with the cell membranes of hemocytes. It is a reasonable speculation (which could be tested experimentally) that the hemagglutinin is produced by the hemocytes, some of it remaining on the cell surface, some being liberated into the hemocele fluid. If the two types of hemagglutinin shown by McKay *et al.* in fresh-water mussel are each produced by distinct clones of hemocytes, the beginnings of a mechanism of adaptive immunity could be in the making.

An alternative approach, suggested to me by Marchalonis (personal communication), is that the complex hemagglutinins (like those in *Limulus* with their eighteen subunits) have this structure to provide possibilities of creating various types of reactive patterns out of a limited number of separately coded subunits. The two approaches are not mutually exclusive, and it should not be outside of the capabilities of modern experimental techniques to establish the actual situation. It must be emphasized, however, that whatever findings are obtained in some suitable invertebrate, they do not necessarily provide a model of some early stage in the evolution of the vertebrate immune system.

If some of the major steps in evolution were made by larval forms taking on adult capacities without the normal metamorphoses, then we must be prepared to accept the possibility that there were periodic losses of great amounts of genetic information. If the protochordates arose from an echinoderm larval form and the true Chordata, in their turn, from some tunicate larva that failed to grow up, transmitted genetic information relevant to para-immunological functions might be very sparse indeed. All that one could justifiably expect to remain constant is some capacity of each cell to recognize that it was in its right place and in contact with genetically proper neighbors — in other words, at least a rudimentary ability to differentiate self from not-self. It is highly probable too that, through all transformations and degenerations, the information coding for some type of elaboration of that capacity to recognize foreignness which is manifested in phagocytic wandering cells would be retained.

If this is a reasonable interpretation of the position, the most important objective for para-immunological investigation of organisms other than vertebrates is to undertake a broad comparative survey of capacity to recognize differences between self and not-self. It would seem reasonable to suggest that more attention should be paid to reactions with cells or proteins from more or less closely related invertebrate forms rather than to those with vertebrate erythrocytes. When appropriate model systems have been developed, the obvious objective will be to elucidate their genetic control and the molecular mechanism of their phenotype expression. In other words, what is needed is precisely analogous to what is now being done at the growing edge of classical immunology. Perhaps the most important decision for any group interested in the general problem is to pick an experimental system which can be conveniently studied at genetic, cytological, and biochemical levels, as well as by the para-immunological methods being used at present.

Even more interesting, though strictly speaking lying outside the scope of this paper, are the pollen reactions of self-incompatibility in flowering plants. The real possibility that pollen allergens are identical with pollen recognition factors adds a certain immunological excitement to a thorough investigation at molecular level of the nature of the interactions between pollen proteins and stylar tissue in plants showing self-incompatibility. There is a major opportunity here for interdisciplinary work by botanists, biochemists, and immunologists.

REFERENCES

Burnet, F. M., 1971, "Self-recognition" in colonial marine forms and flowering plants in relation to the evolution of immunity, *Nature 232*:230-235.

Curtis, A. S. G., 1972, Adhesive interactions between organisms, in: *Functional Aspects of Parasite Surfaces, Symposia of the British Society of Parasitology, Vol. 10*, pp. 1-21 (Angela E. R. Taylor and R. Muller, eds.), Blackwell Science Publishers, Oxford.

Curtis, A. S. G., and Van de Vyver, G., 1971, The control of cell adhesion in a morphogenetic system, *J. Embryol. Exp. Morphol. 26*:295-312.

Knox, R. B., and Heslop-Harrison, J., 1971, Pollen-wall proteins: localization of antigenic and allergenic proteins in the pollen-grain walls of *Ambrosia spp.* (ragweeds), *Cytobios 4*:49-54.

Lewis, D., 1952, Serological reactions of pollen incompatibility substances, *Proc. Roy. Soc. Lond. B140*:127-135.

Linskens, H. F., 1961, Biochemical aspects of incompatibility, *Advances in Botany 2*:1500-1503.

Marchalonis, J. J., and Edelman, G. M., 1968, Isolation and characterization of a hemagglutinin from *Limulus polyphemus, J. Mol. Biol. 32*:453-465.

McKay, D., Jenkin, C. R., and Rowley, D., 1969, Immunity in the invertebrates. I. Studies on the naturally occurring hemagglutinins in the fluid from invertebrates, *Australian J. Exp. Biol. Med. Sci. 47*:125-134.

Moscona, A. A., 1968, Cell aggregation: properties of specific cell-ligands and their role in the formation of multicellular systems, *Develop. Biol. 18*:250-277.

Mukai, H., 1967, Experimental alteration of fusibility in compound ascidians, *Sci. Rep. Tokyo Kyoiku Daigaku, B13*:51-73.

Oka, H., 1970, Colony specificity in compound ascidians, in: *Profiles of Japanese Science and Scientists* (H. Yukawa, ed.), pp. 195-206, Kodansha, Tokyo.

Pollara, B., Benson, S., and Bridges, R. A., 1968, Erythrocyte agglutinins in the sea lamprey *Petromyzon marinus, Federation Proc. 27*:492 (Abstract).

Sabbadin, A., 1971, Self- and cross-fertilization in the compound ascidian *Botryllus schlosseri, Develop. Biol. 24*:379-391.

Salt, G., 1965, Experimental studies in insect parasitism. XIII. The hemocytic reaction of a caterpillar to eggs of its habitual parasite, *Proc. Roy. Soc. (London), B162*:303-318.

Salt, G., 1970, The cellular defence reactions of insects, *Cambridge Monographs in Experimental Biology*, No. 16., Cambridge University Press, Cambridge.

Theodor, J. L., 1966, Les greffes chez les Gorgones: étude d'un système de reconnaissance de tissus, *Bull. Inst. Océanog. 66*:No. 1374.

Theodor, J. L., 1970, Distinction between "self" and "not-self" in lower invertebrates, *Nature 227*:690-692.

Townsend, C. E., 1971, Advances in the study of incompatibility, in: *Pollen: Development and Physiology* (J. Heslop-Harrison, ed.), pp. 281-309, Butterworths Science Publishers, London.

Wilson, E. V., 1907, On some phenomena of coalescence and regeneration in sponges, *J. Exp. Zool. 5*:245-258.

Chapter 2

An Electron Microscope Study of the Fate of Bacteria Phagocytized by Granulocytes of Crassostrea virginica*

Thomas C. Cheng and Ann Cali

Institute for Pathobiology
Center for Health Sciences, Lehigh University
Bethlehem, Pennsylvania

INTRODUCTION

It is well established that the primary line of defense in molluscs, in all invertebrates for that matter, to foreign materials, biotic and abiotic, is what has been generally designated as cellular immunity (see Cheng, 1967, and Cheng and Rifkin, 1970, for reviews), although it could be argued that this may not be "immunity" *sensu strictu* since the involvement of antibodies in the form of immunoglobulins has not been demonstrated (Cheng, 1969, 1973). Nevertheless, as a rule, foreign elements, molecules, or organisms naturally or experimentally introduced into naïve molluscs are phagocytized (Stauber, 1950; Tripp,1958a, b, 1960, 1961; Feng, 1959, 1965; Arcadi, 1968; Cheng *et al.* 1969; Pauley and Krassner, 1972), encapsulated (Drew and De Morgan, 1910; Labbé, 1928, 1929, 1930; Newton, 1952, 1954; Brooks, 1953; Sudds, 1960; Mackin, 1961; Cheng and Rifkin, 1968), or nacrezized (Dubois, 1901, 1907; Perrier, 1903; Jameson, 1902; Giard, 1907; Alverdes, 1913; Nishikawa, 1917; Mikimoto, 1918; Tsujii, 1960). These appear to be highly efficient mechanisms for arresting and eliminating foreign materials, although exceptions are known (Naville, 1926; Goetsch and Scheuring, 1926; Yonge, 1936; Yonge and Nicholas, 1940; Prytherch, 1940; Mackin, 1951; Michelson, 1961; Feng, 1966; Feng and Stauber, 1968). In these instances, the foreign organisms are either not reacted against or are phagocytized but not degraded intracellularly. The reason(s) for these ex-

*This research was supported by Grant FD-00416-02 from the U.S. Public Health Service.

ceptions remains undetermined, although in the case of the organisms not reacted against, it is evident that the hosts do not recognize them as being nonself.

THE PRESENT PROBLEM

The current status of our knowledge relative to the encapsulation phenomenon has already been critically analyzed (Cheng and Rifkin, 1970) and therefore need not be considered here. Similarly, no new significant information pertaining to nacrezation has appeared since the comprehensive treatise by Tsujii (1960). On the other hand, reported herein is some new information pertaining to the fate of bacteria that become phagocytized by granulocytes of the American oyster, *Crassostrea virginica,* as revealed by electron microscopy. Specifically, since it is generally agreed that what Foley and Cheng (1972) have designated as granulocytes among the cellular elements of the hemolymph of *C. virginica* are the principal phagocytic cells (Galtsoff, 1964; Cheng and Rifkin, 1970), it appeared to be of interest to examine the fate of bacteria that have become phagocytized by these cells. Consequently, the following study was carried out.

All of the oysters *(C. virginica)* were obtained from the proximity of Oxford, Maryland, during January, 1972. They were brought into the laboratory and maintained in recirculating seawater tanks kept at 21–22°C and with a salinity of 25‰. The tanks were periodically fortified with bacteria (unidentified) and the molluscs maintained therein for 4 to 6 weeks prior to examination.

A 1-ml sample of hemolymph was collected from the adductor muscle sinus of each of 12 molluscs by employing the technique of Feng *et al.* (1971). The cells, concentrated by centrifugation, were fixed for 2 hr in 2% glutaraldehyde in phosphate buffer at pH 7.2. After being washed in phosphate buffer, the cells were postfixed in 1% osmium tetroxide in phosphate buffer for 4 hr, embedded in Luft's Epon, and sectioned with a diamond knife (DuPont) on a Sorvall MT-2B ultramicrotome. The sections, placed on uncoated copper grids, were stained with a saturated solution of uranyl acetate and lead citrate (Reynolds, 1963) and viewed in a Philips 300 electron microscope operated at 60 kV

DISCUSSION AND CONCLUSIONS

It has been established that the cytoplasmic granules of granulocytes of *C. virginica* as seen with the light microscope are in the form of membrane-delimited vesicles that are ovoid when studied with the transmission and scanning electron microscopes. Detailed descriptions of these vesicles have been presented earlier (Feng *et al.* 1971; Cheng *et al.* 1974; Cheng and Foley, 1973). In following the terminology of Feng *et al.* (1971), the zone of heterogeneous, medium electron density situated mediad to the delimiting, surfacial membrane is known as the cortex. Mediad to the cortex is the electron-lucid vesicular lumen, known as the core (Fig. 1). In the majority of instances, the core is devoid of inclusions; however, as described in detail below, this is the site of active foreign material degradation (digestion) and glycogen synthesis.

As foreign materials, unidentified bacteria in this case, are taken into granulocytes by phagocytosis, they come to lie within cytoplasmic vacuoles (digestive vacuoles or phagosomes) situated between the vesicles. That bacteria are digested within these vacuoles is evidenced by the disorganized and degraded appearance of their fine-structural integrity as well as the appearance of con-

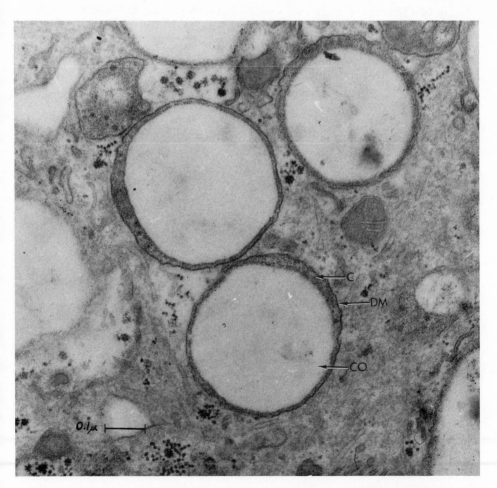

Fig. 1. Electron micrograph showing three secondary phagosomes of *Crassostrea virginica* granulocyte: (C) cortex; (CO) core or vesicular lumen; (DM) delimiting membrane; magnification 168,000 ×.

centric lamellae along their periphery (Hohl, 1965). Although the actual mechanism for the transfer of constituents of partially digested bacterial cells to vesicles is still uncertain, the finding of concentric lamellae enclosing amorphous material of heterogeneous electron density projecting into the lumina of vesicles suggests that this process is in some way associated with the intake of foreign materials.

Not only are concentric lamellated bodies found during the process of uptake into vesicles, but distinct, concentric lamellae also occur within the vesicles. These intravesicular lamellae are comprised of 10 to 20 electron-dense, membranous rings with a lucid zone between the rings. Each membrane appears to be a typical unit membrane with an electron-lucid zone situated between two dense borders. As discussed below, these lamellae are believed to be associated with the intravesicular degradation of the bacteria.

In other vesicles, an amorphous, electron-dense material is sometimes encountered. This is believed to represent degraded material resulting from intravesicular digestion and constitute an intermediate step in the intravesicular

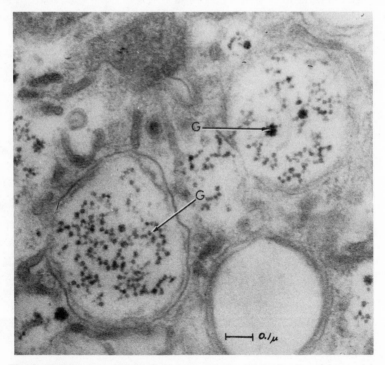

Fig. 2. Electron micrograph of glycogen granules in the lumina of two vesicles (secondary phagosomes). Note the partial disintegration of the phagosomal walls: (G) glycogen granules, magnification 109,000 ×.

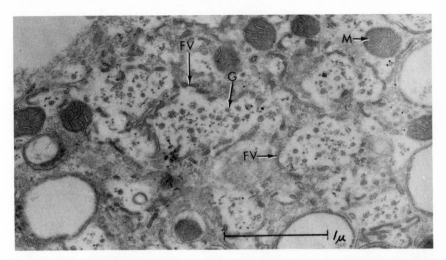

Fig. 3. Electron micrograph showing a portion of the cytoplasm of a granulocyte of *Crassostrea virginica* containing several packets of glycogen, each enveloped by a partially fragmented secondary phagosomal wall: (FV) fragmented vesicular wall, (G) glycogen granules, (M) mitochondrion, magnification 40,000 ×.

synthesis of glycogen. In other words, the glucose resulting from the intravesicular digestion of carbohydrate-containing foreign materials (bacteria in this case) is believed to be a constituent of such an amorphous mass since the sequential event involves the appearance of glycogen particles, both α and β particles, within vesicles (Fig. 2).

Concurrent with the appearance of glycogen particles within vesicles, the delimiting membrane and cortex of each vesicle commences to disintegrate. Specifically, breaks begin to appear in the vesicular wall, i.e., the delimiting membrane and cortex. Furthermore, as disintegration progresses, in some instances the remnant of the vesicular wall becomes singular rather than double. This condition reflects the more rapid disintegration of the cortex. The low-magnification electron micrograph presented in Fig. 3 shows a region of a granulocyte where a number of glycogen-containing vesicles occur with walls which have begun to break down.

Fragmentation of the vesicular wall progresses until eventually no visible lamellar fragments encompass the glycogen granules. This results in the appearance of clumps of glycogen granules free in the cytoplasm of the granulocyte (Fig. 4). Subsequent to this, the free clumps of glycogen coalesce, and larger masses of glycogen become distributed throughout the cytoplasm of the granulocyte. It is of interest that occasionally glycogen granules have been observed in the process of expulsion from granulocytes. This involves enveloping the glycogen by the surface membrane as the granules are discharged into the serum (Fig. 5).

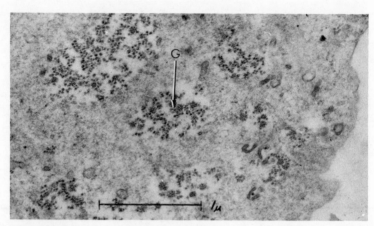

Fig. 4. Electron micrograph showing packets of glycogen in the cytoplasm of a granulocyte of *Crassostrea virginica*. Note the absence of enveloping secondary phagosomal walls: (G) glycogen granules, magnification 40,000 ×.

Apparently two types of vesicles are involved in the uptake and intracellular degradation of nonself materials, bacterial cells in this case. Cells of the first type, which have been referred to earlier as "digestive vacuoles," qualify as phagosomes by modern definition, i.e., membrane-delimited vesicles in which exogenous or autophagic materials are digested. However, cells of the second type, which are much smaller and referred to earlier as "vesicles" (electron microscopy) or as "granules" (light microscopy), also qualify as phagosomes. Therefore, in order not to cause confusion in the subsequent literature, the first type is being designated as primary and the second type as secondary phagosomes

Beginning with the pioneering studies by Yonge (1926) the leukocytes of molluscs are now known to be involved in a variety of physiological processes. These include the arrest of foreign materials by internal defense mechanisms and digestion, although the correlation between these two functions is still unknown. As a result of our electron microscope studies, two functions are indeed a part of a continuous process. Specifically, foreign materials phagocytized by granulocytes of *C. virginica* are partially digested within primary phagosomes. Later the breakdown products are taken up into secondary phagosomes and further degraded. Furthermore, if foreign macromolecules include carbohydrates, the simple sugars (presumably glucose) resulting from digestion within secondary phagosomes are resynthesized into glycogen within these organelles.

Light-microscope cytochemical studies show that oyster leukocytes, specifically granulocytes, include glycogen (Cheng, unpublished). Our electron-microscope studies reveal glycogen situated initially within secondary phagosomes and later, when the phagosomal wall fragments and disappears, the granules become distributed in large clumps throughout the cytoplasm.

Concentric lamellae surrounding partially digested bacteria occur in primary and secondary phagosomes. These lamellae are associated with intracellular digestion in a variety of cells. They have been reported in mammalian cells (Swift and Hruban, 1964) as well as in the food vacuoles of myxamoebae (Gezelius, 1959, 1961; Mercer and Shaffer, 1960; Hohl, 1965). This is the first report of their occurrence in molluscan cells. Furthermore, their presence within secondary phagosomes with hemolymph (or blood) cells is apparently the first for any type of blood cells, vertebrate or invertebrate, although they may not occur in vertebrate blood cells not directly involved in digestion.

Hohl (1965), who presented a detailed account of these lamellae in food vacuoles of the slime molds *Dictyostelium discoideum* and *Polysphondylium pallidum,* expressed the opinion that these organelles are synthesized from products resulting from digested foreign material such as the bacterium *Escherichia coli.* If this proves valid, which seems highly likely, then the concentric lamellae found within the primary phagosomes of *C. virginica* granulocytes may also be

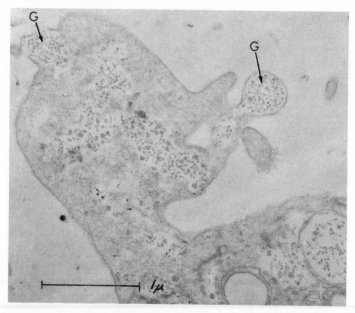

Fig. 5. Electron micrograph showing two packets of glycogen granules in consecutive stages of being expelled into the serum. Note that the one on the right is delimited by the surface membrane of the granulocyte: (G) glycogen granules, magnification 37,500 X.

synthesized from breakdown products of microorganisms phagocytized by these hemolymph cells. In fact, the fine-structural morphology of the lamellae surrounding bacteria in the process of being digested in these vacuoles is almost identical with that surrounding bacteria in the food vacuoles of the slime molds studied by Hohl. However, it is unknown whether the lamellae of secondary phagosomes are totally formed *de novo* after intake of material passed from primary phagosomes, although we suspect that some originate from within primary phagosomes and are transferred along with partially digested exogenous material. This postulation is based on our finding lamellae, along with amorphous exogenous material, protruding into secondary phagosomes.

From the data presented herein, it is now evident that the phagocytic arrest of foreign materials by molluscan granulocytes represents one phase in the continuous process ranging from nonself recognition, i.e., an immunological phenomenon, to intracellular digestion and nutrient (glycogen) storage. Thus, our results further elucidate the subject, treated in earlier reports by Tripp (1958a, b, 1960), of digestible foreign materials (erythrocytes, vegetative bacteria, some yeast cells) being degraded within molluscan phagocytes.

Finally, it is of interest to speculate on the metabolic fate of membrane-bound glycogen that is discharged into the serum. The enveloping membrane may be degraded within the serum, and the released glycogen once again hydrolyzed to glucose and distributed as a nutrient to other cells comprising the mollusc's soma. Indeed, the occurrence of glucose in molluscan serum is known (Holtz and von Brand, 1940; Altman and Dittmer, 1971; Cheng and Lee, 1971).

In conclusion, evidently the recognition of nonself leading to phagocytosis of foreign cells by molluscs, specifically *C. virginica*, eventually gives rise to the synthesis of glycogen within secondary phagosomes. This occurs if the foreign cell includes carbohydrates, hence the internal defense mechanisms of molluscs may also be intimately associated with nutritional processes.

SUMMARY

An electron microscope study of the hemolymph cells of the American oyster *Crassostrea virginica*, exposed to bacteria, has revealed that the foreign cells phagocytized by the mollusc's granulocytes are initially enclosed within digestive vacuoles (or primary phagosomes) where they are subjected to digestion. This is evidenced by the fine-structural decomposition of the bacteria and the appearance of a tunic of membranous lamellae along their periphery.

Subsequent to digestion within primary phagosomes, the degradation products are in some yet undetermined manner transferred to the lumina (or core) of the cytoplasmic vesicles (the granules of light microscopy that are designated herein as secondary phagosomes). Macromolecules that are being transferred are surrounded by concentric lamellae that protrude into the secondary phagosomes. Intraphagosomal digestion ensues, accompanied by the synthesis and deposition of typical concentric lamellae. It is postulated, on the basis of our electron-microscopical evidence, that the carbohydrates constituting the bacterial cells are eventually degraded to simple sugars that become resynthesized to glycogen. Glycogen granules are deposited within secondary phagosomes, and, concurrent with this, the delimiting membrane and cortex of these organelles disintegrate so that eventually the glycogen granules become free in the cytoplasm of granulocytes. Occasionally, glycogen granules have been observed in the process of being extruded from granulocytes into the serum. As this occurs, the unbound granules become delimited by the surface membrane of the granulocyte. Our data indicate that the recognition of nonself, an immunological phenomenon, is but one phase of a continuous process in *C. virginica* of which intracellular digestion and nutrient (glycogen) deposition are subsequent phases.

ACKNOWLEDGMENT

The authors wish to acknowledge the assistance of Mr. William S. Alexander in printing the electron micrographs.

REFERENCES

Altman, P. L. and Dittmer, D. S. (eds.), 1971, *Respiration and Circulation,* p. 930, Fed. Amer. Soc. Exp. Biol. Bethesda.

Alverdes, F., 1913, Ueber Perlen und Perlbildung, *Z. Wiss. Zool. 105*:598-633.

Arcadi, J. A., 1968, Tissue response to the injection of charcoal into the pulmonate gastropod *Lehmania poirieri, J. Invert. Pathol. 11*:59-62.

Brooks, C. P., 1953, A comparative study of *Schistosoma mansoni* in *Tropicorbis havanensis* and *Australorbis glabratus, J. Parasitol. 39*:159-163.

Cheng, T. C., 1966, The coracidium of the cestode *Tylocephalum* and the migration and fate of this parasite in the American oyster, *Crassostrea virginica, Trans. Am. Microscop. Soc. 85*:246-255.

Cheng, T. C., 1967, Marine molluscs as hosts for symbioses with a review of known parasites of commercially important species, in: *Advanced Marine Biology, Vol. 5,* pp. 1-424 (F. S. Russell, ed.), Academic Press, London.

Cheng, T. C., 1969, An electrophoretic analysis of hemolymph proteins of the snail *Helisoma duryi normale* experimentally challenged with bacteria, *J. Invert. Pathol. 14*:60-81.

Cheng, T. C., 1973, *General Parasitology,* Academic Press, New York.

Cheng, T. C. and Cooperman, J. S., 1964, Studies on host—parasite relationships between larval trematodes and their hosts. V. The invasion of the reproductive system of *Helisoma trivolvis* by the sporocysts and cercariae of *Glypthelmins pennsylvaniensis, Trans. Am. Microscop. Soc. 83*:12-23.

Cheng, T. C. and Foley, D. A., 1973, A scanning electron microscope study of the cytoplasmic granules of *Crassostrea virginica* granulocytes, *J. Invert. Pathol. 19*:383-394.

Cheng, T. C. and Lee, F. O., 1971, Glucose levels in the mollusc *Biomphalaria glabrata* infected with *Schistosoma mansoni, J. Invert. Pathol. 18*:395-399.

Cheng, T. C. and Rifkin, E, 1968, The occurrence and resorption of *Tylocephalum* metacestodes in the clam *Tapes semidecussata, J. Invert. Pathol. 10*:65-69.

Cheng, T. C. and Rifkin, E., 1970, Cellular reactions in marine molluscs in response to helminth parasitism, in: *A Symposium on Diseases of Fishes and Shellfishes* (S. F. Snieszko, ed.), Spec. Publ. No. 5, American Fisheries Society, Washington, D.C.

Cheng, T. C., Shuster, C. N., Jr., and Anderson, A. H., 1966, A comparative study of the susceptibility and response of eight species of marine pelecypods to the trematode *Himasthla quissetensis, Trans. Am. Microscop. Soc. 85*:284-295.

Cheng, T. C. Thakur, A. S., and Rifkin, E., 1969, Phagocytosis as an internal defense mechanism in the mollusca with an experimental study of the role of leucocytes in the removal of ink particles in *Littorina scabra,* Linn. *Proc. Symp. Mollusca, Part II,* pp. 546-563, The Bangalore Press, Bangalore, India.

Cheng, T. C., Cali, A., and Foley, D. A., 1974, Cellular reactions in marine pelecypods as a factor influencing endosymbioses, in: *Symbiosis in the Sea* (W. A. Vernberg and F. J. Vernberg, eds.), University of Southern Carolina Press,

Chernin, E., 1962, The unusual life history of *Daubaylia potomaca* (Nematoda: Cephalobidae) in *Australorbis glabratus* and in certain other fresh-water snails, *Parasitology, 52*:459-481.

Drew, G. H. and De Morgan, W., 1910, The origin and formation of fibrous tissue produced as a reaction to injury in *Pecten maximus,* as a type of the Lamellibranchiata, *Quart. J. Microscop. Sci. 55*:595-620.

Dubois, R., 1901, Sur le mécanisme de la formation des perles fines dans le *Mytilus edulis, C.R. Hebd. Séanc. Acad. Sci. (Paris) 133*:603-605.

Dubois, R., 1907, Action de la chaleur sur le distome immature de *Gymnophallus margaritarum, C.R. Séanc. Soc. Biol. 63*:502-504.

Feng, S. Y., 1959, Defense mechanism of the oyster, *Bull. N.J. Acad. Sci. 4*:17.

Feng, S. Y., 1965, Pinocytosis of proteins by oyster leucocytes, *Biol. Bull. 128*:95-105.

Feng, S. Y., 1966, Experimental bacterial infections in the oyster *Crassostrea virginica, J. Invert. Pathol. 8*:505-511.

Feng, S. Y. and Stauber, L. A., 1968, Experimental hexamitiasis in the oyster *Crassostrea virginica, J. Invert. Pathol. 10*:94-110.

Feng, S. Y., Feng, J. S., Burke, C. N., and Khairallah, L. H., 1971, Light and electron microscopy of the leucocytes of *Crassostrea virginica* (Mollusca: Pelecypoda), *Z. Zellforsch. 120*:222-245.

Foley, D. A. and Cheng, T. C., 1972, Interaction of molluscs and foreign substances: The morphology and behavior of hemolymph cells of the American oyster, *Crassostrea virginica, in vitro, J. Invert. Pathol. 19*:383-395.

Galtsoff, P. S., 1964, The American oyster, *Crassostrea virginica* Gmelin. *Fisheries Bull., Fish Wildlife Service U.S., 64*:1-480.

Gezelius, K., 1959, The ultrastructure of cells and cellulose membranes in *Acrasiae, Exptl. Cell Res. 18*:425-453.

Gezelius, K., 1961, Further studies in the ultrastructure of *Acrasiae, Exp. Cell. Res. 23*:300-310.

Giard, 1907, Sur les trématodes margaritigènes du Pas-de-Calais (*Gymnophallus somateriae* Levinsen et *G. bursicola* Odhner), *C.R. Séanc. Soc. Biol. 63*:416-420.

Goetsch, W. and Scheuring, L., 1926, Parasitismus und Symbiose der Algengattung *Clorella, Z. Morphol. Oekol. Tiere 7*:220-253.

Hohl, H. R., 1965, Nature and development of membrane systems in food vacuoles of cellular slime molds predatory upon bacteria, *J. Bacteriol. 90*:755-765.

Holtz, F. and von Brand, T., 1940, Quantitative studies upon some blood constituents of *Helix pomatia, Biol. Bull. 79*:423-431.

Jameson, H. L., 1902, On the origin of pearls, *Proc. Zool. Soc. London 1*:140-166.

Jullien, A., 1940, Sur les reactions des mollusques céphalopodes aux injections de goudron, *C.R. Séanc. Soc. Biol. 210*:608-610.

Labbé, A., 1928, Production expérimentale de tissue conjonctif par les amoebocytes chez *Doris tuberculata* L., *C.R. Hebd. Séanc. Acad. Sci. (Paris) 187*:1073-1075.

Labbé, A., 1929, Reactions expérimentales des mollusques a l'introduction de stylets de celloidine, *C.R. Séanc. Soc. Biol. 100*:166-168.

Labbé, A., 1930, Réaction du tissu conjonctif au goudron chez un mollusque: *Doris tuberculata* Cuvier, *C.R. Séanc. Soc. Biol. 103*:20-22.

Mackin, J. G., 1951, Histopathology of infection of *Crassostrea virginica* (Gmelin) by *Dermocystidium marinum* Mackin, Owen, and Collier, *Bull. Marine Sci. Gulf Caribbean 1*:72-87.

Mackin, J. G., 1961, Oyster leucocytes in infectious disease, *Am. Zool. 1*:371.

Mercer, E. H. and Shaffer, B. M., 1960, Electron microscopy of solitary and aggregated slime mold cells, *J. Biophys. Biochem. Cytol. 7*:353-356.

Michelson, E. H., 1961, An acid-fast pathogen of fresh-water snails, *Am. J. Trop. Med. Hyg. 10*:423-427.

Mikimoto, K., 1918 (Cited in Tsujii, T., 1960), Studies on the mechanism of shell- and pearl-formation in Mollusca, *J. Fac. Fisheries Prefect. Univ. Mie 5*:1-70.

Naville, A., 1926, Notes sur les Eolidiens. Un Eolidien d'eau saumatre. Origine des nématocytes. Zooxanthelles et homochromie. *Rev. Suisse Zool. 33*:251-289.

Newton, W. L., 1952, The comparative tissue reaction of two strains of *Australorbis glabratus* to infection with *Schistosoma mansoni*, *J. Parasitol. 38*:362-366.

Newton, W. L., 1954, Tissue response to *Schistosoma mansoni* in second generation snails from a cross between two strains of *Australorbis glabratus*, *J. Parasitol. 40*:1-4.

Nishikawa, T., 1917 (Cited in Tsujii, T., 1960), Studies on the mechanism of shell- and pearl-formation in Mollusca, *J. Fac. Fisheries Prefect. Univ. Mie 5*:1-70.

Pauley, G. B. and Krassner, S. M., 1972, Cellular defense reactions to particulate materials in the California sea hare, *Aplysia californica, J. Invert. Pathol. 19*:18-27.

Perrier, E., 1903, Remarques de M. Edm. Perrier à propos de la communication de M. Raphaël Dubois, de 19 Octobre dernier, "sur les huîtres perlières vraies," *Compt. Rend. 137*:682.

Prytherch, H. F., 1940, The life cycle and morphology of *Nematopsis ostrearum* sp. nov., a gregarine parasite of the mud crab and oyster, *J. Morphol. 66*:39-64.

Reynolds, E. S., 1963, The use of lead citrate at high pH as an electron opaque stain in electron microscopy, *J. Cell Biol. 17*:208-212.

Stauber, L. A., 1950, The fate of India ink injected intracardially into the oyster *Ostrea virginica* Gmelin, *Biol. Bull. 98*:227-241.

Sudds, R. H., Jr., 1960, Observations on schistosome miracidial behavior in the presence of normal and abnormal snail hosts and subsequent tissue studies of these hosts, *J. Elisha Mitchell Sci. Soc. 76*:121-133.

Swift, H. and Hruban, Z., 1964, Focal degradation as a biological process, *Federation Proc. 23*:1026-1037.

Tripp, M. R., 1958*a*, Disposal by the oyster of intracardially injected red blood cells of vertebrates, *Proc. Nat. Shellfisheries Assoc. 48*:143-147.

Tripp, M. R., 1958*b* Studies on the defense mechanism of the oyster, *J. Parasitol. 44* (Sect. 2): 35-36.

Tripp, M. R., 1960, Mechanisms of removal of injected microorganisms from the American oyster, *Crassostrea virginica* (Gmelin), *Biol. Bull. 119*:210-223.

Tripp, M. R., 1961, The fate of foreign materials experimentally introduced into the snail *Australorbis glabratus, J. Parasitol. 47*:745-751.

Tsujii, T., 1961, Studies on the mechanism of shell- and pearl-formation in Mollusca, *J. Fac. Fisheries Prefect. Univ. Mie 5*:1-70.

Yonge, C. M., 1926, Structure and physiology of the organs of feeding and digestion in *Ostrea edulis, J. Marine Biol. Assoc. U.K. 14*:295-386.

Yonge, C. M., 1936, Mode of life, feeding, digestion, and symbiosis with zooxanthellae in the Tridacnidae, *Sci. Rep. Great Barrier Reef Exped. 1*:283-321.

Yonge, C. M. and Nicholas, H. M., 1940, Structure and function of the gut and symbiosis with zoothanthellae in *Tridacna crispata* (Oerst.), *Bgk. Papers Tortugas Lab. Carnegie Inst. 32*:287-301.

Chapter 3

On the Immediate Fate of Bacteria
in the Land Snail Helix

C. J. Bayne

Department of Zoology
Oregon State University
Corvallis, Oregon 97331

INTRODUCTION

The fate of materials injected into molluscs and other facets of molluscan internal defense mechanisms have been investigated and discussed widely. The unifying vision among the investigators was that they saw in such studies a useful tool for invertebrate immunology. Cheng's (1967b) account of defense mechanisms in molluscs remains an excellent working model. Based largely upon investigations by Stauber (1950), Tripp (1958a,b, 1960, 1961), Feng (1959, 1965a,b), Bang (1961), Michelson (1961, 1963) and last, but not least, his own group (Cheng, 1966, 1967a; Cheng and Cooperman, 1964, Cheng and Snyder, 1962), Cheng (1967b) has shown that a scheme can be drawn up as illustrated in Fig. 1. Studies on a variety of molluscs reveal that when small particles are introduced into the circulation they are rapidly cleared from the hemolymph. We may now ask the question: "What are the agents of clearance?"

CLEARANCE MECHANISMS

The dominant concept has been that hemocytes (blood amebocytes) phagocytose particles, thus eliminating or clearing them from the circulation. Examples of publications lending support to this view are Prowse and Tait (1969), Bayne and Kime (1970), Cheng (1970), Tripp (1970), Feng et al. (1971), and Pauley et. al. (1971). Some details of the process are presented: Tripp and Kent

(1968) reported that hemolymph proteins of *Crassostrea gigas,* an oyster, facilitate phagocytosis by hemocytes. Prowse and Tait (1969) extended this observation to *Helix aspersa,* a garden snail, and even claimed that different opsonins, specific for red blood cells or yeast, were present in the hemolymph. Most of the research has been with bivalves, but recently Bayne and Kime (1970) and Pauley and Krassner (1972) have looked at clearance rates of particles from gastropod hemolymph. Before continuing, let me note that I have referred to the phylum Mollusca as a unit, but our new data indicate that the three Classes so far investigated possess different levels of physiological responses. It is therefore dangerous to extrapolate too freely from bivalve investigations to gastropods which are more complex. And further, as pointed out by Cowden (this volume), the cephalopods, if judged by their tissue involvement, may be even more specialized in internal defense (Stuart, 1968; Bayne, 1973*a*).

Recent investigations have been directed at answering the broad question, "What are the details of *self–nonself* recognition and phagocytosis?" As a first question we asked, "What is the capacity of the *Helix* clearance system?" In 1970 (Bayne and Kime) we demonstrated that *Helix pomatia* eliminates large numbers of bacteria (very rapidly, 90% in the first two hours) from its circulation. More recently, we have repeated this experiment using the bacterium *Serratia marcescens.* The bacteria are grown in nutrient broth for 24 or 48 hr, spun down in a clinical centrifuge, rinsed twice in *Helix* saline (Chiarandini, 1964), and resuspended in this saline. Active adult *Helix pomatia* receive 0.1-ml injections of live bacteria into the cephalopedal sinus or foot. Microcapillaries are used to collect hemolymph samples (approximately 30 μl each time) from the columellar sinus, as described previously (Bayne and Kime, 1970). The samples are measured, then added to 10 ml nutrient agar at 49 ± 1°C. Serial 10X dilutions are prepared and poured into petri plates. The bacteria grow at room tempera-

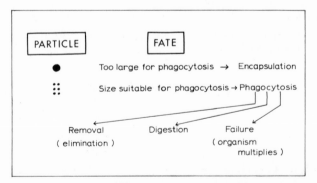

Fig. 1. Theoretical fate of particles entering the body of a mollusc. This diagram does not deal with particles such as compatible parasites which do not elicit any response. (Based largely upon Cheng, 1967*b*.)

Table I. Data from an Experiment with Very Heavy Doses of *Serratia marcescens* Injected into *Helix pomatia*

Name of snail	Bacteria injected	Before injection	Bacteria (in millions) per ml of hemolymph					
			26 min	55 min	80 min	115 min	170 min	260 min
A	11×10^{11}	0.000296	5920^a	41^d	137^d	15.8^d	5.7^d	10.1^d
B	11×10^{10}	0.000723	52^b	9.05	38.5	0.375	0.087	0
C	11×10^9	0.000321	0.054^c	0.005	0.0028	0	0	0

[a] 2.6% of injected dose.
[b] 0.24% of injected dose.
[c] 0.0025% of injected dose.
[d] These samples were taken from the heart, since the snail had withdrawn into its shell.

ture or 30°C, and the colonies can be counted after growth to a suitable size (1–3 days).

In attempting to determine the capacity for clearance, snails received injections of 1.1×10^{11}, 1.1×10^{10}, or 1.1×10^9 *S. marcescens* (Table I). Astonishingly, one snail which received over one trillion bacteria not only cleared them in normal time, but survived for one week and regenerated a hole in its shell (because the snail withdrew into its shell, a hole had to be cut over the heart and hemolymph sampled from the heart). The number of hemocytes in *Helix pomatia* indicate a mean count of 2×10^5/ml (Bayne and Kime, 1970). Calculations based on the number of hemocytes, the number of bacterial cells, and the rate of clearance indicate that in one hour 1×10^6 hemocytes had eliminated $1,099,795 \times 10^6$ bacteria! This rate – more than one million bacteria per hemocyte in one hour – seems outside the realm of possibility. The rate of bacterial phagocytosis in the Sea Hare appears to be of the same order of magnitude (Pauley *et al.* 1971). Larger erythrocytes and yeast cells are, naturally, phagocytosed many orders of magnitude more slowly. *In vitro,* in reportedly suboptimal conditions, less than 40% of oyster hemocytes phagocytosed bacteria, and most hemocytes never contained more than five bacteria (Tripp and Kent, 1968). Recently Foley and Cheng (1972) found that a single clam hemocyte may associate with 15–40 or more *Bacillus megatherium* during 15 min *in vitro*. The staggering number of one million in one hour seems at least in the realm of "highly unlikely."

It becomes necessary to postulate that circulating hemocytes may not be the sole agents responsible for bacterial clearance. Another experimental approach provides supporting evidence, as follows: Specimens of *Helix pomatia* received injections of 1×10^{10} *S. marcescens.* After intervals of 10, 30, or 60 min, hemolymph samples were withdrawn by capillary. Each hemolymph-filled

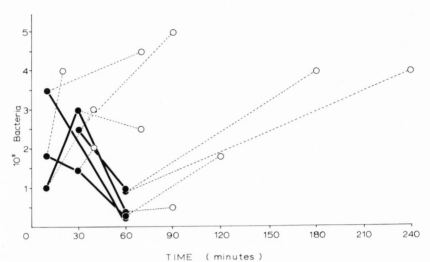

Fig. 2. The numbers of *Serratia marcescens* in halves of capillary tubing directly after hemolymph sampling (solid lines) and after delays of differing duration (dotted lines). Each solid dot ("immediate" value) connects with an open dot (value after *in vitro* incubation). See text.

capillary was broken so that the hemolymph was divided in half. One half was added to sterile water, serially diluted, added to nutrient agar, and poured into petri plates. The other half was retained for either 10, 20, 30, 40, 50, 60, 120, or 180 min before the addition of sterile water, then processed like the first half. In each capillary tube there were hemocytes, bacteria, and hemolymph — supposedly all that is necessary for clearance. If phagocytosis proceeded *in vitro*, then in the capillaries the number of bacteria should fall during incubation, as in intact snails. In Fig. 2, bacterial clearance *in vivo* (solid lines) follows its normal course. (The 30-min rise in one snail is a rare but not unique occurrence, and may be an erroneous datum.) *In vitro*, in the capillary halves retained for various periods, bacteria almost invariably increased in numbers, but bacterial division cannot account for this increase. Bacteria may be somehow revitalized *in vitro*, probably by release from hemocytes. As hemocytes adhere to glass, their shape and surface properties change, and perhaps the bacteria become "unstuck" during this process.

Further evidence that bacteria cleared *in vivo* do not accumulate in circulating hemocytes is revealed in the following information: *S. marcescens* were grown for 12 hr in nutrient broth at $30°C$, centrifuged, the supernatant discarded, and the cells resuspended in 7 ml physiological saline containing 17 μCi of C^{14} amino acid mixture (algal protein hydrolysate, ICN); growth in this medium was allowed to continue for 18 hr. Labeled cells were centrifuged, the supernatant discarded, and the cells resuspended in unlabeled nutrient broth. After 3.5 hr of growth, the bacteria were centrifuged and rinsed in saline twice before resuspension in snail saline. *Helix pomatia* received 0.1 ml of suspension, and were bled from the heart at 10, 30, 60, and 150 min after injection. Portions of the digestive gland were also removed. Hemolymph was collected onto plastic sheet within petri dishes and the area covered by hemolymph measured indirectly. After 60 min (Fig. 3), hemocytes (*A*) became attached to the plastic. On a small area of the plastic sheet, hemocytes were counted microscopically; the hemolymph was removed by syringe, the volume measured, and then filtered through 0.45 μm

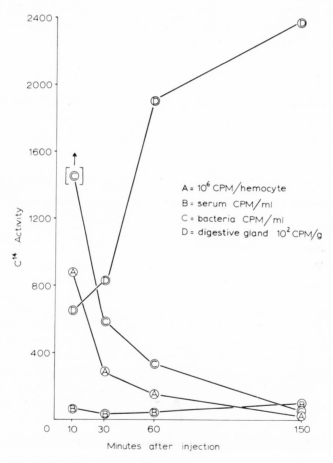

Fig. 3. Abundance of bacteria, reflected by their C^{14} counts, in various fractions of hemolymph and digestive gland. *Note:* the hemocyte value (*A*) is very low in terms of actual counts, and has been multiplied by 10^6 for plotting. The counts in this fraction are probably due to small amounts of serum which was not rinsed away.

millipore filters providing cell-free serum (B); the filter membrane retained the bacteria (C); the digestive gland was denoted as (D).

A, B, C, and D, containing, respectively, the hemocytes, serum, bacteria, and digestive gland portion, were each dried overnight at 80°C. After weighing the dry digestive glands, all samples were combusted in pure oxygen according to the method of Schöniger (Wang and Willis, 1965). The $C^{14}O_2$ was trapped in 10 ml ethanol: ethanolamine (1:1). At 60 min, 10 ml ethanol was added, and after thorough mixing, 5 ml was transferred to a scintillation vial, 10 ml aquasol added, and the disintegrations measured on a Packard Tri Carb scintillation counter. Radioactivity was calculated as (A) CPM per hemocyte; (B) CPM per ml; (C) CPM per ml; and (D) CPM per gram dry weight. Figure 3 illustrates that a small amount of hemolymph remains on the plastic with the cells (not rinsed for fear of dislodging and losing some). At least in part, the presence of radioactivity in the cell portion reflects this contamination. The five salient features of this graph are: (1) The clearance of C^{14} follows the same rate as is found routinely by agar plating methods for viable bacteria. (2) As the C^{14} level drops in the bacterial fraction, it results in no increase in the hemocyte C^{14}, as would occur if phagocytosis by circulating hemocytes were the clearance mechanism. (3) The serum level of C^{14} is always low, but there are signs of a gradual increase after 30 min, possibly due to release of C^{14} metabolites by the bacteria. (4) As bacteria are cleared from the hemolymph, they accumulate in the digestive gland. (5) Bacterial lysis is not important in clearance. If it were, the C^{14} level in the serum would be expected to increase proportionately as the C^{14} level of bacteria decreases. We may assume that adherence of the bacteria to the hemocyte surface precedes phagocytosis. Either fixed phagocytes in the digestive gland, and possibly elsewhere, are responsible for clearance (Reade, 1968), or as hemocytes agglutinate large numbers of bacteria, they leave the circulation in the digestive gland. Briefly then, bacteria are cleared from the circulation and do not accumulate in circulating hemocytes, but in specified tissue(s).

DISCUSSION AND CONCLUSIONS

As is now widely known, most attempts to demonstrate adaptive immune response in molluscs have failed (see Cushing et al., 1971). In one case of apparent evidence of immune responses (Action et al., 1969), the investigators suggested that the response was cellular rather than humoral. In this regard, it now seems evident that the experimental approaches used were not suitable. The methods most widely used: (1) measuring clearance rates from circulation, (2) looking for increased titers of bacteriocides, etc., (3) looking for changes in hemolymph proteins — would be suitable if molluscan immunity were similar in type to vertebrate immunity, where humoral factors (antibodies) are of utmost importance. What now needs to be emphasized is the possibility that molluscs possess an immune capability at a different level. My hypothesis is that intracellular killing and/or body clearance, rather than hemolymph clearance *per se*, may be achieved more efficiently in secondary or later infections.

In conclusion, clearance of bacteria progresses more rapidly than seems possible by phagocytosis. Evidently phagocytosis by circulatory hemocytes is probably *not* the means for clearance of small particles. Agglutination and phagocytosis are associated more with definite tissues and organs, especially the digestive gland (Reade, 1968; Bayne, 1973*b*). Lysis is not important in the clearance of *Serratia marcescens* from *Helix* hemolymph. The evident absence of an *humoral* immune response in molluscs may be due to the presence of a broad range (all nonself), highly efficient, high-capacity opsonization–agglutination system, obviating any induced response. The possibility still exists, however, that an adaptive *cellular* immune response may be present, enabling molluscs to clear foreign material more rapidly on second and subsequent encounters.

ACKNOWLEDGMENTS

It is my pleasure to thank Drs. Leo Parks, C. H. Wang, and F. P. Conte for advice on the radioactive work. Anita Hutchins and Karen Miller provided laboratory assistance, and Mrs. Miller prepared the illustrations.

REFERENCES

Acton, R. T., Evans, E. E., and Bennett, J. C., 1969, Immunological capabilities of the oyster, *Crassostrea virginica, Comp. Biochem. Physiol. 29*:149-160.

Bang, F. B., 1961, Reaction to injury in the oyster (*Crassostrea virginica*), *Biol. Bull. 121*:57-68.

Bayne, C. J., 1973*a*,Internal defense mechanisms of *Octopus dofleini, Malocological Rev. 6*: 13-17.

Bayne, C. J., 1973*b*, Molluscan internal defense mechanism: the fate of C^{14}-labelled bacteria in the Land Snail *Helix pomatia* (L.), *J. comp. Physiol. 86*:17-25.

Bayne, C. J., and Kime, J. B., 1970, *In vivo* removal of bacteria from the hemolymph of the land snail *Helix pomatia* (Pulmonata: Stylommatophora), *Malacological Rev. 3*:103-113.

Cheng, T. C., 1966, Perivascular leucocytosis and other types of cellular reactions in the oyster *Crassostrea virginica* experimentally infected with the nematode *Angiostrongylus cantonensis, J. Invert. Pathol. 8*:52-58.

Cheng, T. C., 1967*a*, The compatibility and incompatibility concept as related to trematodes and molluscs, *Pacific Sci. 22*:141-160.

Cheng, T. C., 1967*b*, Marine molluscs as hosts for symbioses, *Advances in Marine Biology,* Volume 5 (F. R. Russell, ed.), Academic Press, London and New York.

Cheng, T. C., 1969, An electrophoretic analysis of hemolymph proteins of the snail *Helisoma duryi normale* experimentally challenged with bacteria, *J. Invert. Pathol. 14*:60-81.

Cheng, T. C., 1970, Immunity in mollusca with special reference to reactions to transplants, *Transplant. Proc. 2*:226-230.

Cheng, T. C. and Cooperman, J. S., 1964, Studies on host–parasite relationships between larval trematodes and their hosts. V. The invasion of the reproductive system of *Helisoma trivolvis* by the sporocysts and cercariae of *Glypthelmins pennsylvaniensis*, *Trans. Am. Microscop. Soc. 83*:12-23.

Cheng, T. C. and Sanders, B. G., 1962, Internal defense mechanisms in molluscs and an electrophoretic analysis of a naturally occurring serum hemagglutinin in *Vivparus malleatur* Reeve, *Proc. Penn. Acad. Sci. 36*:72-83.

Cheng, T. C. and Snyder R. W., Jr., 1962, Studies on host–parasite relationships between larval trematodes and their hosts. I. A review. II. The utilization of the host's glycogen by the intramolluscan larvae of *Glypthelmins pennsylvaniensis* Cheng, and associated phenomena, *Trans. Am. Microscop. Soc. 81*:209-228.

Chiarandini, D. J., 1964, A saline solution for pulmonate molluscs, *Life Sci. 3*:1513-1518.

Cushing, J. E., Evans, E. E., and Evans, M. L., 1971, Induced bactericidal responses of Abalones, *J. Invert. Pathol. 17*:446-448.

Feng, S. Y., 1959, Defense mechanism of the oyster, *Bull. N.J. Acad. Sci. 4*:17.

Feng, S. Y., 1965a, Pinocytosis of proteins by oyster leucocytes, *Biol. Bull. Marine Biol. Lab., Woods Hole 128*:95-105.

Feng, S. Y., 1965b, Heart rate and leucocyte circulation in *Crassostrea virginica* (Gmelin), *Biol. Bull. Marine Biol. Lab., Woods Hole 128*:198-210.

Feng, S. Y., 1966, Experimental bacterial infections in the oyster, *Crassostrea virginica*, *J. Invert. Pathol. 8*:505-511.

Feng, S. Y., 1967, Responses of molluscs to foreign bodies, with special reference to the oyster, *Federation Proc. 26*:1685-1692.

Feng, S. Y., Feng, J. S., Burke, C. N., and Khairallah, L. H., 1971, Light and electron microscopy of the leucocytes of *Crassostrea virginica* (Mollusca: Pelecypoda), *Z. Zellforsch. 120*:222-245.

Foley, D. A. and Cheng, T. C., 1972, Morphology and phagocytic behavior of hemolymph cells of *Mercenaria mercenaria*. Presented at the *Fifth Annual Meeting of the Society for Invertebrate Pathology*, Minneapolis, 1972.

Michelson, E. H., 1961, An acid-fast pathogen of fresh-water snails, *Am. J. Trop. Med. Hyg. 10*:423-427.

Michelson, E. H., 1963, Development and specificity of miracidial immobilizing substances in extracts of the snail *Australorbis glabratus* exposed to various agents, *Ann. N.Y. Acad. Sci. 113*:486-491.

Pauley, G. B. Krassner, S. M., and Chapman, F. A., 1971, Bacterial clearance in the California sea hare, *Aplysia californica*, *J. Invert. Pathol. 18*:227-239.

Pauley, G. B., and Krassner, S. M., 1972, Cellular defense reactions to particulate materials in the California sea hare, *Aplysia californica*, *J. Invert. Pathol. 19*:18-27.

Prowse, R. H., and Tait, N. N., 1969, *In vitro* phagocytosis by amoebocytes from the hemolymph of *Helix aspersa* (Muller). I. Evidence for opsonic factor(s) in serum, *Immunology 17*:437-441.

Reade, P. C., 1968, Phagocytosis in invertebrates, *Australian. J. Exp. Biol. Med. Sci. 46*:219-229.

Stauber, L. A., 1950, The fate of India ink injected intracardially into the oyster, *Crassostrea virginica* Gmelin, *Biol. Bull. 96*:401-402.

Stuart, A. E., 1968, The reticulo-endothelial apparatus of the lesser octopus, *Eledone cirrosa*, *J. Pathol. Bacteriol. 96*:401-412.

Tripp, M. R., 1958a, Disposal by the oyster of intracardially injected red blood cells of vertebrates, *Proc. Nat. Shellfisheries Assoc. 48*:143-147.

Tripp, M. R., 1958b, Studies on the defense mechanism of the oyster, *J. Parasitol. 44* (Sect. 2):35-36.

Tripp, M. R., 1960, Mechanisms of removal of injected microorganisms from the American oyster, *Crassostrea virginica* (Gmelin), *Biol. Bull. Marine Biol. Lab., Woods Hole 119*:210-223.

Tripp, M. R., 1961, The fate of foreign materials experimentally introduced into the snail *Australorbis glabratus*, *J. Parasitol. 47*:745-751.

Tripp, M. R., 1963, Cellular responses of mollusks, *Ann. N. Y. Acad. Sci. 113:*467-474.
Tripp, M. R., 1970, Defense mechanisms of mollusks, *J. Reticuloendothel. Soc.* 7:173-182.
Tripp, M. R. and Kent, V. E., 1968, Studies on oyster cellular immunity, *In Vitro* 3:129-135.
Wang, C. H. and Willis, D. L., 1965, *Radiotracer Methodology in Biological Sciences,* p. 382, Prentice Hall Inc., New Jersey.

Chapter 4

Metabolism of Insect Hemocytes During Phagocytosis

Robert S. Anderson

Sloan-Kettering Institute for Cancer Research
Donald S. Walker Laboratory
Rye, New York 10580

INTRODUCTION

Phagocytosis by ameboid blood cells is a protective mechanism generally ascribed to both vertebrate and invertebrate animals. In simplest terms, this process involves ingestion of a particle recognized as foreign by a phagocytic cell. The exact basis for the phenomenon of recognition of foreignness is of central importance to immunology but is not within the scope of this review. Phagocytosed microorganisms are enclosed in intracellular vacuoles to which other membrane-bound cytoplasmic granules (lysosomes) fuse. These lysosomes release bactericidal products and hydrolytic enzymes into the phagocytic vacuoles. Thereafter microorganisms may be killed and digested; however, for a variety of reasons, cellular bactericidal capacity may be incomplete in some cases. Certain pathogenic bacteria can remain viable within the phagocyte; others may survive because of cellular or biochemical defects.

THE PRESENT PROBLEM

Considerable information has been obtained recently on normal and abnormal human leukocyte metabolism during phagocytosis and the subsequent events of degranulation, killing, and digestion. This knowledge has been expanded by detailed studies of leukocytes from patients with histories of repeated, chronic bacterial infections. A striking example of this work is the correlation between defects in metabolism of leukocytes from patients with chronic granulomatous disease and their failure to kill certain microorganisms which ultimately results in the expression of the disease (Holmes *et al.* 1967). In this disease, uptake of bacteria proceeds normally, but a number of characteristic postphagocytic metabolic alterations are abnormal and the cells are deficient in bactericidal action (Holmes and Good, 1972).

While many details are known about the metabolism and antimicrobial processes in higher vertebrates, such information is incomplete for the invertebrates. This paper reports preliminary investigations concerning metabolism of phagocytosing *Blaberus craniifer* hemocytes maintained *in vitro*. The observations on cockroach cells will be contrasted with those obtained from higher vertebrate leukocytes.

Blaberus hemolymph contains three major blood cell types: prohematocytes, or immature blood cells; coagulocytes, which release substances triggering coagulation; and plasmocytes, the primary phagocytic hemocytes. These cells were maintained in short-term culture in a glucose-containing balanced salt solution similar to that employed by Landureau and Jollès (1969) for embryonic cells from *Periplaneta americana*. The hemocytes are capable of killing many bacterial species, including: *Staphylococcus aureus, Staphylococcus albus, Streptococcus faecalis, Serratia marcescens,* and *Proteus mirabilis* (Anderson *et al.*, 1973).

HUMAN PHAGOCYTOSIS

Phagocytosis in normal human polymorphonuclear leukocytes is accompanied by a burst of metabolic activity. The most marked changes are a considerable stimulation of respiration and an increase in the amount of glucose oxidized via the hexose-monophosphate pathway. Other changes include lactic acid production, intracellular glycogen breakdown, utilization of extracellular glucose, and hydrogen peroxide formation. These changes occur rapidly during phagocytosis; the respiratory burst takes place immediately after cell-particle contact, before extensive phagocytosis and degranulation (Klebanoff, 1971). It is known that glycolytic inhibitors will also inhibit phagocytosis (Cohn and Morse, 1960; Sbarra and Karnovsky, 1959). However, inhibition of cytochrome-linked respiration, Krebs cycle activity, or oxidative phosphorylation has no effect on particle uptake or the accompanying metabolic activity (Iyer *et al.*, 1961). Therefore, glycolysis appears to be a necessary requirement for the phagocytic process. Increased H_2O_2 produced as a consequence of increased O_2 uptake is thought to participate directly in bactericidal mechanisms in the presence of myeloperoxidase and a halide. The increment in respiration, direct oxidation of glucose, and production of H_2O_2 is greatly reduced in the bactericidally defective leukocytes from patients with chronic granulomatous disease

(Holmes *et. al.*, 1967) and is therefore thought to be linked to abnormal intracellular bactericidal activity.

While the exact chain of events leading to the observed alterations in leukocyte biochemistry is not as yet totally defined, the following scheme is one currently favored (Holmes *et al.*, 1970):

(1) Increase in respiration

$$NADH + H^+ \quad + \quad O_2 \xrightarrow[\text{oxidase}]{\text{flavoprotein}} H_2O_2 + NAD^+$$
$$NADPH + H^+ \qquad\qquad\qquad\qquad\qquad NADP^+$$

(2) Removal of peroxide

$$H_2O_2 + 2GSH \xrightarrow[\text{peroxidase}]{\text{glutathione}} GSSG + 4H_2O$$
$$\text{(reduced}\qquad\qquad\qquad\qquad \text{(oxidized glutathione)}$$
$$\text{glutathione)}$$

$$GSSG + NADPH + H^+ \xrightarrow[\text{reductase}]{\text{glutathione}} 2GSH + NADP^+$$

Sum of (1) and (2):

$$H_2O_2 + NADPH + H^+ \longrightarrow NADP^+ + 2H_2O$$

(3) Stimulation of hexose-monophosphate pathway by increase in available $NADP^+$.

In the first step, the formation of H_2O_2 is mediated by flavoprotein oxidases present in human leukocytes. Baehner and Karnovsky (1968) suggest that leukocytes from patients with chronic granulomatous disease lack NADH oxidase; however, Holmes *et al.* (1970) were unable to confirm this finding. The second step involves a glutathione pathway which participates in the reduction of H_2O_2 and the generation of $NADP^+$. $NADP^+$ functions, in the third step, to stimulate activity of the hexose-monophosphate pathway by stimulating dehydrogenases in the pathway. Holmes *et al.* (1970) have reported that leukocyte glutathione peroxidase is deficient in two female patients with chronic granulomatous disease, while the enzyme is apparently normal in male patients. Their male patients have an unusually heat labile, but functionally normal, glucose-6-phosphate dehydrogenase, the first dehydrogenase of the hexose-monophosphate pathway.

PHAGOCYTOSIS BY COCKROACH HEMOCYTES

Comparable data obtained from *Blaberus* phagocytic hemocytes indicate that many of the previously described metabolic alterations do not accompany phagocytosis and antimicrobial activity in these cells. Comparative information cited from studies on normal leukocytes were obtained from Holmes *et al.* (1967), unless otherwise designated.

Oxygen consumption was measured using a Biological Oxygen Monitor (Yellow Springs Instrument Co.). Cell suspensions ($1-2.5 \times 10^6$ cells/ml) were incubated at $26°C$, with constant mixing, for 10 min to obtain resting levels of respiration. Particles (heat-killed *S. aureus* 502 A or latex) were injected into the incubation chamber and the rate of respiration during phagocytosis recorded. The average calculated resting rate of oxygen uptake for *Blaberus* hemocytes was $6.88 \mu l O_2/10^7$ cells/hr; the average rate during phagocytosis was $7.46 \mu l O_2/10^7$ cells/hr, indicating a stimulation of about 8.3%. Human leukocytes, on the other hand, showed greater than 400% increase in oxygen utilization during phagocytosis of latex particles. The resting level of O_2 uptake for human leukocytes was $7.35 \mu l O_2/10^7$ cells/hr, which is comparable to that recorded for *Blaberus* cells.

Glucose metabolism was assayed by measuring the release of $C^{14}O_2$ by phagocytosing hemocyte suspensions after the introduction of specifically labeled C^{14} glucose. The $C^{14}O_2$ was absorbed on filter paper saturated with 20% NaOH suspended from the stopper of a 15 ml flask containing 1 ml of reaction mixture. After the incubation period, the filter papers were air-dried and placed in scintillation vials containing 10 ml of scintillation fluid (0.4% PPO and 0.01% POPOP in toluene) and the radioactivity was assayed in a Packard tricarb counter. About 1 μCi of C^{14}-glucose/10^7 cells was added to the vials. When uniformly labeled glucose was used, a slight (about 18%) increase in glucose oxidation was observed during latex phagocytosis by *Blaberus* hemocytes. Trehalose (a glucose disaccharide) is the natural blood sugar of many insects; therefore, uniformly C^{14}-labeled trehalose was introduced into the reaction mixture. Again, only a slight increase in $C^{14}O_2$ release accompanied phagocytosis. We are confident that significant phagocytosis occurred in the hemocyte suspensions on the basis of the examination of stained blood smears and/or the spectrophotometric quantitation of latex uptake after dioxane extraction from hemocytes. Similar determinations of active phagocytosis were performed in all series of experiments. The production of $C^{14}O_2$ from C^{14}-1-glucose indicates the level of hexose-monophosphate shunt activity. *Blaberus* hemocytes phagocytosing latex or heat-killed bacteria produced slightly less (9% decrease in d.p.m.) $C^{14}O_2$ from C^{14}-1-glucose than did the same cells in the resting condition. Normal human leukocytes showed an almost 1000% increase in C^{14}-1-glucose oxidation, indicating marked hexose-monophosphate pathway stimulation.

For the measurement of glycogen breakdown, glucose utilization, and lactate production, hemocyte suspensions were incubated in glucose-enriched balanced salt solution on a reciprocating water bath shaker at $26°C$. After 20 min incubation, they were deproteinized with 70% perchloric acid (0.05 ml

PCA/ml suspension). After centrifugation, the supernatant was neutralized with 5 M K_2CO_3 and aliquots were analyzed for glucose (by the glucose oxidase method using Glucostat reagent, Worthington Biochemical Co.), lactic acid (by the method of Holzer and Söling, 1965), and glycogen (by the method of Seifter, 1950). The average glycogen content in 10^7 *Blaberus* hemocytes, before stimulation with latex particles, was 139.3 μg and dropped to 130.1 μg (about 7% decrease) 20 min after the addition of particles. The glycogen content of human leukocytes was roughly comparable, and latex stimulation brought about a 4% decrease in glycogen concentration in 20 min. Glucose consumption in resting *Blaberus* cells averaged 211.1 nmol/10^7 cells and increased about 9.5% during phagocytosis. Glucose consumption increased 13% during phagocytosis of latex by human leukocytes. Lactate production increased 12% (from 244.4 to 273.7 nmol/10^7 cells) after the addition of latex particles to *Blaberus* cell suspensions. Latex stimulation caused a 25.6% increase in lactate production by human leukocytes. *Blaberus* phagocytes consumed 18.9 nmol glucose/10^7 cells while producing 29.3 nmol lactate/10^7 cells; from these data it may be calculated that 4.25 nmol of the glucose utilized does not appear as lactic acid.

We have previously shown that phagocytosis does not stimulate direct oxidation of glucose via the hexose-monophosphate shunt in *Blaberus,* and data from uniformly C^{14}-labeled glucose oxidation experiments indicate that there is little stimulation of Krebs cycle activity. Therefore, it is possible that some of the glucose is being channeled into other metabolic routes, such as lipid metabolism. However, the data indicate that glycolysis is the only pathway of carbohydrate metabolism in *Blaberus* hemocytes stimulated significantly by phagocytosis.

To examine further the role of glycolysis, the effect of various metabolic inhibitors on the antimicrobial activity of insect hemocytes was tested. In these experiments, suspensions of hemocytes, inhibitors, and living *S. aureus* 502 A were incubated for 60 min at 26°C. The percent of bacteria killed was determined by plating diluted aliquots of the reaction mixture on nutrient agar, incubating 24 hr at 37°C, and counting the viable colonies. The respiratory-chain inhibitor KCN had no effect on hemocyte bactericidal capacity at concentrations that usually inhibit respiration (such as $8 \times 10^{-4} M$), and only at the extremely high concentration of $2.4 \times 10^{-3} M$ was bactericidal capacity slightly reduced. Arsenite uncouples oxidation and phosphorylation at the triose oxidation step of glycolysis; no high-energy phosphate group is generated by the dehydrogenase, although overall oxidation takes place. Iodoacetate (CH_2ICOOH) also inhibits this enzyme (glyceraldehyde-3-phosphate dehydrogenase) by functioning as an alkylating agent. More than one half of the bactericidal capacity of *Blaberus* hemocytes was abolished by $4 \times 10^{-4} M$ $NaAsO_2$, while $1 \times 10^{-3} M$ arsenate almost totally protected *S. aureus* from being killed by hemocytes. Only about 11% of total bactericidal capacity was expressed in $2 \times$

$10^{-4}M$ CH$_2$ICOOH, and $6 \times 10^{-4}M$ inhibited bactericidal activity entirely. Similar data were reported for rabbit polymorphonuclear leukocytes by Cohn and Morse (1960). They found that $8 \times 10^{-4}M$ KCN had little effect on the killing of *S. albus* while $2 \times 10^{-4}M$ arsenite or iodoacetate markedly inhibited intracellular killing, due to inhibition of bacterial uptake.

One of the events in the metabolic burst, following phagocytosis by mammalian cells, is the production of H_2O_2 by the action of flavoprotein oxidase. NADH oxidase has been shown to reduce nitroblue tetrazolium (NBT) by Cagan and Karnovsky (1964). If NBT and zymosan particles are phagocytosed by human leukocytes, the dye will be reduced, coloring the ingested particles a deep blue. Preliminary studies indicate that NBT is not reduced after zymosan ingestion by *Blaberus* hemocytes.

A potent antimicrobial system in mammalian cells consists of hydrogen peroxide, a halide, and myeloperoxidase (Klebanoff, 1968). Myeloperoxidase (MPO) of lysosomal origin and H_2O_2 (formed by the ingested microorganisms and/or formed by the phagocytosing cell) react with an introcellular halide causing the halogenation of the microorganisms and adjacent leukocyte material. MPO is not bactericidal by itself, but acts in synergism with H_2O_2 and a halide. If human leukocytes are examined histologically after staining for MPO, the enzyme is associated with lysosomal granules throughout the cytoplasm of every cell. *Blaberus* hemocytes also contain many lysosomal granules, but only about 1 cell in 50 shows the presence of some MPO. If human leukocytes are placed in a medium containing NaI[125] and stimulated with zymosan particles, they will iodinate the particles by the action of MPO and H_2O_2. The iodide is converted into a TCA (trichloroacetic acid) precipitable form, which may be quantitated by detection of the isotopically labeled halide (Pincus and Klebanoff, 1971). Since *Blaberus* cells have small amounts of MPO, a quantitative iodination test was run to see if they could iodinate particulates. Little or no iodination occurred in the *Blaberus* hemocytes, while marked iodination took place in normal human leukocytes run at the same time.

SUMMARY OF THE METABOLIC EVENTS IN PHAGOCYTOSIS

In summary, it is clear that many of the characteristic alterations in metabolism of phagocytosing mammalian leukocytes are absent in phagocytosing *Blaberus craniifer* hemocytes. As in mammalian cells, the process of ingestion is accompanied by stimulated glycolysis, but the subsequent metabolic burst is absent. This rush of activity typically includes increased respiration, hexosemonophosphate shunt stimulation, and H_2O_2 production. The only metabolic alterations detected in phagocytosing *Blaberus* cells are those associated with glycolysis. Since glycolysis is also normal in chronic granulomatous disease, it is apparently not related directly to intracellular killing; uptake of bacteria is normal in these cells, although bactericidal activity is diminished. Glycolytic inhibitors are inhibitors of bacterial killing by virtue of inhibiting uptake rather than postphagocytic events. The myeloperoxidase-halide-hydrogen peroxide antibacterial system of mammalian leukocytes apparently does not function in insect hemocytes. Despite the absence of metabolic events similar to those observed in mammalian systems, it has been demonstrated that *Blaberus* hemocytes in these *in vitro* systems are phagocytically active and capable of killing many bacterial species.

ACKNOWLEDGMENTS

I am indebted to Robert A. Good for his guidance and encouragement during these studies. This investigation was carried out at the University of Minnesota in the laboratory of Beulah Holmes (an established investigator of the American Heart Association), who supplied invaluable information aiding experimental design, and who critically examined the manuscript. Technical assistance was contributed by Susan Buron, Judy Haseman, and Jean Rodgers. Marion A. Brooks supplied a breeding colony of *Blaberus craniifer.*

This investigation was supported by grant GB-16835 from the National Science Foundation, grant 70-711 from the American Heart Association, The National Foundation-March of Dimes, and Public Health Service Cardiovascular Training Grant HE-0522 from the National Heart and Lung Institute.

REFERENCES

Anderson, R. S., Holmes, B., and Good, R. A., 1973, *In vitro* bactericidal capacity of *Blaberus craniifer* hemocytes, *J. Invert. Path. 22*:127-135.

Baehner, R. L. and Karnovsky, M. L., 1968, Deficiency of reduced nicotinamide adenine dinucleotide oxidase in chronic granulomatous disease, *Science 162*:1277.

Cagan, R. H. and Karnovsky, M. L., 1964, Enzymatic basis of the respiratory stimulation during phagocytosis, *Nature 204*:255-257.

Cohn, Z. A. and Morse, S. I., 1960, Functional and metabolic properties of polymorphonuclear leukocytes, *J. Exp. Med. 111*:667-687.

Holmes and Good, 1972, Laboratory models of chronic granulomatous disease, *R.E.S.— J. Reticuloendothelial Soc. 12*:216-237.

Holmes, B., Page, A. R., and Good, R. A., 1967, Studies of the metabolic activity of leukocytes from patients with a genetic abnormality of phagocytic function, *J. Clin. Invest. 46*:1422-1432.

Holmes, B., Park, B. H., Malawista, S. E., Quie, P. G., Nelson, D. L., and Good, R. A., 1970, Chronic granulomatous disease in females. A deficiency of leukocyte glutathione peroxidase, *New Engl. J. Med. 283*:217-221.

Holzer. H. and Söling, H., 1965, Determination of lactic acid with lactic dehydrogenase and the 3-acetylpyridine analogue of DPN, *Methods of Enzymatic Analysis,* p. 275, Academic Press, New York.

Iyer, G. Y. N., Islam, M. F., and Quastel, J. H., 1961, Biochemical aspects of phagocytosis, *Nature 192*:535.

Klebanoff, S. J., 1968, Myeloperoxidase-halide-hydrogen peroxide antimicrobial system, *J. Bacteriol. 95*:2131-2138.

Klebanoff, S. J., 1971, Intraleukocytic microbicidal defects, *Ann. Rev. Med. 22*:39-62.
Landureau, J. C. and Jollès, P., 1969, Étude des exigences d'une lignée de cellules d'insects. I. Acides Amines, *Exp. Cell Res. 54*:391-398.
Pincus, S. H. and Klebanoff, S. J., 1971, Quantitative leukocyte iodination, *New Engl. J. Med. 284:*744-750.
Sbarra, A. J. and Karnovsky, M. L., 1959, The biochemical basis of phagocytosis. I. Metabolic changes during the ingestion of particles by polymorphonuclear leukocytes, *J. Biol. Chem. 234:*1355-1362.
Seifter, S., 1950, The estimation of glycogen with the anthrone reagent, *Arch. Biochem. 25:*191.

Chapter 5

The Coelomocytes of Nereid Polychaetes

Denis G. Baskin

Department of Zoology
Seaver Laboratory, Pomona College
Claremont, California

INTRODUCTION

The coelomic fluids of most polychaetes, or marine annelids, contain numerous mobile cells which have phagocytic abilities. Many investigators have observed that coelomocytes of several species of polychaetes take up foreign matter and have suggested that they probably remove particulate wastes. This applies equally to nereids (Dehorne, 1922*a,b*; Romieu, 1923; Fretter, 1953; Kermack, 1955; Dales, 1961, 1964; Marsden, 1963, 1966). Recent fine-structural studies support the view that coelomocytes of nereid polychaetes have a phagocytic role, which has still to be defined adequately in terms of cellular defense mechanisms. Nevertheless, investigations of their phagocytic responses are important in view of current ideas on the significance of the relationship of primitive phagocytic cells to origins of immune mechanisms (Burnet, 1968, 1970).

FINE STRUCTURE OF COELOMOCYTES

The most abundant and distinctive cells of coelomic fluids have an irregular shape and contain one or more large vacuoles. These are usually referred to as *eleocytes* (Fig. 1). Their name is derived from the presence of numerous cytoplasmic lipid droplets (up to 4 μ in diameter in nereids). The vesicular nucleus is usually situated in an eccentric position. The large, characteristic vacuoles of nereid eleocytes often contain a uniformly distributed, flocculent, electron-dense substance of unknown composition. Prominent globules of electron-dense material adhere to the vacuolar inner surface and a thin layer of similar material fre-

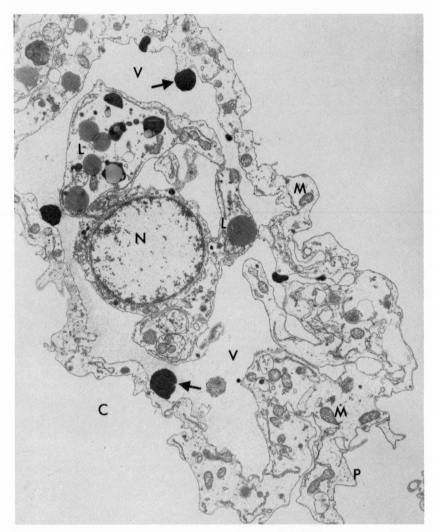

Fig. 1. Electron micrograph of an eleocyte showing nucleus (N), vacuole (V), lipid droplets (L), mitochondria (M), coelomic fluid (C), and pseudopodia (P). Note electron-dense
globules attached to vacuole membrane (arrows) (magnification 5200×), *Nereis succinea.*

quently lines this vacuole. Vacuoles of nereid eleocytes contain fragments of
muscle fibers, apparently in various stages of digestion (Figs. 2, 3), and are a
feature which characterizes nereid eleocytes (Schroeder, 1967; Dhainaut,
1966*a*). This fact led earlier investigators to assume that eleocytes are involved in
phagocytosis of free muscle fibers, or sarcolytes, which are present in the coelomic fluid (Dehorne, 1922*a,b*; Dales, 1950). Sarcolytes are presumably derived
from body-wall muscle which undergoes histolysis during later stages of re-

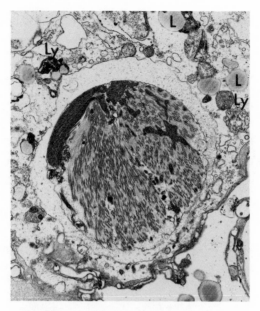

Fig. 2. Electron micrograph of a muscle fiber (sarcolyte) engulfed by eleocyte. Note lyso-somelike inclusions (Ly) and lipid droplets (L) (magnification 5300×), *Nereis succinea.*

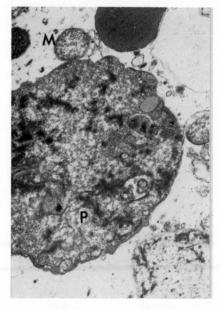

Fig. 3. Electron micrograph of eleocyte phagolysosome (P) containing partially digested muscle fibers. Note mitochondrion (M) for scale (magnification 11,500×), *Nereis succinea.*

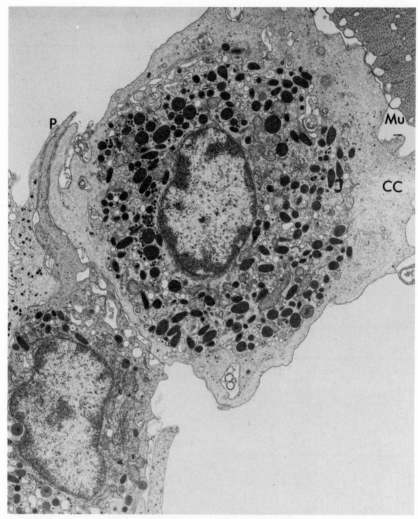

Fig. 4. Electron micrograph of granulocyte in coelomic fluid, showing perinuclear zone of granules and other organelles, and cortical cytoplasm (CC) devoid of organelles but exhibiting pseudopods (P) and surface infoldings. Note muscle cell (Mu) (magnification 9900×), *Nereis succinea.*

productive maturation (Defretin, 1949). Therefore, current electron microscopic evidence strongly reinforces older ideas that nereid eleocytes engulf and digest free muscle cells.

Phagocytosis of muscle is probably related to nutrition of gametes. Studies of polychaetes belonging to several families indicate that coelomocytes contain substantial amounts of the total glycogen and lipid reserves of the worm's body;

such reserves are utilized by developing oocytes (Dales, 1961, 1964; Dhainaut, 1966b). Of particular interest here is the choice made by eleocytes; only free muscle cells are engulfed. Apparently *in situ* muscle cells and even other tissues are not affected in *Nereis diversicolor* (Dales, 1950) or in other nereids. This provides at least circumstantial evidence that eleocytes recognize a change in some quality of the worm's own muscle cells and that they respond like macrophages by phagocytosing effete sarcolytes. The cellular basis for this apparent self-recognition is not understood and it remains an outstanding problem.

One interesting and related observation is provided by Smith (1950), who worked on the reproduction of a viviparous polychaete, *Nereis limnicola* (as *Neanthes lightii*). Eggs and larvae of this worm develop in the adult coelomic fluid but are not normally attacked by coelomocytes. However, Smith occasionally found that deteriorating eggs and larvae were invested by layers of small cells. Furthermore, parasitic gregarines were also encapsulated by coelomic cells.

The coelomic fluids of nereids also have smaller, ovoid cells that contain numerous membrane-delimited, electron-opaque granules resembling lysosomes (Figs. 4, 5, 6). The nucleus is centrally located and contains more electron-opaque chromatin than does the typical eleocytic nucleus. The granules (as well as abundant microtubules, microfilaments, endoplasmic reticulum, glycogen rosettes, and other inclusions) are usually concentrated in a perinuclear zone. Peripheral to this is an area of cytoplasm largely devoid of organelles. This

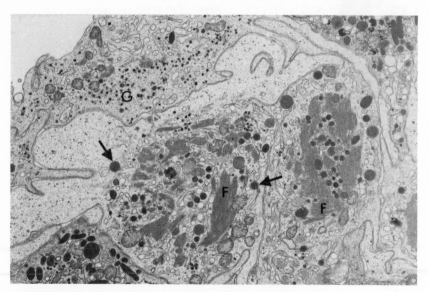

Fig. 5. Electron micrograph showing dense bundles of microfilaments (F) in several closely-packed granulocytes. Note membrane-delimited granules (arrow) and glycogen (G) (magnification 9900×), *Nereis succinea*.

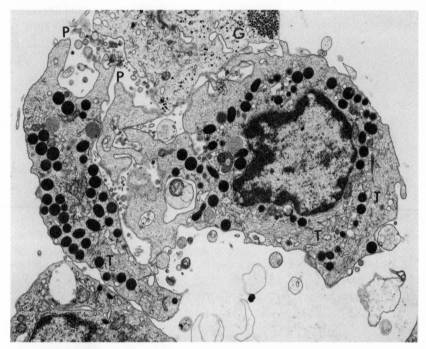

Fig. 6. Electron micrograph of granulocyte showing numerous microtubules (T). Also note characteristic glycogen accumulation (G) and pseudopodia (P) (magnification 6900×), *Nereis succinea.*

cortical region exhibits pseudopodia, surface pockets and folds, and small vesicles with electron-lucent contents. Some granulocytelike cells lack this distinctive zonation, and in such cells the endoplasmic reticulum and Golgi apparatus are more prominent, but relatively few granules are present (Fig. 7). In nereids, granulocytes are frequently found between body-wall muscle cells (Fig. 8) and among neuroglial cells in the central nervous system, where they are interpreted as being neuroglial elements (Baskin, 1971). These granulocytes (as well as those described in this paper) are similar in fine structure to vertebrate granulocytic leucocytes (Anderson, 1966; Bainton and Farquhar, 1966; Scott and Horn, 1970), a resemblance suggesting that nereid granulocytes also possess phagocytic abilities.

DISCUSSION

Much of the confusion that exists regarding polychaete coelomocytes is a consequence of the inconsistent nomenclature employed by various investigators. A bewildering variety of cell "types" has been described: leukocytes, phagocytes, amoebocytes, lymphocytes, chloragogen cells, eleocytes, etc. (see

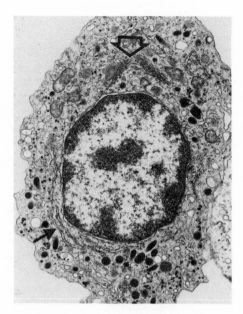

Fig. 7. Electron micrograph of granulocyte with relatively few granules. Note absence of organelle-free cortical zone but presence of endoplasmic reticulum (small arrow) and Golgi apparatus (large arrow) (magnification 9400×), *Nereis succinea*.

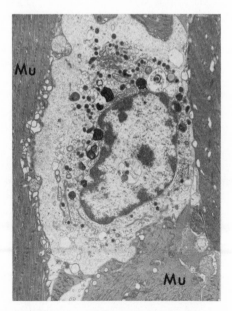

Fig. 8. Electron micrograph of granulocyte situated between muscle cells (Mu) of body wall (magnification 4700×), *Nereis succinea*.

synopsis by Beauchamp, 1959, p. 59). Where terms with functional meaning have been employed, it is frequently impossible to be certain of actual coelomocyte identity (for example, eleocytes have been called phagocytes, amoebocytes, and leukocytes). Some synthesis in terminology is provided by Dales (1961, 1964), who concludes that the various coelomocytes in *Sabella* (Sabellidae) and *Amphitrite* (Terebellidae) are different stages in the life of one cell type. Eleocytes are considered as "amoebocytes transformed by uptake of oil and other substances"; smaller coelomocytes (amoebocytes) are thought to be more "actively phagocytic."

There is additional evidence that nereid eleocytes may undergo a similar morphological transformation during the period of active gametogenesis. One aspect of this transformation is the appearance of the prominent eleocyte nucleolus (Schroeder, 1967). Furthermore, Dhainaut (1966*a*, 1972) reports that eleocytes of immature female nereids contain numerous granules of presumed protein content and abundant granular endoplasmic reticulum, but the granules disappear by the time the worms are fully mature. In summary, therefore, at the present a distinction between granulocytes and eleocytes in nereids seems valid only on morphological grounds, since they may represent different developmental or functional phases of one cell type.

It may be conceptually useful for future investigators of annelid coelomocytes to consider current views about insect hemocytes, where diversity in structure may reflect division of labor and functional diversity of one basic cell type. This obviates a strict classification adhering to distinctly separate cellular types (Scharrer, 1972). I wish to emphasize that before the role of coelomocytes in polychaete cellular defense mechanisms can begin to be explored and understood, we must have more information about coelomocyte identity, genealogy, interconvertibility, and paths of differentiation.

CONCLUSIONS

Recent studies strongly implicate coelomocytes in specific immune responses of oligochaete annelids. Thus, investigations of annelid coelomocytes may provide insights into the evolution of cellular defense mechanisms (Cooper, 1968, 1969; Bailey *et al.,* 1971). Although there is good reason to believe that mobile cells of polychaetes are phagocytic, whether these coelomocytes respond to antigens in a specific and adaptive fashion still remains to be determined. Nevertheless, Burnet (1968, 1970) suggests that cells of the vertebrate defense and immune systems are evolutionary equivalents and, in a sense, descendants of many invertebrate wandering phagocytic cells. Nereid coelomocytes resemble such hypothetical "ancestral cells" and the coelomocytes of nereid polychaetes could, therefore, influence our understanding of the cellular basis of primitive immune responses.

ACKNOWLEDGMENTS

Part of this study was carried out while the author was a Post-doctoral Trainee in the Department of Anatomy, Albert Einstein College of Medicine, Bronx, New York, and was supported by grants NIH 5P01 NS-7521, NIH 2T01 GM-00102, and NB-00840 from the U.S. Public Health Service. I am indebted to Mrs. Sarah Wurzelmann and Mr. Stanley Brown for their excellent technical assistance, and to Dr. Berta Scharrer and Dr. Edwin L. Cooper for stimulating discussions. I gratefully acknowledge the support and facilities provided by the Department of Zoology and the Seaver Science Center, Pomona College.

REFERENCES

Anderson, D. R., 1966, Ultrastructure of normal and leukemic leukocytes in human peripheral blood, *J. Ultrastruct. Res. 9*(Suppl):1-42.
Bailey, S., Miller, B. J., and Cooper, E. L., 1971, Transplantation immunity in annelids. II. Adoptive transfer of the allograft reaction, *J. Immunol. 21*:81-86.
Bainton, D. F. and Farquhar, M. G., 1966, Origin of granules in polymorphonuclear leukocytes, *J. Cell. Biol. 28*:277-301.
Baskin, D. G., 1971, The fine structure of neuroglia in the central nervous system of nereid polychaetes, *Z. Zellforsch. 119*:295-308.
Beauchamp, P. de, 1959, Annélides Polychètes, in: *Traité de Zoologie,* Vol. V, Fasc. 1, pp. 1-196, Masson, Paris.
Burnet, F. M., 1968, Evolution of the immune process in vertebrates, *Nature 218*:426-430.
Burnet, F. M., 1970, *Immunological Surveillance,* Pergamon Press, New York.
Cooper, E. L., 1968, Transplantation immunity in annelids. I. Rejection of xenografts exchanged between *Lumbricus terrestris* and *Eisenia foetida, Transplantation 6*:322-337.
Cooper, E. L., 1969, Specific tissue graft rejection in earthworms, *Science 166*:1414-1415.
Dales, R. P., 1950, The reproduction and larval development of *Nereis diversicolor* O. F. Müller, *J. Marine Biol. Assoc. U.K. 29*:321-360.
Dales, R. P., 1961, The coelomic and peritoneal cell systems of some sabellid polychaetes, *Quart. J. Microscop. Sci. 102*:327-346.
Dales, R. P., 1964, The coelomocytes of the terebellid polychaete *Amphitrite johnstoni, Quart. J. Microscop. Sci. 105*:263-279.
Defretin, R., 1949, Recherches sur la musculature des Néréidiens au cours de l'épitoquie, sur les glandes parapodiales et sur la spermiogenèse, *Ann. Inst. Océanogr, 24*:117-257.
Dehorne, A., 1922*a*, Histolyse et phagocytose musculaire dans le coelome des néréides à maturité sexuelle, *Comp. Rend. Acad. Sci. Paris 174*:1043-1045.
Dehorne, A., 1922*b*, Destruction et phagocytose des fibres musculaires à la fin de la maturation des ovocytes chez *Hediste diversicolor, Comp. Rend. Soc. Biol. 87*:1305-1307.

Dhainaut, A., 1966a, Étude ultrastructurale de l'évolution des éléocytes chez *Nereis pelagica* L. (Annélide Pólychète) a l'approache de la maturité sexuelle, *Comp. Rend. Acad. Sci. Paris, Ser. D 262*:2740-2743.

Dhainaut, A., 1966b, Étude ultrastructurale de l'évolution cytoplasmique au cours des premiers stades de l'ovogenèse chez *Nereis pelagica* L., *Comp. Rend. Acad. Sci. Paris, Ser. D 262*:2616-2619.

Dhainaut, A., 1972, Influence de la diminution du taux d'hormone cérébrale sur l'évolution éléocytaire et les processus de gametogénèse chez *Nereis pelagica* (Annélide Polychète), *Gen. Comp. Endocrinol. 18*:586.

Fretter, V., 1953, Experiments with radioactive strontium (90 Sr) on certain mollusca and polychaetes, *J. Marine Biol. Assoc. U.K. 32*:367-384.

Kermack, D. M., 1955, The anatomy and physiology of the gut of the polychaete *Arenicola marina, Proc. Zool. Soc. London 125*:347-381.

Marsden, J. R., 1963, A preliminary report on digestive enzymes of *Hermodice carunculata, Can. J. Zool. 41*:159-164.

Marsden, J. R., 1966, The coelomocytes of *Hermodice carunculata* (Polychaeta: Amphinomidae) in relation to digestion and excretion, *Can J. Zool. 44*:377-389.

Romieu, M., 1923, Recherches histophysiologiques sur le sang et sur le corps cardiaque des Annélides Polychètes. Contribution à l'histologie comparée du sang, *Arch. Morphol. Exp. Gén. 17*:1-336.

Scharrer, B., 1972, Cytophysiological features of hemocytes in cockroaches, *Z. Zellforsch. 129*:301-319.

Schroeder, P. C., 1967, Eleocyte nucleolus formation in relation to development of female nereid polychaetes, *Am. Zool. 7*:724.

Scott, R. E. and Horn, R. G., 1970, Fine structural features of eosinophil granulocyte development in human bone marrow, *J. Ultrastruct. Res. 33*:16-28.

Smith, R. I., 1950, Embryonic development in the viviparous nereid polychaete, *Neanthes lighti* Hartman, *J. Morphol. 87*:417-465.

Chapter 6

On the Ultrastructure of Invertebrate Hemocytes: An Interpretation of Their Role in Comparative Hematology

Christiane Stang-Voss

Anatomical Institute
University of Freiburg
Freiburg, B. D. R.

INTRODUCTION

The comparative, morphological investigation of blood cells is restricted mainly to experiments with vertebrates. Statements about structure, origin, and functions of invertebrate blood cells are extremely fragmentary and are mostly based upon light microscopic findings. There exists very little information about the course of blood cell development and functional relationships in different animal species. However, there are several trends in· cell differentiation: formation of erythrocytelike cells (Figs. 1--6), appearance of coagulation cells (Figs. 7, 8), and the formation of amebocytes, which phagocytose foreign bodies (Figs. 9, 10). My investigations add some electron microscopic data on invertebrate blood cells to comparative hematology with the intention of contributing something to the morphology and the development of "blood" within phylogeny.

THE BLOOD

According to Herzog (1933), the designation "blood" means the liquid content of the body cavities which provides nourishment, exchange of gases, the elimination of waste products, and transmission of hormonal information (cit.

65

according to Undritz, 1946). With increasing differentiation and size, a vascular system develops which allows regulated blood circulation. The blood, which will henceforth be called hemolymph, consists of a liquid portion, the plasma and formed elements, the blood cells, called hemocytes. Primitive metazoa, for example certain Plathelminthes, possess neither a functional vascular system separated from the widely branched digestive tract, nor a hemolymph distinguishable from the chyme. They have in their parenchyme tissue cells, which correspond to phagocytes in the hemolymph of advanced Plathelminthes (Prenant, 1922). This suggests that these cells, in phylogeny, have migrated from the surrounding connective tissue into the liquid hemolymph. Since the fundamental functions of the hemolymph are similar throughout the animal kingdom, blood cells develop in different animal species which are not homologous but analogous in function. In erythrocytelike cells, the pigments hemoglobin, hemerythrin, hemocyanin, or echinochrome are synthesized to bind oxygen, in spite of their different molecular structure and metallic components. Also, the processes of coagulation and wound closure are effected in different ways. The more varied and complicated the hemolymph functions, the more comprehensive is the number of hemocyte types (Undritz, 1946).

MOLLUSCAN HEMOCYTES

The morphology and behavior of molluscan hemocytes resemble the condition in Plathelminthes (Prenant, 1922). *Lymnea stagnalis L.* (Stang-Voss, 1970c) possesses only one type of hemocyte in the hemolymph, in the open vascular system, and in the connective tissue. This cell occurs in two morphologic forms, however: One is characterized by the presence of extensive storage cisterna in the granular ER and the other is without such organelles.

These ameboid cells possess long pseudopodia and glycogen deposits. The cytoplasm also contains numerous lysosomes whose acid phosphatase activity and characteristic structure suggest endocytosis. The cells are found in various numbers in the connective tissue (Fig. 1) and in the hemolymph. These cells can assemble to form reversible syncytial cell assemblages by dissolving the limiting plasmalemma (Müller, 1956), a distinct advantage in wound closure as the hemolymph contains no coagulant (George and Ferguson, 1950). In connection with hemocyte differentiation, the fine structure of the so-called *Leydig-cells* in the connective tissue was examined. Assembled, hexagonally arranged microtubuli in the cisterna of the granular ER show a remarkable similarity to the hemocyanin of blood cells of *Limulus polyphemus* (Chelicerata) described by Fahrenbach (1970). Moreover, I have also been able to trace microtubular aggregations in the free hemocytes of *Anodonta cygnea L.* (Lamellibranchiata). If this tubular system is also a product of hemocyanin synthesis, then the following conclusion is probable: In *Lymnea stagnalis L.*, pigment synthesis occurs in cells which are closely bound to the connective tissue. In *Anodonta cygnea L.*, the step to free, movable, pigment-forming cells in the hemolymph appears (Fig. 2). In both cases, however, the pigment is not stored, but is released in hemolymph by cell breakdown.

ANNELID HEMOCYTES

Most annelids have a closed vascular system. *Eisenia foetida (Sav.)* (Lumbricidae) possesses two types of cells in the hemoglobin-containing hemolymph (Stang-Voss, 1971a): the eleocytes which originate from the chloragogen tissue (Fig. 3), and the phagocytic amebocytes (Fig. 10) which are derived from undifferentiated cells of the septal and parietal peritoneum (Liebmann, 1942). Both types of cells are of mesodermal origin. In addition to other various functions, the eleocytes, once free from the chloragogen, play the role of simple erythrocytelike cells. Their protein-vacuoles sometimes reveal the presence of typical hemoglobin crystals and deposits of ferritin, also present in chloragogen (Lindner, 1965). As in the Molluscs, the occurrence of perishing, highly vacuolated eleocytes in Annelids suggests that the pigment is released into the hemolymph by these cells. Ochi (1969) found that some marine annelids possess real erythrocytes corresponding to those of vertebrates. Therefore, one can assume that the erythrocytelike cells of *Eisenia foetida (Sav.)* are an intermediate evolutionary stage similar to that of the Molluscs.

The amebocytes of *Eisenia foetida (Sav.)* possess extensive glycogen deposits, show acid phosphatase activity by light microscopy (Stang-Voss, 1971a), and contain especially characteristic electron-dense granules from which bundlelike cytoplasmic filaments emanate. These cells appear in two morphologic forms. The *petaloid* form or phagocyte (Liebmann, 1942) possesses a cytoplasm, rich in organelles; the outer ectoplasm is free of organelles. The transportation form is characterized by long finger-shaped pseudopodia (Fig. 10). These types are particularly important because agglutination is best achieved by aggregations of these cells. They are crucial to wound closure and therefore function partially in excluding foreign bodies.

SIPUNCULID HEMOCYTES

The Sipunculids, whose systematic position is often disputed, are usually classified as close relatives of the annelids. In Sipunculids, the step to real erythrocyte formation (Stang-Voss, 1970b), as in some marine annelids (Ochi, 1969), has already been accomplished (Fig. 6). In *Golfingia gouldi*, two types of cells

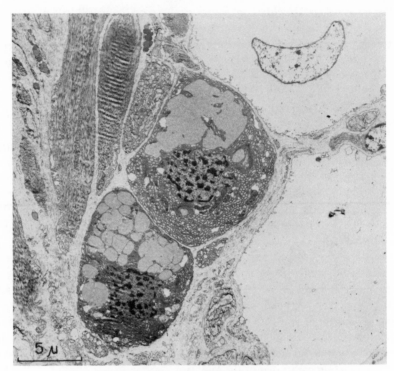

Fig. 1. *Lymnea stagnalis L.* (Mollusca): Erythrocytelike cells.

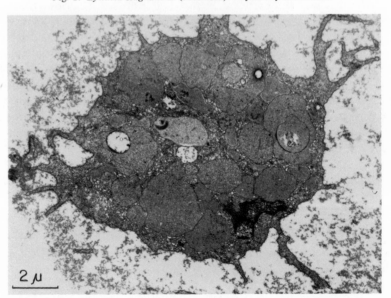

Fig. 2. *Anodonta cygnea L.* (Mollusca): Erythrocytelike cell.

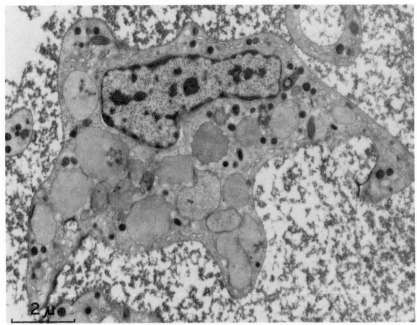

Fig. 3. *Eisenia foetida (Sav.)* (Annelida): Erythrocytelike cell.

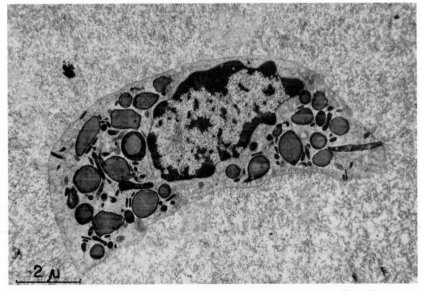

Fig. 4. *Astacus astacus L.* (Arthropoda: Crustacea): Erythrocytelike cell.

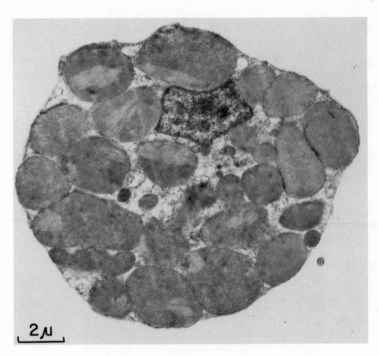

Fig. 5. *Psammechinus miliaris* (Echinodermata): Erythrocytelike cell.

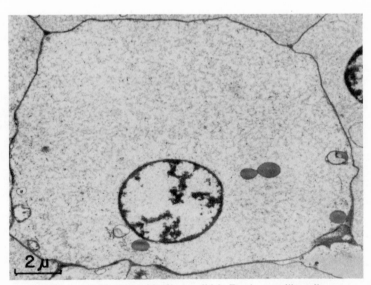

Fig. 6. *Golfingia gouldi* (Sipunculida): Erythrocytelike cell.

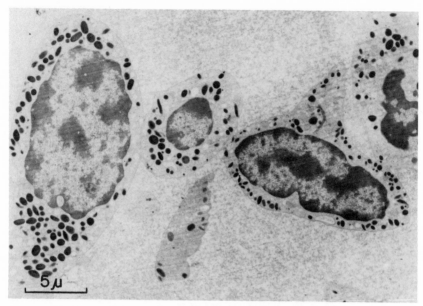

Fig. 7. *Astacus astacus L.* (Arthropoda: Crustacea): Coagulation cells.

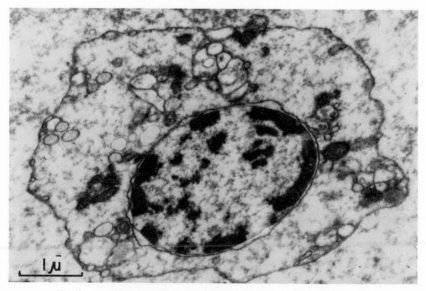

Fig. 8. *Tenebrio molitor L.* (Arthropoda: Insecta): Coagulation cell.

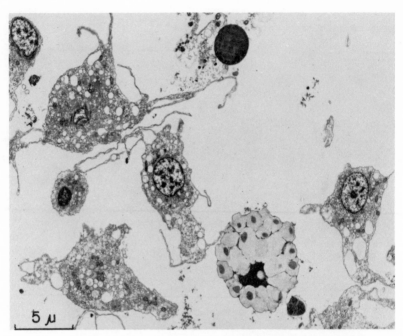

Fig. 9. *Psammechinus miliaris* (Echinodermata): Phagocytes.

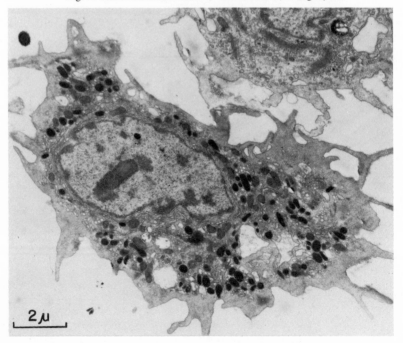

Fig. 10. *Eisenia foetida (Sav.)* (Annelida): Phagocytes.

are derived from peritoneal cells: hemerythrin-containing erythrocytes and phagocytic amebocytes. The erythrocytes develop from prohemocytes which still bear cinocilia in early stages. In the course of their maturation, cell organelles degenerate and reduction of nuclear volume takes place gradually. In the mature state, they show a remarkable similarity to the hemoglobin-containing erythrocytes of primitive vertebrates which contain only rudiments of cell organelles but have deposits of ferritin. The amebocytes originate from prohemocytes bearing cinocilia, many of which already show electron-dense inclusions at this stage. These electron-dense granules later become the dominant element of structure, as in the amebocytes of *Eisenia foetida* (*Sav.*). Long pseudopodia and multivesicular cytoplasmic bodies suggest endocytosis.

ARTHROPOD HEMOCYTES

With regards to the highly organized Arthropods, the number of hemocyte types developed in each class is so great that, in spite of a large number of light microscopic and electron microscopic investigations, few statements concerning common characteristic structures and functional correlations are possible. The hemocytes of *Astacus astacus* (Crustacea) and *Tenebrio molitor L.* (Insecta) share certain properties previously observed by other authors. In the Crustacea, hematopoetic organs appear for the first time (Andrew, 1965). The foci of cell formation are, especially in the insects, variable in position (Wigglesworth, 1959). In the decapod crabs, hemocytes are set free from a pharyngeal gland. In the hemolymph of *Astacus astacus L.*, hemocytes appear in three age-dependent functional forms (Stang-Voss, 1971*b*): coagulation inducing cells, phagocytic amebocytes, and probable hemocyanin-synthesizing granular amebocytes. *Tenebrio molitor* L. seems to possess only the first two cell types named (Stang-Voss, 1970*a*). In both species coagulation is caused by an explosionlike destruction of young hemocytes (Fig. 7, 8).

This process of hemocyte destruction liberates a "hemagglutinin" bound previously in characteristic granules. It induces skeinlike precipitations in the hemolymph, which form a network; other hemocytes can then become entrapped in these meshes (Grégoire, 1951). Thus, the Arthropods have developed a cell-bound mechanism of coagulation which is superior to the reversible cell assemblage in the Molluscs. It occurs rapidly. The interior structure of the coagulation-inducing granules is the same in all species examined so far. These granules are produced by the Golgi apparatus, as one can demonstrate in *Tenebrio molitor L.*

The phagocytic amebocytes of *Tenebrio molitor L.* are rich in lysosomes and seem to participate mainly in wound-healing, regeneration, and destruction of foreign bodies. The granular amebocyte (Fig. 4) in *Astacus astacus L.* appears as a third cell type (Stang-Voss, 1971*b*). It is probably a simple form of the erythrocytelike cyanoblast developed in *Limulus polyphemus* (Chelicerata)

(Fahrenbach, 1970). They synthesize hemocyanin and release it into the hemolymph. This cell type in *Astacus astacus L.* still probably corresponds to the eleocytes of the Annelids or the ameboid pigment formers of molluscs. *Tenebrio molitor L.*, like other species of insects, does not possess this cell type, a fact related to the formation of a richly branched trachea system, making oxygen bearers unnecessary.

HEMOCYTES OF ECHINODERMS AND UROCHORDATES

The question of the site of blood pigment synthesis remains to be elucidated in Echinoderms and Urochordates. *Psammechinus miliaris* (Echinoidea) possesses a hemolymph corresponding to sea water in its composition. It contains cells which originate from the coelomic endothelium and which bear, in young forms, cinocilia (Liebmann, 1950). From these cells arise ameboid phagocytes (Fig. 9), which often assume a petaloid form, and eleocytes with red or colorless vacuoles (Stang-Voss, 1971c). The phagocytes correspond functionally to the amebocytes of other species: They eliminate impurities and, by aggregating, function in agglutination. Beyond that, they show a peculiarity not observed until now. They often phagocytose whole eleocytes (Stang-Voss, 1971c), by cell "cannibalism" (Liebmann, 1950). It seems more probable that the amoebocytes, analogous to RES cells of vertebrates, "recognize" and phagocytose already damaged eleocytes before their autolysis. A similar behavior has been observed by Overton (1966) in phagocytes of *Perophora viridis,* a tunicate belonging to the Urochordata.

The inclusions of the "white" eleocytes are located on a netlike structure (Stang-Voss, 1971c). According to experiments of Jacobson and Millott (1953), these cells synthesize preliminary stages of melanin which are then transported to the epidermis. Thus we have melanin formers in the hemolymph of mesodermal origin. The "red" eleocytes (Fig. 5) synthesize and store echinochrome, which can bind a small amount of oxygen (Lederer, 1940). Large granular structured vacuoles gradually replace the basic cytoplasm and cell organelles. The nucleus degenerates as the cell grows in size and advances in age.

CONCLUSIONS

In agreement with the findings of other authors, my investigations propose the following conclusions: In the course of phylogeny, morphologically and functionally convergent hemocyte types have been developed. The tendency for highly specialized erythrocyte development occurs first by cells still localized in the connective tissue. These synthesize an oxygen binding pigment, which is set free into the hemolymph. These fixed cells of the connective tissue are replaced in the course of evolution by cells which are ameboid. In the Sipunculidae, some marine Annelidae, and Echinodermatae, one encounters erythrocytes which not only synthesize but also store and retain their own pigment. The ultrastructure of all these cells is similar to that of vertebrate erythrocytes. These mutually shared criteria of structure seem to be generated as functional and morphological parallelisms in evolution. Still other hemocyte types, called amebocytes, with a marked activity for phagocytosis, are able to destroy and remove foreign bodies. Analogous to the granulocytes of vertebrates, they sometimes show acid phosphatase activity. Amebocytes replace the often nonexisting ability of coagulation by aggregation and formation of reversible syncytical tissues. In the Arthropods, they contain a hemagglutinin in characteristic granules which may be set free by the explosionlike cell autolysis enabling accelerated wound closure. One first observes amebocyte behavior in the Echinoderms and Urochordates, i.e., phagocytosis of whole eleocytes, reminiscent of RES cells of vertebrates. Undoubtedly invertebrate blood cells play an important role in immune reactions.

REFERENCES

Andrew, W., 1965, *Comparative Hematology*, Grune & Stratton, New York and London.

Fahrenbach, W. H., 1970, The cyanoblast: Hemocyanin formation in *Limulus polyphemus*, *J. Cell Biol. 44*:445-453.

Fernandez-Morán, H., Marchalonis, J. J., and Edelman, G. H., 1968, Electron microscopy of a hemagglutinin from *Limulus polyphemus, J. Mol. Biol. 32*:467-469.

George, W. C. and Ferguson, J. H., 1950, The blood of gastropod molluscs, *J. Morphol. 86*:315-327.

Grégoire, C., 1951, Blood coagulation in Arthropods. II. Phase contrast microscopic observations on hemolymph coagulation of sixty-one species of insects, *Blood 6*:1173-1198.

Herzog, D., 1933, *Handbuch der allgemeinen Haematologie, I*, p. 1299, Urban & Schwarzenberg, Berlin–Wien.

Jacobson, F. and Millott, N., 1953, Phenolases and melanogenesis in the coelomic fluid of *Diadema, Proc. Roy. Soc.* (London), Ser. *B 141*:231-247.

Lederer, E., 1940, Les pigments des invertebrés, *Biol. Rev. 15*:273-306.

Liebmann, E., 1942, The coelomocytes of Lumbricidae, *J. Morphol. 71*:221-245.

Liebmann, E., 1950, The leucocytes of *Arbacia punctulata, Biol. Bull. 98*:46-59.

Lindner, E., 1965, Ferritin und Hämoglobin im Chloragog von Lumbriciden (Oligochaetae), *Z. Zellforsch. 66*:891-913.

Müller, G., 1956, Morphologie, Lebenslauf und Bildungsort der Blutzellen von *Lymnea stagnalis L., Z. Zellforsch. 44*:519-556.

Ochi, O., 1969, Blood pigments and erythrocytes found in some marine Annelida, *Mem. Ehime Univ., Ser. B 6*:23-131.

Overton, J., 1966, The fine structure of blood cells in the Ascidian *Perophora viridis, J. Morphol. 119*:305-326.

Prénant, C. T., 1922, Recherches sur le parenchyme des Plathelmintes, *Arch. Morphol. Exp. Gén. 5*:12-165.

Prosser, C. L. and Brown, F. A., 1965, *Comparative Animal Physiology*, 2nd ed, Saunders, Philadelphia.

Stang-Voss, C., 1970a, Zur Ultrastruktur der Blutzellen wirbelloser Tiere. I. Über die Hämocyten der Larve des Mehlkäfers *Tenebrio molitor L.*, *Z. Zellforsch.* *103*:589-605.

Stang-Voss, C., 1970b, Zur Ultrastruktur der Blutzellen wirbelloser Tiere. II. Über die Blutzellen von *Golfingia gouldi* (Sipunculidae), *Z. Zellforsch.* *106*:200-208.

Stang-Voss, C., 1970c, Zur Ultrastruktur der Blutzellen wirbelloser Tiere. III. Über die Hämocyten der Schnecke *Lymnea stagnalis L.* (Pulmonata), *Z. Zellforsch.* *107*:142-156.

Stang-Voss, C., 1971a, Zur Ultrastruktur der Blutzellen wirbelloser Tiere. IV. Die Hämocyten von *Eisenia foetida L.* (Sav.) (Annelidae), *Z. Zellforsch.* *117*:451-462.

Stang-Voss, C., 1971b, Zur Ultrastruktur der Blutzellen wirbelloser Tiere. V. Über die Hämocyten von *Astacus astacus* (L.) (Crustacea), *Z. Zellforsch.* *122*:68-75.

Stang-Voss, C., 1971c, Zur Ultrastruktur der Blutzellen wirbelloser Tiere. VI. Über die Hämocyten von *Psammechinus miliaris* (Echinoidea), *Z. Zellforsch.* *122*:76-84.

Stang-Voss, C. and Staubesand, J., 1971, Mikrotubuläre Formationen in Zisternen des endoplasmatischen Retikulums. Elektronenmikroskopische Untersuchungen an Bindegewebszellen von *Lymnea stagnalis L.* (Pulmonata), *Z. Zellforsch.* *115*:69-78.

Undritz, E., 1946, Les cellules sanguines de l'homme et dans la série animale, *J. Suisse Med.* *76*:1-32.

Wigglesworth, V. B., 1959, Insect blood cells, *Ann. Rev. Entomol.* *4*:1-16.

Chapter 7

The Octopus White Body:
An Ultrastructural Survey

Ronald R. Cowden and Sherill K. Curtis

Department of Anatomy
Albany Medical College
Albany, New York

INTRODUCTION

While much has been written about immunity in molluscs, the only serious attempts at studying immune competence have produced conflicting results. Tripp (1963) and others have demonstrated repeatedly that oysters do not clear microorganisms at any greater rate or efficiency after secondary or subsequent exposures. Similarly Cheng (1969) was unable to show the presence of new proteins or shifts in amounts of hemolymph proteins in snails injected with bacteria. Still other evidence from multiple sources covering three taxonomic classes indicates that molluscs are able to produce vigorous and effective defenses against potential pathogenic organisms or foreign substances. However, only one line of evidence, reviewed by Cheng and Rifkin (1970), suggests that this is some form of cellular immunity. This is directly related to the acceptance of appropriate helminth larval forms by a molluscan intermediate host and the vigorous tissue rejection mechanism that develops when inappropriate ones are introduced. Cheng and Galloway (1970) found tissue rejection reactions in gastropods; the response to xenogeneic transplants is similar in principle to encapsulation and destruction of "foreign" larval forms. It seems certain that representatives of all molluscan classes have some capacity to reject or isolate "foreign" material like the gastropods, a capacity not studied extensively in cephalopods.

The results of several research groups actively studying defense or immunity in molluscs suggest that substantial differences in the forms and capacities for

*This research was supported by an institutional grant, GRS-FR-5394.

defense reactions do exist among the classes. The lamellibranchs present a relatively primitive situation in which phagocytosis of "foreign" substances or particulates plays an important role. As Bayne and Kime (1970) have recently shown, cells in the digestive gland of *Helix pomatia* are responsible for rapid removal of most injected particulates – bacteria in this instance. Gastropod hemocytes possess *some* phagocytic capacities. In cephalopods, Stuart (1968) found very little phagocytosis of carbon particles in the white body cells (mature hemocytes) of the lesser octopus. By contrast, particles are quickly removed from the circulation by cells in the gills. Similar observations for another cephalopod species are reported in this symposium by Bayne.

Cephalopods represent, unquestionably, the most specialized group of molluscs, and they therefore offer several challenges and experimental advantages for studying immunity. A single type of cell predominates in the circulating hemolymph, and its site of origin is and has been known for some time. Hemocytes appear to possess trivial phagocytic capacities but they can rapidly form cell-to-cell associations (cellular clots) and accumulate around "foreign" substances or at sites of inflammation. Adding to the concept of specialization, molluscs, in general, and cephalopods, in particular, possess a complex level of tissue organization balanced against a restricted capacity for regeneration.

THE LEUKOPOIETIC ORGANS OF CEPHALOPODS

The modern exploration of leukopoietic organs, the so-called "white bodies," of cephalopods began with the publication of two relatively long studies by Bolognari (1949, 1951). His monographs include a literature review on these organs and hemocytes, extending back into the 19th century. His 1951 paper presents a definitive account of the histology and some aspects of the cytology and histochemistry of cephalopod leukopoiesis.

The white bodies are located in the orbital pits behind the eyes, and their name is derived from their resemblance to the color and texture of a vertebrate thymus. Each organ usually consists of several interconnected lobes. The surface is covered with a connective tissue sheet which stains for collagen and contains fibers displaying the characteristic periodic pattern of collagen at the ultrastructural level. The leukopoietic elements are disposed toward the surface, which is thrown into a series of folds that extend deeply into the lumen of the organ. These folds form the leukopoietic cords. The lumen is filled with mature leukocytes or proleukocytes, and because of extensive surface folding, the lumen is considered to be a series of interconnecting sinusoids.

Since mitotic activity occurs normally in the white body, certainly there may be relatively rapid turnover of hemocytes. However, mitosis is abundant only among cells that will become secondary leukoblasts. Necco and Martin (1963) were able to develop a maintenance medium from TC-199 which sustained life for a limited time and allowed cell division but not propagation of cell lines. Cowden (1972) reviewed the histology of *Octopus vulgaris* white bodies. Since then, examination of white bodies from another octopus species and from two squid species disclosed no major differences in organization. The lumens appear larger in *Octopus briareus* than in *Octopus vulgaris* and the folding is emphasized, but the fundamental histological organization is consistent with earlier comparative observations of Bolognari (1951).

In Cowden's (1972) study, a slightly different hemopoietic cell classification scheme was proposed for cephalopods. It differs from that of Bolognari (1949, 1951) in recognizing the most primitive cell type as a hemocytoblast or reticulum cell rather than as a "primary leukoblast." These cells are large and have a large vesicular nucleus with an extensive nucleolus and an abundance of basophilic cytoplasm. The cells recognized as primary leukoblasts possess a substantially lower cytoplasmic to nuclear ratio. Another leukoblast type, the secondary leukoblast, is even smaller and has a more compact nucleus with a thin rim of cytoplasm. It is conceivable that a third type exists, but in most species this distinction must depend on quantitative criteria. Since dimensional differences would probably overlap within the cell cycle, it is of no use to extend classification schemes beyond the secondary leukoblasts. Of these cell types, only secondary leukoblasts divide actively. Thus at this level in cell development, a substantial increase in cell numbers occurs. Secondary leukoblasts are the smallest cells.

A transitional form, the proleukocyte, between secondary leukoblasts and mature hemocytes is also recognized. Transformation from secondary leukoblasts into proleukocytes involves cytoplasmic enlargement, alteration in nuclear organization, and reorganization of cytoplasmic organelles involved in synthesis. In short, transformation from a leukoblast to the terminal cell probably requires profound shifts in metabolic functions.

HEMOCYTOBLASTS

The changes during various stages of differentiation are probably best appreciated by examination of cell ultrastructure. The hemocytoblast or reticulum cell possesses a large amount of cytoplasm with a significantly different organization from that of leukoblasts. The cell shown in Fig. 1 contains abundant rough endoplasmic reticulum, an extremely granular ground substance, mitochondria, and the vesicular portion of a Golgi complex containing electron-dense secretory material. Another type of inclusion particularly characteristic of this stage is best described as a moderately electron-transparent, irregularly shaped, complex vesicle. The inclusion shown in Fig. 1 appears to be membrane-bound and seems to contain some internal fibrillar material condensed more in some surface zones than in others. The nucleus is enclosed in a typical nuclear envelope, and the chromatin displays some margination along the nuclear envelope. The nucleus apparently possesses the "extended" pattern of chromatin organization. Nucleoli occur always in these cells, and nucleolar zonation is usually obvious. The most striking feature of these cells' nuclei, at the ultrastructural level, is the presence of electron-opaque accumulations of material in the *extrachromosomal* nucleoplasm. These dense regions are a consistent feature in all cells of this series, including the mature leukocytes.

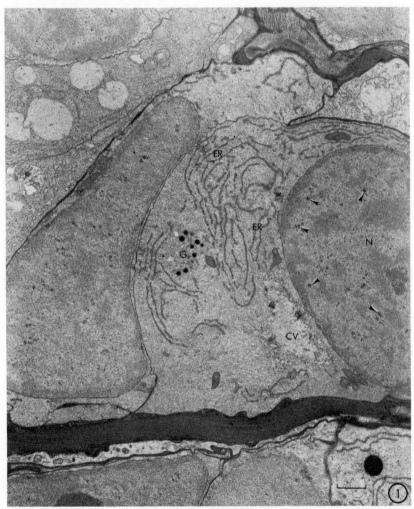

Fig. 1. Section through part of a hemocytoblast (reticulum cell) containing an abundance of rough endoplasmic reticulum (ER), some mitochondria, a Golgi complex (G) with dense secretory droplets, and an irregularly shaped, complex vesicle (CV). The nucleus (N) is large and rounded and possesses electron-dense accumulations of material in the extrachromosomal nucleoplasm (arrows) (magnification 12,000X). Line scale = 1 μm.

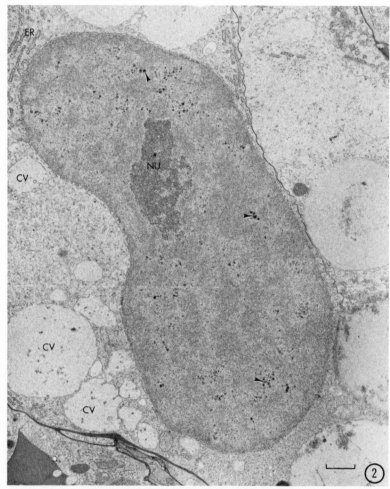

Fig. 2. Section through part of a hemocytoblast containing more abundant complex vesicles (CV). The nucleolus (NU) and extrachromosomal aggregates of dense
material (arrows) are particularly conspicuous. Strands of rough endoplasmic reticulum (ER) are also visible in the cytoplasm (magnification 12,000×). Line scale =
1 μm.

The hemocytoblast seen in Fig. 2 differs from the one just described in
possessing a substantial number of relatively electron-transparent, complex cytoplasmic inclusions. These inclusions are clearly surrounded by membranes and
contain a fine filamentous substructure and multiple foci where the filaments
apparently aggregate forming small irregular electron-dense zones. Rough endoplasmic reticulum is evident, although it does not appear to be particularly
abundant in this plane of section near the cell center. The cell seen in Fig. 3

possesses nearly all of the features of a typical octopus hemocytoblast: an abundance of rough endoplasmic reticulum, large complex inclusions, electron-dense inclusions, mitochondria, and a nucleus containing the irregular electron-dense extrachromosomal inclusions and a large multicomponent nucleolus.

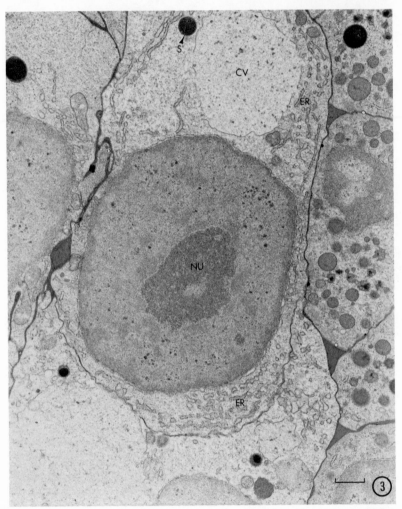

Fig. 3. Hemocytoblast with many of the features of the cells shown in Figs. 1 and 2: rough endoplasmic reticulum (ER), a complex vesicle (CV), several mitochondria, dense extrachromosomal accumulations in the nucleus, and a complex nucleolus (NU). An electron-dense, rounded inclusion (S) is also apparent in the cytoplasm (magnification 12,000×). Line scale = 1 μm.

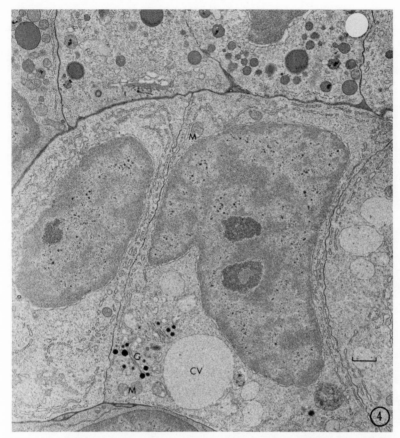

Fig. 4. Two cells possibly in the process of transforming into primary leukoblasts. Both of the cells display most of the features of hemocytoblasts. The complex vesicles (CV), Golgi complex (G), and mitochondria (M) are particularly conspicuous in one of the cells (magnification 9000×). Line scale = 1 μm.

HEMOCYTOBLASTS TO LEUKOBLASTS

In the transformation from hemocytoblast to leukoblast, the relative amount of cytoplasm is reduced substantially. Both of the cells in Fig. 4 display most of the cytoplasmic characteristics of the hemocytoblast, including a Golgi complex containing secretory material, rough endoplasmic reticulum, and typical hemocytoblast complex vesicles. The reduction in nuclear size, so apparent by light microscopy in cells of this kind, is not so obvious at the ultrastructural level unless the chromatin thickness associated with the nuclear envelope is

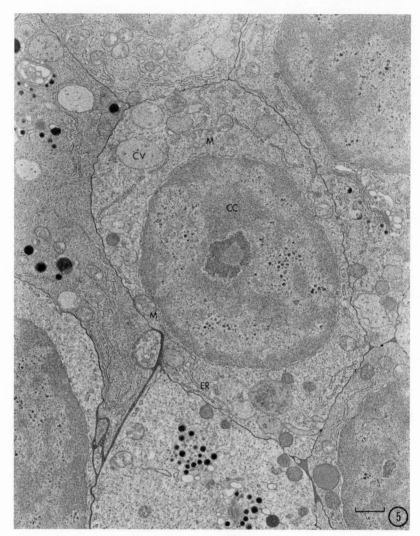

Fig. 5. Possible late primary leukoblast or early secondary leukoblast showing an increase in the amount of condensed chromatin (CC) in the nucleus and a reduction in the amount of cytoplasm. Strands of rough endoplasmic reticulum (ER), complex vesicles (CV), and mitochondria (M) are visible in the cytoplasm (magnification 12,000×). Line scale = 1 μm.

considered. With progressive differentiation from hemocytoblast to primary leukoblast to secondary leukoblast, this zone of chromatin, associated with the nuclear membrane, thickens, reflecting progressive chromatin condensation

LEUKOBLASTS

Since it is somewhat difficult to identify transitional stages at the ultrastructural level, the cell shown in Fig. 5 may represent either a late primary leukoblast or an early secondary leukoblast. While the nucleus does display substantial condensation and the cytoplasm is reduced, the derivatives of the electron-dense secretory inclusions found in later stages are not visible here. This is the only type of actively mitotic cell in the leukopoietic series encountered at the light microscopic level (Bolognari, 1951; Cowden, 1972). These cells are usually found in small groups and thus appear to develop in synchrony. At the ultrastructural level, they are joined by intercellular bridges which provide a probable structural basis for synchrony. These connections, as shown in Fig. 6, closely resemble those first described by Burgos and Fawcett (1955) in the testis of the cat, in various synchronously differentiating cell types (Fawcett *et*

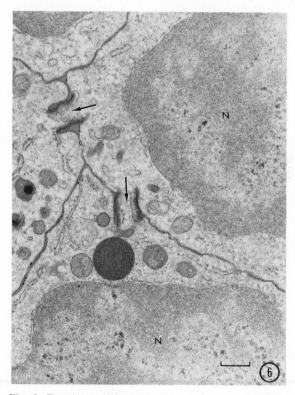

Fig. 6. Two intercellular bridges (arrows) connecting three contiguous cells. Portions of two nuclei (N) are also visible (magnification 24,000×). Line scale = 0.5 μm.

al., 1959), and, more recently, in vertebrate oogenesis (Ruby *et al.,* 1970). The cytoplasm is substantially reduced in these cells, but all normal organelles are represented despite some overall reduction in the amount of endoplasmic reticulum. The principal type of inclusion found in mature leukocytes is the dense, rounded secretory inclusion together with an apparent derivative distinguished by its irregular shape and central electron-dense core zone. The derivative form of the dense secretory inclusions is first seen in secondary leukoblasts.

SECONDARY LEUKOBLASTS TO MATURE LEUKOCYTES

The transformation of relatively small secondary leukoblasts into mature leukocytes or transitional forms, proleukocytes, requires substantial growth and

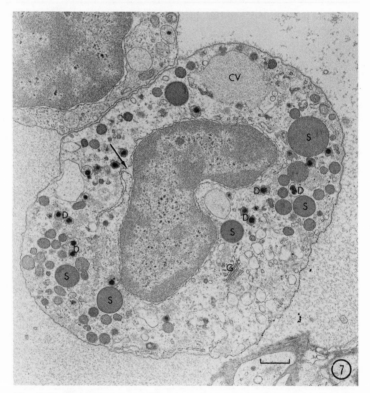

Fig. 7. Proleukoblast containing a small Golgi complex (G), a complex vesicle (CV), abundant electron-dense, rounded inclusions (S), and a number of irregularly shaped inclusions with dense cores (D). The irregularly shaped inclusions are possible derivatives of the electron-dense, rounded inclusions. A site of continuity between the nuclear membrane and the endoplasmic reticulum is marked with an arrow. The nucleus of the cell is folded and contains a number of dense extrachromosomal aggregates (magnification 12,000×). Line scale = 1.0 μm.

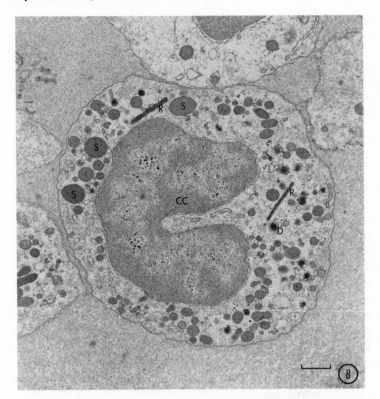

Fig. 8. Mature leukoblast with a folded nucleus containing an abundance of condensed chromatin (CC) and dense extrachromosomal aggregates. The cytoplasm contains a number of electron-dense, rounded inclusions (S), a few irregularly shaped inclusions with dense cores (D), and two unusual rod-shaped inclusions (R) (magnification 12,000X). Line scale = 1.0 μm.

reorganization of both cytoplasm and nucleus. Figure 7 represents a transitional form. This state can be recognized by the presence of a well developed Golgi complex, the remnants of a rough endoplasmic reticulum, and residual complex vesicles derived from (or similar to) those characteristic of secondary luekoblasts. In addition, both uniformly electron-dense inclusions and their probable derivatives — i.e., irregularly shaped inclusions with electron-dense core zones — are found in reasonable numbers.

The folded appearance of the nuclei of proleukocytes is even more evident in the mature leukocyte shown in Fig. 8. In this particular cell, the complex vesicles of hemocytoblast types are substantially reduced in number and there is an abundance of uniformly electron-dense inclusions. The ground substance of the cell shows a general reduction in granularity and electron density, and only a few remnants of the rough endoplasmic reticulum remain. In addition, there are several rod-shaped inclusions. Inclusions of this type were not observed in cells at earlier stages of development, and these appear to be typical of only later stages of differentiation. Finally, Cowden (1972) found glycogen in the cytoplasm of mature hemocytes of *Octopus vulgaris,* but neither cytochemical nor ultrastructural evidence for glycogen in *Octopus briareus* hemocytes. This points to a rather fundamental difference in metabolic patterns within hemocytes at the species level.

FINAL COMMENT

The observations made at all levels, whether light microscopic, cytochemical, *in vitro,* or electron microscopic, are consistent with the hypothesis that initial stages in the developmental pathway have three principal functions: to elaborate ribosomes, to initiate the synthesis of cell-specific products, and to increase the number of cells available for transformation into terminal forms. The second stage appears to be directed toward production of definite leukocytes. Presumably, the synthetic machinery inherited from precursor leukoblasts suffices to sustain and direct this second phase of differentiation since the nucleolus is absent in proleukocytes despite an obvious need for the synthesis of an enlarged cytoplasm. Protein synthesis apparently occurs in these cells in the absence of new RNA synthesis, or at least of new ribosomal RNA synthesis.

With respect to all parameters, the present report must still be considered a preliminary one: the details of synthetic patterns are being inferred on sound morphological and cytochemical grounds, nevertheless they are inferred, rather than demonstrated. Further autoradiographic, quantitative cytochemical, and ultrastructural studies will be required to clarify these matters. Because the cephalopod hemocyte contains granules homologous to those found in cells of other molluscs (Foley and Cheng, 1972), it has been called granulocyte. It seems more confusing that vertebrate hematological nomenclature and homologies should be extended without reservation into invertebrate hematology. Cephalopod leukocytes and vertebrate heterophile leukocytes *may* share common roles, but this, too, has yet to be critically demonstrated.

Mature leukocytes function primarily to establish cell-to-cell aggregations or cellular clots. The mechanism of this reaction still remains obscure, and it has not been established what role, if any, in this process is assigned to intracellular inclusions. Because each tentacle in *Octopus briareus* possesses a demonstrable autotomy joint, hemolymph clotting is particularly important to species survival. It has been known for decades that the hemocytes of cephalopods respond to irritants and accumulate at sites of injuries (see Bolognari, 1949; 1951). It now seems certain that these cells are not involved primarily in conventional phagocytosis. The possibility must be considered that cellular clots simply wall off any foreign or irritating material or contribute toward dissolution of foreign tissue by release of enzymes. This role, however, is potential and has not been demonstrated. Whatever the case, the host is protected.

As information develops relative to invertebrate immunity, it becomes increasingly clear that before any grand designs concerning the evolution of immunity finally emerge, substantially more detailed information must be established for particular species. Adaptive immunity, either cellular or humoral, has certainly not been demonstrated in cephalopods. Unlike many other invertebrate animals and molluscan classes, the cephalopods do offer the experimental advantages of a known single type of hemocyte and a known site or organ of origin for these cells. Much is now known about hemocytes and white bodies so that the serious study of defense mechanisms and immunity in this group can go forward. The very high degree of specialization and tissue complexity within this group could be deceiving. While it *is* necessary for organisms to have efficient defense mechanisms beyond the routine recognition and eventual expulsion of "foreign" material, this need not be an immune mechanism with the necessary components of specificity and anamnesis.

REFERENCES

Bayne, C. J. and Kime, J. B., 1970, *In vivo* removal of bacteria from the hemolymph of the land snail *Helix pomatia* (Pulmonata: Stylommatophora), *Malacological Rev.* *3*:103-113.

Bolognari, A., 1949, Morfologia, struttura e funzione del "corpo bianco" dei Cefalopodi. I. Morfologia, *Arch. Zool. Ital. 34*:79-97.

Bolognari, A., 1951, Morfologia, struttura e funzione del "corpo bianco" dei Cefalopodi. II. Struttura e funzione, *Arch. Zool. Ital. 36*:253-285.

Burgos, M. H. and Fawcett, D. W., 1955, Studies on the fine structure of the mammalian testis. I. Differentiation of the spermatids in the cat. *J. Biophys. Biochem. Cytol.* *1*:287-300.

Cheng, T. C. 1969, An electrophoretic analysis of hemolymph proteins of the snail *Helisoma duryi normale* experimentally challenged with bacteria, *J. Invertebr. Pathol. 14*:60-81.

Cheng, T. C. Galloway, P. C., 1970, Transplantation immunity in mollusks: the histoincompatibility of *Helisoma duryi normale* with allografts and xenografts, *J. Invertebr. Pathol. 15*:177-192.

Cheng, T. C. and Rifkin, E., 1970, Cellular reactions in marine molluscs in response to helminth parasitism, in: *A Symposium on Diseases of Fishes and Shellfishes,* Spec. Pub. No. 5, pp. 443-496 (S. F. Snieszko, ed.). American Fisheries Society, Washington, D.C.

Cowden, R. R., 1972, Some cytological and cytochemical observations on the leukopoietic organs, the "white bodies," of *Octopus vulgaris, J. Invertebr. Pathol. 19*:113-119.

Fawcett, D. W., Ito, S., and Slatterback, D. L., 1959, The occurrence of intercellular bridges in groups of cells exhibiting synchronous differentiation, *J. Biophys. Biochem. Cytol.* *5*:453-460.

Foley, D. A. and Cheng, T. C., 1972, Interaction of molluscs and foreign substances: the morphology and behavior of hemolymph cells of the American oyster, *Crassostrea virginica, in vitro, J. Invertebr. Path. 19*:383-394.

Necco, A. and Martin, R., 1963, Behavior and estimation of the mitotic activity of the white body cells in *Octopus vulgaris,* cultured *in vitro, Exp. Cell Res. 30*:588-590.

Ruby, J. R., Dyer, R. F., Skalko, R. G., and Volpe, E. P., 1970, Intercellular bridges between germ cells in the developing ovary of the tadpole, *Rana pipiens, Anat. Rec.* *167*:1-10.

Stuart, A. E., 1968, The reticulo-endothelial apparatus of the lesser octopus, *Eledone cirrosa, J. Pathol. Bacteriol. 96*:401-412.

Tripp, M. R., 1963, Cellular responses of molluscs, *Ann. N.Y. Acad. Sci. 113*:467-474.

Chapter 8

Earthworm Coelomocyte Immunity *

Russell K. Hostetter † and Edwin L. Cooper ‡

Department of Anatomy
School of Medicine, University of California
Los Angeles, California

---

*"Man is certainly stark mad; he cannot make a worm, and yet he will
be making gods by dozens."*

"Apology for Raimond Sebond"

Michael de Montaigne (1533-1592)

INTRODUCTION

The coelomic cavity of *Lumbricus terrestris* may be considered a hypothetical precursor of the vertebrate immune system. It is in contact with all organs, allowing communication with the coelomic fluid, and with coelomic cells, obviating a specialized lymphatic vascular system. The coelom is equipped with septa positioned perpendicularly to the flow of coelomic fluid, forming an efficient filtering organ, which together with the coelomic epithelial lining may be analogous to the vertebrate reticulo-endothelial system. Earthworm coelomocytes respond to pathogenic organisms and effect tissue graft rejection, both reactions are characteristics of vertebrate lymphoid cells.

*Supported by NSF Grant GB17767, The California Institute for Cancer Research, and The Brown-Hazen Corporation.
†Present address: Department of Anatomy, School of Medicine, Ohio State University. Supported by Training Grant GM616.
‡Send requests for reprints to: Edwin L. Cooper, Ph.D.

91

Earthworms are capable of distinguishing sharply between self and non-self tissue. Autografts heal promptly and never show signs of rejection or incompatibility. However, allografts are destroyed but require longer times for rejection than xenografts. Xenografts exchanged between different genera and species within the same family, or between members of different families, heal but are always eventually destroyed. The response to xenografts is characterized by specificity and anamnesis. If second-set grafts are transplanted five days after first-set grafting, hosts respond with an accelerated reaction to both the first and second set. A third independent first-set graft from a different genus does not influence the other rejection times. It is rejected independently, confirming specificity of the response.

The coelomocyte is thought to be the major mediator of graft destruction. If coelomocytes are harvested from worms previously immunized with allografts or xenografts and injected into naive nonimmune or uneducated worms, accelerated rejection of the first graft occurs, similar to a normal second-set reaction. How coelomocytes effect graft rejection is open to conjecture. With regard to phylogeny of immune competence the earthworm coelomocyte may thus emerge as a model immunocyte for understanding the early evolutionary events in the development of cellular immunity (Cooper, 1965a,b, 1966a,b, 1968a,b; Cooper and Baculi, 1968; Cooper 1969a,b,c; Cooper and Rubilotta, 1969; Winger and Cooper, 1969; Cooper, 1970, 1971, 1973a,b; Hostetter and Cooper, 1973; Lemmi, et al., 1973). This account takes the liberty of speculating on earthworm coelomocyte activities in what, for now, remains the only clear, acceptable description of specific immune recognition accompanied by a memory component among invertebrates.

HISTORICAL OBSERVATIONS

Earthworm coelomocytes have been a curiosity since the late 1800's when Metchnikoff first reviewed their defense functions against gregarine and nematode parasites (Metchnikoff, 1891). Thereafter only a few investigators studied annelid coelomic cells and they formulated varying opinions with regard to type, number, function, and origin (Keng, 1895; Rosa, 1896). Observations by Joseph (1942), Degrone (1925), and Faure-Fremiet (1927) added many more categories and classification schemes, causing complications and confusion in identifications. The more recent works of Cameron (1932) and Liebman (1942) yielded a simplification of coelomic cell nomenclature. Cameron classified coelomic cells as basophilic or acidophilic. Liebman referred to them as eleocytes and true leukocytes.

THE PRESENT PROBLEM

According to Burnet (1968), vertebrate immunocytes may be derived phylogenetically from the amoeboid wandering cell of invertebrates, which, when presented with an antigen, is capable of reacting to it. The earthworm coelomocyte conforms to this hypothetical ancestral cell. During reactions to tissue allografts (Cooper and Rubilotta, 1969, 1969a) and xenografts (Cooper, 1968b) coelomocytes congregate at graft sites where they can adoptively transfer the response from previously grafted worms to nongrafted recipients and can show an anamnestic response. With increasing implications of coelomocytes in the graft rejection process, reevaluation of coelomocyte classification schemes and functional characteristics is appropriate.

THE COELOMOCYTES

"Transitional" cells (20 μ) contain coarse cytoplasmic acidophilic granules (Fig. 1). The granules, surrounded by a light blue cytoplasm, are less dense in acidophilic cells. The nucleus is round (14 μ) and contains clumped chromatin which is less dense than that in the nuclei of acidophilic or basophilic cells. Transitional cell nuclei are more centrally located than those of acidophilic coelomic cells.

Large and small acidophilic cells occur in coelomic fluid smears (Fig. 2). The smaller cells measure 9 μ to 11 μ and contain coarse acidophilic granules. Larger cells contain fine acidophilic granules and range from 20 μ to 30 μ in diameter. The nucleus is located peripherally in large acidophilic cells, but varies in position in smaller acidophilic coelomocytes. Large acidophilic cell nuclei stain lighter than basophilic cell nuclei and measure only 5 μ in diameter (Fig. 3).

Total coelomocytes for normal *Lumbricus* range from 2500/mm^3 to 6075/mm^3 (mean = 5640/mm^3 ± 300 cells/mm^3). This background or normal cell count appears to vary among *Lumbricus*, but it can be categorized into three general groups: 2500 cells/mm^3; 5000 cells/mm^3; and 6000 cells/mm^3, depending upon which group of *Lumbricus* is sampled.

Examination of centrifuge-packed coelomic cell pellets at low magnification (25X) reveals three general regions. The upper portion contains lightly staining cells of 9 μ to 11 μ with a large nucleo-cytoplasm ratio. The central area consists of acidophilic and basophilic coelomocytes ranging from 10 μ to 15 μ. Nuclei are equivalent in size (7 μ) to those of 9 μ to 11 μ cell types from the upper third of the pellet. The lower portion is composed of clumps of acidophilic and basophilic coelomocytes which are mixed with chloragogen cells and debris. These coelomocytes range from 15 μ to 25 μ in diameter.

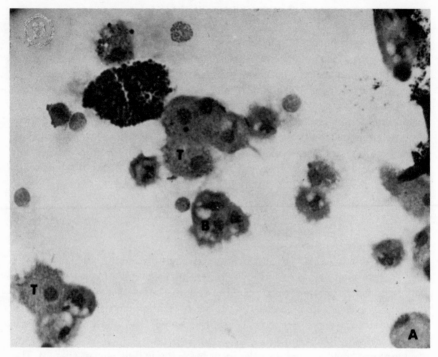

Fig. 1. "Transitional cells (T) were observed in a ten-minute hanging drop preparation (magnification 500×).

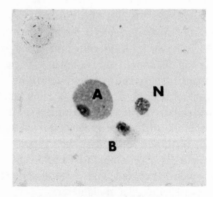

Fig. 2. Coelomic fluid contains three cell types: basophilic (B), neutrophilic (N), and acidophilic (A). Smear preparation stained with Wright's blood stain (magnification 300×).

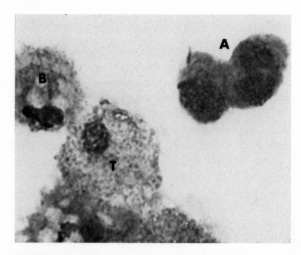

Fig. 3. Small acidophilic cells (9 μ to 11 μ) stained with Wright's blood stain (A). T = transitional coelomic cell; B = basophilic coelomic cell (magnification 500×).

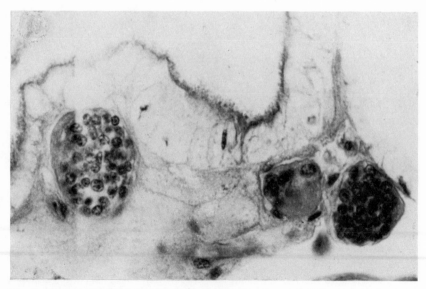

Fig. 4. Clusters of cell nuclei can be demonstrated in the area of the nephridial tubules. Stained with Harris' hematoxylin and eosin (magnification 500×).

COELOMIC CAVITY

Cross sections of *Lumbricus* stained with May-Greunwald Giemsa or PAS show aggregations of rod bacteria in the septa, nephridia, peritoneal lining, and circular muscle layers of the body wall. A closer inspection of the septal regions reveals acidophilic and basophilic cells surrounded by a matrix which stains homogeneously. The cellular network is interwoven among septal connective tissue and muscle fibers in close association with the blood supply. Observations of the alimentary canal reveal cellular accumulations in the gut lining near the anterior end. These cells stain blue with Meyer's hematoxylin and eosin. Such small aggregations of 5 to 20 cells are located immediately below the visceral peritoneum in close association with blood vessels. Numerous cellular aggregates are also present in the nephridia. Large cellular masses measuring 50 μ to 70 μ in diameter are formed apparently by free nuclei or nuclei surrounded by thin rims of cytoplasm. These nuclei measure 7 μ in diameter and contain large clumps of chromatin (Fig. 4). The entire cell mass is surrounded by a "capsule" which is PAS positive and apparently formed by a single endothelial cell type (Figs. 5, 6).

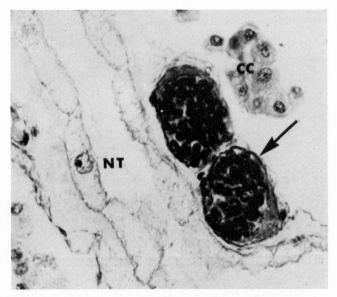

Fig. 5. A PAS-positive structure surrounds the nuclear aggregations found in the nephridia (arrow). NT = nephridial tubules; CC = coelomic cells (magnification 500×).

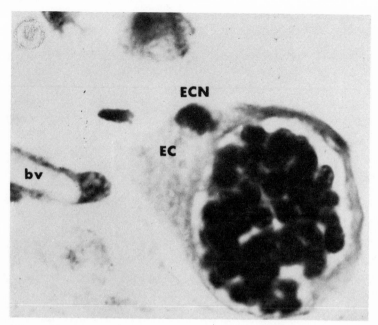

Fig. 6. An endothelial-like cell surrounds the nuclear accumulations associated with the nephridia. EC = endothelial cell; ENC = endothelial cell nucleus; bv = blood vessel.

PHAGOCYTOSIS

After five minutes, coelomic cells from carbon injected worms contain carbon particles in the cytoplasm. Ten minutes after injection, coelomic cells clump around large (300 μ) carbon particles. Cell masses become larger, and fewer free floating cells are observed in the coelomic cavity. Most of the free floating cells are of the round variety without phagocytized carbon. Stained preparations show that cellular clumps are composed mainly of basophilic cells and carbon, with a few acidophilic cells scattered throughout the clump. Small (9 μ to 11 μ), round acidophilic and basophilic cells are free of clumps and contain no carbon.

At the end of ten minutes, coelomic fluid clumps after setting at room temperature. Clumps are composed of coelomic cells and various particles of debris, but unclumped portions contain free, round coelomic cells; cells with pseudopodia are few. This same suspension appears homogenous after mild centrifugation, containing only round cell forms (Fig. 7).

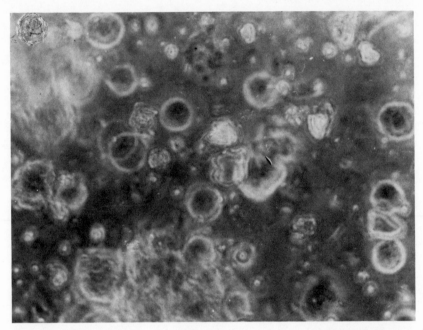

Fig. 7. Unclumped portion of coelomic fluid after centrifugation. Phase-contrast (magnification 500×).

ORIGIN

The epithelial lining of the coelomic cavity may be the prime source of coelomic corpuscles (Cameron, 1932; Liebman, 1942; Jones, 1962). With regard to cell division, Cameron believed that coelomocytes are capable of mitosis, but Liebman reported lack of any mitotic figures and believed that coelomocytes are effete cells. During this study, we found few, if any, mitotic figures. Thus, until more rigorous analysis, coelomocytes may still be incapable of mass reproduction.

The morphological and functional characteristics of coelomic corpuscles in *Lumbricus* and other invertebrates strongly suggest that these cells are protective and function like vertebrate leukocytes (Cameron, 1932; Liebman, 1942; Cowden, 1968; Johnson, 1969*a,b*; Cameron, 1934; Huff, 1940; Salt, 1967; Dawe, 1967; Scott, 1971; Fänge, 1966). If these cells are true leukocytes, then they may originate from regions or discrete organs analogous to those of vertebrates. Fänge (1966) employs the term "lymphocyte tissue" as tissue where lymphocytes, or similar cells, are produced and stored. Usually, the general anatomical sites associated with lymphoid tissue include connective tissue, the alimentary canal, and the kidney (Good *et al.* 1966). If Fänge's hypothesis is correct, then it may be possible to locate coelomocytes in such sites.

Coelomic cell aggregations are found in the anterior portion of the alimentary canal, the septa, and in blood vessels of the nephridia. Lymphoid tissue associated with gut has been discussed by several investigators (Good *et al.,* 1966; Ackerman and Knouff, 1959; Crabbe *et al.,* 1965). The presence of lymphoid tissue in association with an excretory organ in poikilothermic vertebrates was reviewed by Fänge, but the interrelationships between lymphoid and excretory tissues in invertebrates are unknown. The evidence which is presented here for the earthworm suggests that coelomocytes may, at least in part, be formed in blood vessels associated with the nephridia; the results of Stang-Voss (this volume) show that *Eisenia* possesses blood coelomocytes. The presence of an endothelial-like cell and PAS positive material surrounding clusters of nuclei support the hypothesis that this structure is a capillary which contains nuclei. This may not be a multinucleated giant cell as described by Hancock (1965) and Cooper (1968c). Further support for this reasoning is offered by Benham (1891) and Beddard (1890):

". . . it is a well-known fact that in the nephridia of *Lumbricus* the capillaries are here and there dilated,...being filled with free nuclei. These...are comparable to the blood-glands of other species. They are scattered here and there among the coils of the nephridium. The fact that the dilations are always crowded with small cells, which seem to be just like the free corpuscles of the blood, suggests that they might be the seat of formation of the latter."

Thus the nephridia or associated blood vessels may be an important site for the production of coelomic corpuscles in *Lumbricus.* The nuclear size within these nephridial-tubule blood vessels corresponds to the small 9μ to 11μ coelomocytes. Moreover, smaller coelomocytes are immature forms and may serve as precursors for other cells found in the coelom. This is consistent with the observations of cell or nuclear clusters being associated with nephridial blood vessels. Finally, before any serious conclusions can be supported, a series of autoradiographic studies must be performed to determine the dynamic characteristics of cells located within nephridial vessels. Is cellular division occurring there, and do the cells actually migrate out into the coelom? Only careful labeling studies or other such approaches can give the answers. Cellular aggregations found in the anterior gut may likewise be coelomic corpuscle precursors. The location of these cells in the alimentary canal is such that they are positioned close to the intestinal blood supply but are also in contact with the coelomic cavity.

INTERRELATIONSHIPS OF COELOMOCYTES

Considering the above information, we can present a hypothetical outline of coelomic cell interrelationships (Fig. 8). The small basophilic cells grow and

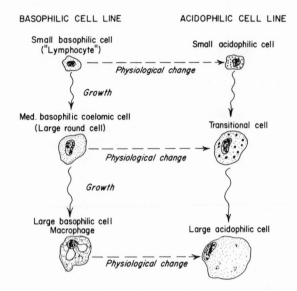

Fig. 8. The interrelationships of *Lumbricus terrestris* coelomic cells.

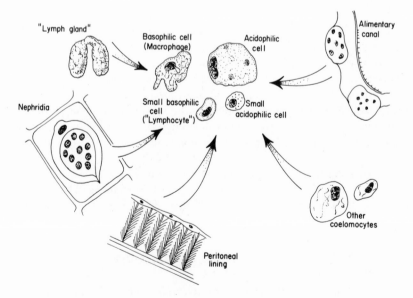

Fig. 9. Possible origins of coelomic cells in *Lumbricus terrestris.*

become large phagocytic amoebocytes. Acidophilic granular cells may represent an independent cell line developing from small acidophilic granular cells (Fig. 8). In the transitions from small basophilic cells to large basophilic cells, the cells could be modified to acidophilic cells. Several structures have been suggested as sites for the production of *Lumbricus* coelomic cells. The epithelial lining of the coelomic cavity, the lymph glands, other coelomic cells, the nephridia, and the alimentary canal may all be involved (Fig. 9).

COELOMIC CELL RESPONSES TO TISSUE GRAFTS

In responding to autografts and xenografts, *Lumbricus* coelomocytes may utilize similar or even the same mechanisms as those observed during cellular reactions against bacteria and parasites. Phagocytosis and encapsulation result in the clearing of dead and injured tissue from graft or injury sites (Figs. 10, 11). Once this material is removed, the stimulus for coelomic cell accumulation near the area is minimal (Fig. 10). After repair of graft or injury sites, the stimulus for the attraction of coelomic cells no longer exists (Fig. 10).

During the primary stages of cellular reactions to xenografts, the sequence of events is similar to that described for autografts or injury (Fig. 11). The major difference in the coelomic cell response to xenografts is continued cellular infiltration into the grafts after the removal of all dead or injured tissue (Fig. 11).

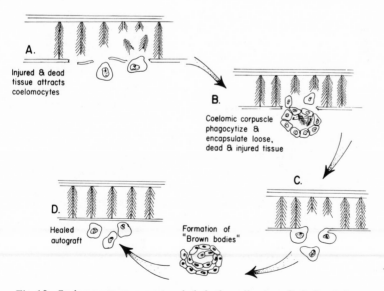

Fig. 10. Coelomocyte response to whole body wall autografts in *Lumbricus*.

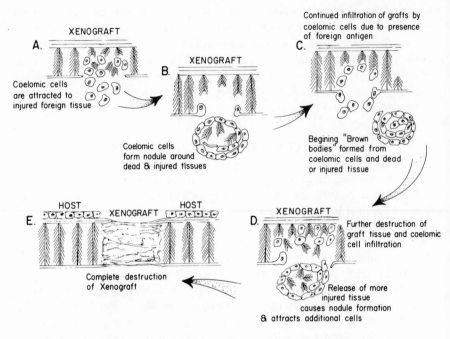

Fig. 11. Coelomocyte responses to whole body wall xenografts in *Lumbricus*.

Coelomic cells appear in response to loose muscle fibers, and the presence acid phosphatase deposited in a linear fashion under xenografts suggests release of hydrolytic enzymes by coelomic cells. These enzymes act on connective tissue elements of xenografts, resulting in the formation of loose muscle fibers. These fibers provide a continued stimulus for encapsulation by coelomic cells (Fig. 11). The process of tissue erosion and removal of debris progresses until a xenograft is destroyed (Fig. 11).

Two major populations of coelomic cells may act in a synergistic manner to destroy xenografts. The basophils (macrophages) remove and encapsulate loose, injured, or dead tissues. Later, acidophils release hydrolytic enzymes which finally destroy foreign tissues. Such a combination of cell types constitutes a powerful defense or immunologic mechanism against foreign agents.

EVOLUTION OF DELAYED HYPERSENSITIVITY AND THE ANAMNESTIC RESPONSE

Previous experiments reveal that *Lumbricus* coelomic cells destroy xenografts and are capable of an anamnestic reaction to second-set xenografts

(Cooper, 1969c; Hostetter and Cooper, 1972, 1973). Coelomocytes do not react intensely to autografts.

Upon contact with a foreign antigen, coelomocytes become immobilized (Fig. 12) and then release various humoral factors such as opsonins, lysins, agglutinins, and substances similar to mammalian migration inhibitory factor (MIF) (Fig. 12). The presence of antigen or the release of humoral agents causes additional coelomocyte formation by stimulation of coelomic cavity leukopoietic organs. These substances also lead to accumulations around foreign antigens; thus, phagocytosis ensues and is followed by encapsulation and release of hydrolytic enzymes (Fig. 12) which results in antigen destruction (Fig. 12). Once foreign antigens are degraded, the stimulus for coelomocytes is removed (Fig. 12). Excess coelomic cells produced because of antigen stimulation become attached to surrounding organs, and the total coelomocyte population returns to normal (Fig. 12).

Upon second challenge with a foreign antigen, the following events take place: (1) coelomic cells in the free circulating pool come in contact with antigen, are immobilized, and release humoral factors (Fig. 13); (2) these factors stimulate and cause local accumulations and movement of coelomocytes that are

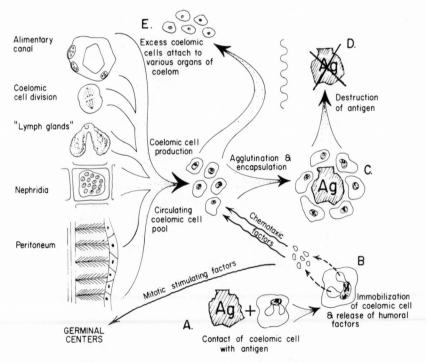

Fig. 12. Coelomocyte responses during a first-set reaction to xenografts.

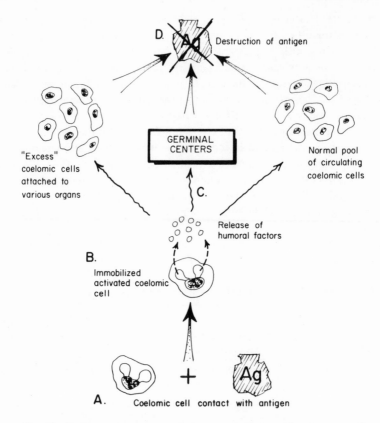

Fig. 13. Coelomocyte responses during a second-set reaction to xenografts.

attached to various organs (Fig. 13); (3) this results in a rapid coelomocyte accumulation at the antigen site and, because of greater numbers of coelomocytes, a more rapid destruction of foreign antigens takes place (Fig. 13).

Recognition of foreignness and destruction of nonself without sequestering self tissues is a basic necessity if the above reactions are to occur. Presupposing the absence of antibodies but assuming a mammalian-type foreignness recognition system, how can invertebrate coelomic cells be capable of distinguishing self from nonself? Some investigators believe that invertebrate tissues are coated with selfmarkers that cause no stimulation of coelomic cells (Phillips, 1966; see Hilgard et al., this volume). Tissues without such markers produce irritation of circulating coelomocyte membranes, a mechanism which is analogous to activation of mammalian blood platelets. Self-marked tissues are unresponsive to opsonins or agglutinins in coelomic fluid, but foreign materials attract these factors to coelomocyte surfaces.

An alternative hypothesis relies on the action of hydrolytic enzymes that might be secreted by coelomic cells (Phillips, 1966). As coelomic cells come into contact with foreignness, enzymes are released. If an enzyme attacks the antigen, utilizing it as a substrate, the reaction products may act to stimulate coelomocytes; all self-tissue is not subject to enzyme action. Invertebrates could, therefore, utilize such "nonimmunologic," nonspecific processes as those used for defense against bacteria and parasites. Such reactions do not explain differences in primary and secondary xenograft rejection times as described by Cooper (1969c). Perhaps a mechanism utilizing immunoglobulins must be formulated to explain this specificity. This could be restricted to factors with functional characteristics similar to mammalian complement as well as immunoglobulins, and they would conform to the evolutionary precursors of vertebrate antibodies, as discussed by Burnet (1968). Such precursor molecules, for example, may be similar to the variable portion of vetebrate immunoglobulins. Incorporations of such a protein into the cell membranes of invertebrate coelomocytes renders them capable of reacting specifically toward antigens according to the clonal selection theory.

We argue about insufficient numbers of coelomic cells to afford variations for dealing with diverse numbers of antigens, or that such a potential is absent from the coelomocyte genome. Either large numbers of cells derived by multiple reproductions may not be necessary, or a high rate of cell recruitment may be marshalled to provide the required variety and number of cells. A final alternative is that an extremely large number of receptors are not required or even possible in invertebrates. Specificity, based upon the clonal selection theory, may be operative in organisms with a compartmentalized structure, causing partial "isolation" of various tissues from the total leukocyte population. Thus, cells in contact with foreign antigens are incapable of interacting with other circulating leukocytes, producing a focused antigen attack. Such a total concerted attack could occur in the earthworm coelomic cavity, which is relatively uncompartmentalized. Stimulation of cells possessing receptor sites leads to cellular accumulating mechanisms and concentration of receptor cells near the antigen. Thus, expression of antigen specificity, from an evolutionary viewpoint, may be influenced by an organism's structure.

FINAL COMMENT

The above observations strongly support the theory of the coelomic cavity of *Lumbricus terrestris* as a functional equivalent of advanced immunological systems. This earthworm system, although much different from its mammalian counterpart, is efficient in dealing with foreign material and offers strong defense mechanisms for the earthworm. The cells comprising this invertebrate immunologic system are morphologically similar to the leukocyte series of mammals. Finally, they play a decisive role in the specific memory response to transplants, the only invertebrate system, to date, possessing two characteristics of vertebrate immune systems.

REFERENCES

Ackerman, G. A., and Knouff, R. A., 1959, Lymphocytopoiesis in the bursa of *Farbricius*, *Am. J. Anat. 104*:163.

Bang, F. B., 1967, Defense reactions in invertebrates, Federation Proc. *26*:1713-1715.

Beddard, F. E., 1890, Contributions to the anatomy of earthworms, *Quart. J. Microscop. Sci., 30*:460.

Benham, W. B., 1891, The nephridium of *Lumbricus* and its blood supply, *Quart. J. Microscop. Sci. 32*:293-334.

Burnet, F. M., 1968, Evolution of the immune process in vertebrates, *Nature, 218*:426-430.

Cameron, G. R., 1932, Inflammation in earthworms, *J. Pathol. 35*:934.

Cameron, G. R., 1934, Inflammation in the caterpillars of Lepidoptera, *J. Pathol. and Bacteriol. 38*:441-466.

Cooper, E. L., 1965a, A method of tissue grafting in the earthworm *Lumbricus terrestris*, *Am. Zool. 5*:754.

Cooper, E. L., 1966a, Algunos aspectos de immunidad en invertebrados, peces, y anfibios, *Acta Medica 2*:1-5.

Cooper, E. L., 1966b, Rechazo de tejidos en la lombriz de tierra. Una Respuesta immunologica? *Arch. Mex. Ant. 7*:21.

Cooper, E. L., 1968a, Transplantation immunity in earthworms, *Am. Zool. 8*:815.

Cooper, E. L., 1968b, Transplantation immunity in Annelids. I. Rejection of xenografts exchanged between *Lumbricus terrestris* and *Eisenia foetida*, *Transplantation 6*:322-337.

Cooper, E. L., 1968c, Multinucleate giant cells, granulomata and "myoblastomas" in annelid worms, *J. Inverebr. Pathol. 11*:123-131.

Cooper, E. L., 1969a, Chronic allograft rejection in *Lumbricus terrestris*, *J. Exp. Zool. 171*:69-73.

Cooper, E. L., 1969b, Neoplasia and transplantation immunity in annelids, *J. Nat. Cancer Inst. 31*:655-669.

Cooper, E. L., 1969,c, Specific tissue graft rejection in earthworms, *Science 166*:1414-1415.

Cooper, E. L., 1970, Transplantation immunity in helminths and annelids, *Transplant. Proc. 2*:216-221.

Cooper, E. L., 1971, Phylogeny of transplantation immunity. Graft rejection in earthworms, *Transplant. Proc. 3*:214-216.

Cooper, E. L., 1973a, Earthworm coelomocytes: Role in understanding the evolution of cellular immunity. I. Formation of monolayers and cytotoxicity, in: *Proceedings of the Third International Invertebrate Tissue Culture Colloquium, Czechoslovakian Academy of Science*, pp. 381-404.

Cooper, E. L., 1973b, Evolution of cellular immunity, in: *Symposium on Non-specific Factors in Immunity*, Berne, pp. 11-23.

Cooper, E. L. and Baculi, B. S., 1968, Cell responses during xenograft rejection in Annelids, *Anat. Rec. 160*:335.

Cooper, E. L. and Rubilotta, L. M., 1969, Allograft rejection in *Eisenia foetida*, *Transplantation, 8*:220-223.

Cowden, R. R., 1968, Cytological and histochemical observations on connective tissue cells in the sea cucumber, *J. Invertebr. Pathol. 10*:151-159.

Crabbe, P. A., Carbonara, A., and Heremans, J. F., 1965, The normal human intestinal mucosa as a major source of plasma cells containing γA-Immunoglobulins, *Lab. Invest.* *14*:235.

Dawe, C. J., 1967, Cellular response of a cockroach *Leucophaea maderae* to transplants, *Federation Proc. 26:*1698-1706.

Degrone, A., 1925 (see Liebman, E.), The Coelomocytes of Lumbricidae. *J. Morphol. 71*:221-248, 1942.

Faure-Fremiet, 1927 (see Cameron, G. R., 1932), Inflammation in earthworms, *J. Pathol. 34*:934.

Fänge, R., 1966, in: *Phylogeny of Immunity*, pp. 141-145 (R. T. Smith, P. A. Miescher, and R. A. Good, eds.), University of Florida Press, Gainesville.

Good, R. A., Finstad, F., Pollara, B., and Gabrielsen, A. E., 1966, in: *Phylogeny of Immunity*, pp. 149-170 (R. T. Smith, P. A. Miescher, and R. A. Good, eds.), University of Florida Press, Gainesville.

Hancock, R. L., 1965, Irradiation induced neoplastic and giant cells in earthworms, *Experientia, 21*:33-34.

Hostetter, R. K. and Cooper, E. L., 1972, Coelomocytes as effector cells in earthworm immunity, *Immunol. Communications 1*:155-183.

Hostetter, R. K. and Cooper, E. L., 1973, Cellular anamnesis in earthworms, *Cellular Immunol. 9*:384

Huff, C. G., 1940, Immunity in invertebrates, *Phys. Rev. 20*:68-85.

Johnson, P. T., 1969*a*, The coelomic elements of sea urchins. I. The normal coelomocytes, *J. Invertebr. Pathol. 13*:25-41.

Johnson, P. T., 1969*b*, The coelomic elements of sea urchins. II. Cytochemistry of the coelomocytes, *Histochemie 17*:213-231.

Jones, J. C., 1962, Current concepts concerning insect hemocytes, *Am. Zool. 2*:209-246.

Joseph, H., 1942 (see Liebman, E., 1942), The coelomocytes of *Lumbricidae, J. Morphol. 71*:221-248.

Keng, L. B., 1895 (see Cameron, G. R., 1932), Inflammation in earthworms, *J. Pathol. 35*:933-972.

Lemmi, C., Cooper, E. L., and Moore, T. C., 1973, An approach to studying evolution of cellular immunity (this volume).

Liebman, E., 1942, The coelomocytes of *Lumbricidae, J. Morphol. 71*:934.

Metchnikoff, E., 1891, *Lectures on the Comparative Pathology of Inflammation,* Dover Publications, Inc., New York.

Phillips, J. H., 1966, in: *Phylogeny of Immunity*, pp. 133-140 (R. T. Smith, P. A. Miescher, and R. A. Good, eds.), University of Florida Press, Gainesville.

Rosa, P., 1896 (see Stephenson, J., 1930), in: *The Oligochaeta*, pp. 58-71, Oxford Press, Oxford.

Salt, G., 1967, Cellular defense mechanisms in insects, *Federation Proc. 26*:1671-1674.

Scott, M. T., 1971, Recognition of Foreignness in invertebrates, *Transplantation 11*:78-86.

Winger, L. A., and Cooper, E. L., 1969, Effect of temperature on the first-set xenograft rejection in the earthworm, *Eisenia foetida, Am. Zool. 9*:1132.

Chapter 9

An Approach to Studying Evolution
of Cellular Immunity

C. A. Lemmi

Department of Anatomy
School of Medicine, University of California
Los Angeles, California
and
Transplantation Laboratory
Department of Surgery, Harbor General Hospital
Torrance, California

E. L. Cooper

Department of Anatomy
School of Medicine, University of California
Los Angeles, California

and

T. C. Moore

Transplantation Laboratory
Department of Surgery, Harbor General Hospital
Torrance, California

"I would not enter on my list of friends (though graced with polish'd manners and fine sense, yet wanting sensibility) the man who needlessly sets foot upon a worm."

Line 560, Book VI,
"Winter Walk at Noon"
The Task
William Cooper (1731-1800)

*Research supported by NSF Grant GB 17767; two grants from The California Institute for Cancer Research, and a grant from The Brown-Hazen Corporation to Edwin L. Cooper, and grants from the John A. Hartford Foundation and NIH (AM10373-01) to Thomas C. Moore.

INTRODUCTION

Transplantation of integument between earthworms is an important model for studying the evolution of immune mechanisms involved in tissue rejection. The lamprey and hagfish are the most primitive vertebrates in which immunoglobulins are found (Thoenes and Hildeman, 1969; Linthicum and Hildeman, 1970). In invertebrates immunoglobulins are not yet demonstrable in the blood, hemolymph, or coelomic fluids. Nevertheless, invertebrate agglutinins are involved in complex reactions to foreign materials. Still, cellular immunity is a reality as evidenced by the destruction of allografts and xenografts in one group, the annelids, best represented by the earthworms.

Although inbred species of earthworms are not available, some general rules of transplantation are operative. Autografts are not rejected, but allo- and xenografts are destroyed with increasing frequency as the degree of genetic difference is increased (Cooper, 1969a). Several basic characteristics of earthworm cellular immunity identify the nature of the phenomenon as definitely immunological. Among them, accelerated rejection of a second graft from the original donor and simultaneous independent rejection of a third, unrelated graft are strong evidence of memory and specificity (Cooper, 1968).

Coelomocytes participate in the rejection process by infiltrating foreign grafts (Cooper, 1968). As another important property, coelomocytes can adoptively transfer typical accelerated second-set reactions from a previously grafted worm to a normal worm (Bailey et al., 1970).

CELLULAR IMMUNITY IN AN INVERTEBRATE

Activity of ^{51}Cr Labeled Earthworm Coelomocytes

One approach to determine the specific role of coelomocytes is to follow the fate of primed cells to foreign grafts after a second exposure. A variety of cells have been tagged with ^{51}Cr to study distribution of the label after introduction into a proper recipient (Bunting et al., 1963; Gesner and Woodruff, 1969; Perlman and Holm, 1969). We decided to study the fate of normal and primed labeled coelomocytes from Lumbricus terrestris in normal, wounded, and previously grafted hosts.

Behavior of Labeled Normal Coelomocytes in Normal Hosts

To study whether labeled coelomocytes remain fixed in one segment of the earthworm or migrate in the coelomic cavity from segment to segment, labeled allogeneic coelomocytes (Fig. 1) from normal Lumbricus were injected into

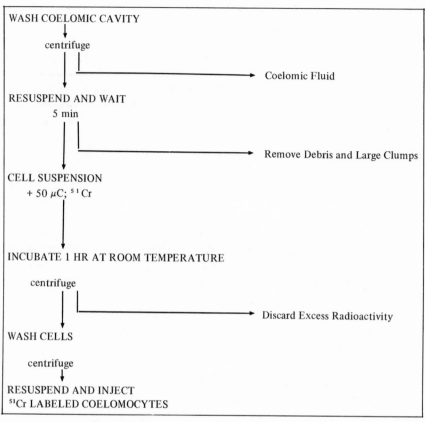

WASH COELOMIC CAVITY
↓
centrifuge

→ Coelomic Fluid

RESUSPEND AND WAIT
5 min

→ Remove Debris and Large Clumps

CELL SUSPENSION
+ 50 μC; ^{51}Cr

INCUBATE 1 HR AT ROOM TEMPERATURE

centrifuge

→ Discard Excess Radioactivity

WASH CELLS

centrifuge
↓
RESUSPEND AND INJECT
^{51}Cr LABELED COELOMOCYTES

Fig. 1. Technique of ^{51}Cr labeling of coelomocytes.

Table I. Behavior of ^{51}Cr Labeled, Normal Coelomocytes in Normal *Lumbricus*

Area of accumulation	Percent labeled coelomocyte
Stationary	
Site of injection (clitellum)	67
Migrating	
Anterior to clitellum	21
1st inch posterior to clitellum	8
2nd inch posterior to clitellum	2
Remaining posterior of earthworm	2
Total % migrated	33

normal recipients. The coelomocytes were introduced under the clitellum area, and, after a period of two hours, the recipients were sacrificed and different areas of the entire earthworm were counted for radioactivity.

We found 67% of the radioactivity at the injection site, and 33% was distributed in the rest of the body. 21% anterior to the clitellum, 8% was found in the second inch behind the injection site and 4% in the remaining posterior portion of the worm (Table I). Cell stability was checked at 48 hrs. We found only 9.4 ± 2.2% radioactivity released into the supernatant after that period. In the cellular pellet, 90.6 ± 2.2% was still present after centrifugation. After an initial short time of 2 hr was allowed for the distribution of coelomocytes and even while earthworms were still partially anesthetized, a considerable amount of movement occurred, considering the distance from the injection site to the posterior regions.

To allow more time for distribution in another experiment, we injected, one inch posterior to the clitellum, labeled, normal *Lumbricus* coelomocytes into recipients and determined the distribution of radioactivity after 16 hr. By that time, 86.7% of the radioactivity emanated from the site of injection, and only 13.3% remained at the injection site (Table II). Apparently more coelomocytes migrate toward the anterior end of earthworms than toward the posterior end. Although the difference was not statistically significant, in all future experiments we alternated graft orientation to compensate for any nonspecific unidirectional flow of coelomocytes (Table II).

Behavior of Labeled Normal Coelomocytes in Wounded Hosts

Simultaneously with the last study, we preformed a wound in another group of worms to test for nonspecific migration. This consisted of a three-sided cut, or flap, one-half inch behind the injection site. The distribution of radioactivity after 16 hr showed considerable differences when compared with normal hosts. This wound area showed 21.6% radioactivity, in contrast to a similar area on the

Table II. Distribution of [51]Cr Labeled, Normal Coelomocytes in Normal and Wounded *Lumbricus*

	Normal, %	Wounded, %	P value
Anterior to clitellum	26.8	6.3	
Anterior to injection site	12.2 ± 5.5	12.9 ± 5.2	
Injection site (I.S.)	13.3 ± 1.9	48.2 ± 6.1	<0.01
Posterior to I.S. or wound	5.7 ± 2.2	21.6 ± 10.7	0.05/0.1
Posterior to wound	5.9 ± 1.9	3.3 ± 1.2	
Posterior end	36.1	7.6	
Total % migrated	86.7	51.8	

previous, nonwounded group with only 5.7% radioactivity. A greater difference was found at the injection site with 48% radioactivity in the wounded group and 13.3% in normal controls, a result due to close proximity of injection and wound sites, making both sites subject to some injury. In other earthworm areas only 51.8% radioactivity was found (Table II).

Behavior of Normal and Sensitized Coelomocytes in Grafted Hosts

To define the behavior of normal and primed coelomocytes, we injected them into worms bearing both auto- and xenografts. To obtain primed cells, we performed multiple xenografts of *Eisenia* on *Lumbricus* recipients. Five days after grafting, we collected coelomocytes from hosts at points closest to the grafted area. Normal *Lumbricus* were used to collect normal, unprimed, control coelomocytes. Both normal and primed coelomocytes were labeled separately. After resuspension, labeled cells were injected into the coelomic cavity midway between the grafts of recipients bearing both auto- and xenografts which were separated by a distance of approximately one inch (Fig. 2). The distribution of radioactivity after two hours suggested considerable cellular migration. The autograft site (Table III) showed a higher concentration of radioactivity, but, surprisingly, the xenograft area showed almost equal radioactivity to the other regions. Furthermore, we found no difference between normal and primed coelomocytes.

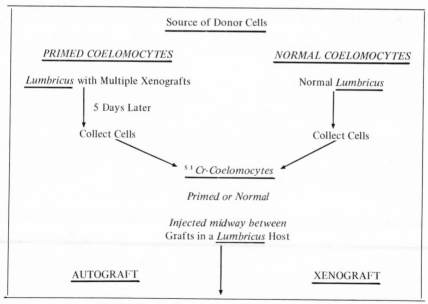

Fig. 2. Source of primed and normal coelomocytes.

Table III. Behavior of Normal and Primed Coelomocytes[a]
in Double Grafted Hosts[b]

	Normal, %[c]	Primed, %[c]
Anterior to clitellum	8.2	12.3
Posterior to posterior graft	9.3	19.1
Injection site	49.7	27.7
Autograft area	24.2 ± 10.7	29.6 ± 6.8
Xenograft area	8.6 ± 3.5	11.3 ± 3.6
Auto- vs. xenograft: P value	0.05	0.05 – 0.1

[a] Labeled coelomocytes were resuspended in saline solution.
[b] Recipient grafts were placed 5 days prior to injection.
[c] Animals were sacrificed 2 hr after injection.

We studied another group of earthworms similarly but modified three parameters. Coelomocytes injected into the first group were suspended in Rushton's
ringers. Since some soluble factors in the coelomic fluid might affect coelomocyte
distribution, thus, after separating cells from donor coelomic fluid, we labeled
and resuspended them in the original coelomic fluid. In the first group, both
recipient grafts were 5 days old, but to minimize the possibility that migration
may be different at earlier stages, grafts were only one day old in the second
group. Coelomocytes were allowed to migrate for two hours in the first group
and sixteen hours in the second group. We demonstrated previously that the
label was stable for at least 48 hr. The distribution of radioactivity in this second
group showed a decrease at the injection site, consistent with the longer period
that coelomocytes were allowed to distribute (Table IV). The higher values
anterior and posterior to the second graft were apparently a reflection of the
greater amount of tissue present. The distribution in autografts and xenografts

Table IV. Distribution of ^{51}Cr Coelomocytes[a]
after 16 hr (Group 2)[b]

	Normal, %[c]	Primed, %[c]
Anterior to clitellum	29.6	33.1
Posterior to posterior graft	49.0	38.4
Injection site	5.2	10.6
Autograft area	11.3 ± 1.8	10.9 ± 6.4
Xenograft area	4.9 ± 0.9	7.0 ± 1.4
Auto- vs. xenograft: P value	0.01 – 0.025	0.05

[a] Labeled coelomocytes were resuspended in their own coelomic fluid.
[b] Recipient grafts were placed 1 day prior to injection.
[c] Animals were sacrificed 16 hr after injection.

followed the same patterns described previously with a higher radioactive concentration to autografts than xenograft. Again, we found no difference between normal and primed coelomocyte distribution.

Summary of Labeled Coelomocyte Studies

Allo- and xenograft destruction, specific accelerated rejection of a second graft, cellular anamnesis, and adoptive transfer by coelomocytes can be demonstrated in the earthworm, *Lumbricus terrestris.* Coelomocytes appear after injury, but greater cell accumulations occur in association with grafts; later these become infiltrated by cells. By labeling coelomocytes with ^{51}Cr, we studied their migration in allogeneic recipients bearing wounds, an autograft, and/or xenografts. Two hours after injection into ungrafted recipients, 33% of labeled, normal allogeneic cells migrated from the injection site. After 15 hr, a value of 86.7% migration was found. From normal recipients injected with labeled allogeneic coelomocytes, with a wound 1 in. posterior to the injection site, 21.6% of the label was found in the wounded area after 16 hr. At a comparable time only 5.7% of the label was detected in normal, nonwounded earthworm controls. Normal or primed cells injected midway between auto- and xenografts at 1 and 5 days showed greater accumulations of labeled cells in association with autografts at 2 and 16 hr than with xenografts. Suspensions of coelomocytes in original donor coelomic fluid or saline did not affect cell migration.

The above results suggest considerable coelomocyte migration in earthworms. Greater accumulations occur in areas of nonspecific reactions such as wounds and autografts. Lack of pronounced accumulations of injected coelomocytes in xenograft areas suggests that specific primed cells are not the final effector cells leading to graft infiltration and ultimate destruction. Conversely, primed cells may recognize *nonself* and initiate event(s) of communication and cooperation necessary for triggering unknown effector cell(s). These distinctions may be apparent after 5 days.

DISCUSSION

Cameron (1932) found longer survival of allogeneic spermatozoa in *Lumbricus terrestris* than xenogeneic cells, and, as an extension, Cooper reported rejection of body wall xenografts in *Lumbricus terrestris* (Cooper, 1965a). This was followed by a series of papers describing the phenomenon in more detail (Cooper, 1965b, Cooper, 1968, Cooper, 1969a, Cooper, 1969b, Cooper, 1970, Cooper, 1971), and, finally, in 1971 Bailey *et al.* reported adoptive transfer of the xenograft reaction by primed coelomocytes. These reports clearly identify the earthworm as an invertebrate capable of recognition of nonself. Moreover, the response to nonself is highly specific (Fig. 3).

(a)   Accelerated Rejection of 2nd Graft
(b)   Simultaneous 1st and 2nd Set Rejection and Independent 1st Set Rejection
(c)   Adoptive Transfer by Coelomocytes
(d)   Cellular Infiltration of Graft
(e)   Cellular Anamnesis

Fig. 3. Evidence of specific immune rejection in earthworms.

Cellular accumulation in response to grafts is one aspect of early reactions to both auto- and xenografts. Coelomocytes do not invade autografts. However, after coelomocytes accumulate in the area of xenografts, the cells actively invade the graft until total destruction is accomplished (Cooper, 1968).

Previous cellular studies of skin grafts in mammals reveal that if cells are labeled *in situ* by administration of radioactive precursor to lymph nodes which drain the grafted area, labeled, primed cells are later found in the area of the second graft. However, this occurs to the same degree whether the graft is from the same donor or from one unrelated to the original skin graft (Prendergast, 1964). When transfer of labeled, primed cells to a normal recipient is performed, there is no detectable accumulation of these cells in the recipient at the challenge site, although a definite cellular infiltration occurs (Najarian and Feldman, 1961, 1962, 1963). Our results are in agreement with these mammalian studies. We found no increased accumulation in xenografts of labeled, primed cells when compared with labeled, normal cells.

The use of ^{3}H-thymidine reveals that the majority of cells in a rejecting mammalian skin graft are not random accumulations of circulating cells; rather, these are accumulations of newly formed cells (Cohen and Feldman, 1970; McClusky et al., 1963; Turk and Oort, 1963). Earthworms are also known to isolate foreign materials – a coelomocyte defense reaction (Cameron, 1932). Lack of accumulation of *labeled cells* at the site of xenografts is due to early isolation of the graft or to a different population of cells. Still, there is histological and kinetic evidence of definite increases in cellular involvement (Cooper, 1968; Hostetter and Cooper, 1972a, b). Finally, the time of coelomocyte injection in relation to the time of graft transplantation is undoubtedly crucial.

Autografts occupy areas of injury and require repair, but they are certainly self-tissue derived from the same earthworm; thus, no incompatibility ever occurs. A normal inflammatory reaction to injury may result in the liberation of chemotactic substances that attract cells from the circulation. This may explain the higher concentration of cells in wounded and autografted areas. Polypeptides of molecular weight ranging from 1000 to 30,000, probably formed as products of collagenolysis by proteolytic enzymes released from injured tissues, are strongly chemotactic in small amounts (Houch et al., 1971). These nonspecific substances attract normal and primed cells.

In Bloom's (1971) review, two mechanisms are proposed for the participation of primed cells in the destruction of foreign tissue. Primed cells may be attracted by antigenic material and participate as final effector cells in graft destruction, or sensitized cells can only recognize nonself material and set in motion other unknown mechanisms that eventually destroy grafts through the participation of other nonprimed cells. Soluble factors found in tissue culture studies have been proposed as mediators between the primed cells and the nonprimed effector cells in mammals. Our results are more in agreement with the last mechanism. There is no doubt that specificity is a property of primed cells, but the lack of massive accumulations at the site of rejecting grafts seems to indicate that they are not the final effector cells. Their function must be one of re-cognizer of nonself and initiator of other, unknown mechanisms that result in infiltration and final graft destruction.

We offer one rationalization for such a mechanism. If all primed co-elomocytes were to accumulate at the site of a foreign graft to effect destruction, the body would be deficient in these valuable and slowly obtainable cells at a time when repeated invasion by foreign materials occurs. By wandering through the earthworm, all areas are checked for nonself, and, after recognition of nonself occurs by a few primed cells, cellular communication activates other coelomocytes to proceed for final infiltration and graft destruction.

Apparently, cell attraction to autografts behaves differently from coe-lomocyte attraction to xenograft sites. Autografts and injury areas may have free communication to the interior of the earthworm, since both cause cells to be attracted to these areas during repair. In xenografts, cells might be attracted early after grafting but after foreignness is recognized, and by the time we study the areas they may be isolated from the interior of the earthworm. The coe-lomocytes might accumulate by division *in situ*, although the scarcity of mitotic figures does not, for now, support this explanation. Perhaps newly formed cells or some special population of recruited cells are attracted differently to grafts, or injected coelomocytes belong to a population not specifically attracted to the graft after initial recognition. In any case, injected coelomocytes behave differently in response to xeno- and autografts.

The basis for vertebrate T-cell specificity is still undefined, and molecular mechanisms operating for plant lectins, invertebrate agglutinins and lysins, *etc.*, are suggested by Good (1972). Agglutinins similar to those of other invertebrates were recently found in earthworms (Cooper et al., 1973). These humoral sub-stances may be involved in the phenomenon of graft rejection. Repeated mutation and natural selection can produce invertebrates equipped with substances able to react against foreign determinants. The importance of these substances for defense was reported, among others, for the marine spider crab (Bang, 1962, 1967). The opsonin properties (Tripp and Kent, 1967) link these humoral substances to hemocytes or coelomocytes of invertebrates. Mutations producing substances interfering with an organism's own self may be classified as antiself and will either kill or decrease the survival capability of the invertebrate producing it.

The price of developing these primitive defense systems of anti-nonself agglutinins is twofold. It requires the death of those mutations producing antiself substances. It also requires a very long time, millions of years perhaps, to produce and preserve the right type of mutation by natural selection. A striking similarity emerges when we compare this long process with the activities normally taking place in the vertebrate thymus. Here we see that many new lymphocytes are produced by division every 6–8 hr, faster than in any other lymphoid organ. Of these cells, 95% are short-lived and probably die in the thymus. It was suggested that they may provide the genetic diversity necessary for clonal selection (Weiss, 1972). It could be possible that the same biological forces that gathered the scattered nephridia into a single encapsulated kidney may have also been responsible for gathering the diffuse (agglutinin producing) cells into a single encapsulated thymus. If these comparisons with more developed systems are proven at all plausible by future investigations as this study seems to suggest, a more universal mechanism for tissue rejection and cellular communication can be extended to the invertebrate phylum.

REFERENCES

Bailey, S., Miller, B., and Cooper, E. L., 1970, Transplantation immunity in earthworms. II. Adoptive transfer of the xenograft reaction, *Immunology* 21:81-86.
Bang, F. B., 1962, Serological aspects of immunity in invertebrates, *Nature* (London) 196:88-89.
Bang, F. B., 1967, Serological responses among invertebrates other than insects, *Federation Proc.* 26:1680-1684.
Bloom, B. R. and Chase, M. W., 1967, Transfer of delayed-type hypersensitivity, *Prog. Allergy* 10:151.
Bloom, B. R., 1971, *In vitro* approaches to the mechanisms of cell mediated immune reactions, *Adv. Immunol.* 13:101.
Bunting, W. L., Kiely, J. M., and Owen, C. A., 1963, Radiochromium labeled lymphocytes in the rat, *Proc. Soc. Exp. Biol. Med.* 113:370.
Cameron, G. R., 1932, Inflamation in earthworms, *J. Pathol. Bacteriol.* 35:933.
Cohen, J. R. and Feldman, M., 1970, The lysis of fibroblasts by lymphocytes sensitized *in vitro:* specific antigen activates a nonspecific affect, *Cell Immunol.* 1:521.
Cooper, E. L., 1965a Rejection of body wall xenografts exchanged between *Lumbricus terrestris* and *Eisenia foetida, Am. Zool.* 5:665.
Cooper, E. L., 1965b, Method of tissue grafting in the earthworm, *Lumbricus terrestris, Am. Zool.* 5:254.
Cooper, E. L., 1968, Transplantation immunity in annelids. I. Rejection of xenografts exchanged between *Lumbricus terrestris* and *Eisenia foetida, Transplantation* 3:332.

Cooper, E. L., 1969*a*, Chronic allograft rejection in *Lumbricus terrestris, J. Exp. Zool. 171*:69.

Cooper, E. L. 1969*b*, Specific tissue graft rejection in earthworms, *Science 166*:1414.

Cooper, E. L., 1970, Transplantation immunity in helminths and annelids, *Transplant. Proc. 2*:216.

Cooper, E. L., 1971, Phylogeny of transplantation immunity: graft rejection in earthworms, *Transplant. Proce. 3*:214.

Cooper, E. L., Lemmi, C. A., and More, T. C., 1974, Agglutinins and cellular immunity in annelids, *Ann. N.Y. Acad. Sci.* (in press).

Gesner, B. M. and Woodruff, J. J., 1969, *Cellular Recognition*, pp. 79-90, Appleton-Century-Crofts (Meredith Corporation), New York.

Good, R. A., 1972, Structure function relations in the lymphoid system, *Clin. Immunobiol. 1*:13-15.

Gowans, J. L., 1965, The role of lymphocytes in the destruction of homografts, *Brit. Med. Bull. 21*:106.

Hostetter, R. K. and Cooper, E. L., 1972*a*, Coelomocytes as effector cells in earthworm immunity, *Immunological Communications 1*:155.

Hostetter, R. K. and Cooper, E. L., 1972*b*, Earthworm cellular immunity, (this symposium).

Houch, J. C., Barnes, S. G., and Chang, C., 1971, *Immunopathology of Inflammation*, pp. 39-51, Excerpta Medica Foundation, Amsterdam.

Linthicum, D. S. and Hildeman, W. H., 1970, Immunological responses of Pacific hagfish. III. Serum antibodies to cellular antigens, *J. Immunol. 105*:912.

McClusky, R. T., Bennacerraf, B., and McClusky, J. W., 1963, Studies on the specificity of the cellular infiltrate in delayed hypersensitivity reactions, *J. Immunol. 90*:466.

Najarian, J. S. and Feldman, J. D., 1961, Passive transfer of tuberculin sensitivity by tritiated thymidine labeled lymphoid cell, *J. Exp. Med. 114*:779.

Najarian, J. S. and Feldman, J. D., 1962, Passive transfer of transplantation immunity. I. Tritiated lymphoid cells. II. Lymphoid cells in millipore chambers, *J. Exp. Med. 115*:1083.

Najarian, J. S. and Feldman, J. D., 1963, Passive transfer of transplantation immunity. III. Inbred guinea pigs, *J. Exp. Med. 117*:440.

Perlman, P. and Holm, G., 1969, Cytotoxic effects of lymphoid cells *in vitro, Adv. Immunol. 11*:124.

Prendergast, R. A., 1964, Cellular specificity in the homograft reaction, *J. Exp. Med. 119*:377.

Thoenes, G. H. and Hildeman, W. H., 1969, *Developmental Aspects of Antibody Formation and Structure*, pp. 711-726, Czechoslavakian Academy of Science, Praque.

Tripp, M. R. and Kent, V. E., 1967, Studies on oyster cellular immunity, *In Vitro 3*:129-135.

Turk, J. L. and Oort, J. A., 1963, A histological study of the early stages of the development of the tuberculin reaction after passive transfer of cells labeled with ^{3}H-thymidine, *Immunology, 6*:140-147.

Weiss, L., 1972, *Cells and Tissues of the Immune System*, pp. 88-89, Prentice-Hall, Inc.

Weiss, L., 1972, *Cells and Tissues of the Immune System*, pp. 88-89, Prentice-Hall, Inc. Englewood Cliffs, N. J.

Wilson, D. B., 1970, *Biology of the Immune Response*, pp. 444-466, McGraw-Hill Company, New York.

Chapter 10

Cellular Aspects of Graft Rejection in Earthworms and Some Other Metazoa

Pierre Valembois

*Laboratoire de Zoologie de l'Université de Bordeaux I
et Centre de Morphologie Expérimentale du C.N.R.S.
Institut de Biologie Animale
33405 Talence, France*

INTRODUCTION

Knowledge concerning the immune response of invertebrates is relatively obscure when compared to vertebrates. Many authors believe that invertebrates cannot achieve specific reactions characteristic of acquired immunity. According to the approaches of Ehrlich (1900), Jerne (1955), and Burnet (1959), adaptive immunity requires the presence of leukocytes which recognize various antigenic structural patterns. The molecular basis of this recognition is the production of cell-bound receptors which combine specifically with antigens. Each immunocyte carries only one receptor pattern, and one type of injected antigen must select from among the different cells those which have appropriate receptors. Cell division is stimulated and produces leukocytes which exhibit specific immunity against a stimulating antigen. Studies of protein uptake by cells of invertebrates, and especially by echinoderm coelomocytes (Hilgard and Phillips, 1968; Hilgard *et al.*, this symposium) have argued strongly that some of these cells possess specific receptor molecules. However, according to Burnet (1968) and Hilgard (1970), contact with antigen may not produce any permanent proliferation in echinoderm coelomocyte populations which synthesize receptors.

The conclusions made by Hilgard are only based upon data collected in echinoderms. Recently, simultaneous investigations performed by French and American workers (Valembois, 1963, 1971*a*, 1971*b*; Duprat, 1964, 1967; and Cooper, 1968, 1969) showed specific graft rejection in earthworms. Moreover, earthworms develop immunologic memory. In order to provide a basis for evolutionary comparisons, this paper reviews the cellular aspects of graft rejection in earthworms. Moreover, these results are discussed with respect to both invertebrate and vertebrate adaptive immune mechanisms. I shall use the terms lumbricids and earthworms interchangeably.

GRAFT REJECTION IN LUMBRICIDS

We studied the histoincompatibility of *Eisenia foetida* bearing xenografts from *Allolobophora caliginosa*. Generally, xenografts exchanged between lumbricids of different genera or between different species of the same genus are rejected. Allografts between worms of the same geographical location remain intact, but allografts exchanged between worms of different regions often are rejected (Duprat, 1964; Cooper, 1969). A comparative study using the light microscope revealed that the behavior of xenografts is similar to that of certain incompatible allografts studied by Duprat (1967).

The electron microscope revealed that rejection of foreign tissue involves a succession of two events. During the first week following transplantation, the implanted tissues apparently undergo self-destruction without any activity by host leukocytes. Afterward, the graft is destroyed by host coelomocytes. The relative importance of these two successive reactions is altered during the second-set response (Valembois, 1971a) to test for memory.

Self-Destruction of Grafts

In the few hours following graft transplantation, both host and transplant epidermis connect to each other and healing is accomplished by somatic leukocytes. About two days after transplantation, the grafted tissues show damages which precede increased cellular activity in the muscle fibers of the graft. This is characterized by an increase in mitochondria, an abundant rough-surfaced endoplasmic reticulum organized in flattened cisternae, and a prominent Golgi complex in the muscle cells. Various vesicular coated vesicles or multivesicular bodies are frequently observed on the periphery of the Golgi apparatus. At the same time, the Gomori method shows an increased acid phosphatase activity in muscular fibers. Reaction products accumulate in the sarcoplasm. Deposits of lead phosphate occur adjacent to the cisternae of the rough-surfaced endoplasmic reticulum, or they may be found concentrated in vesicular bodies. Besides this heavy deposit, isolated precipitated granules are situated along the H lines of the myofibrils (Chapron and Valembois, 1967). These changes in acid phosphatase activity and probably in the content of other lysosomal enzymes suggest autolysis of graft musculature. In fact, the release of hydrolytic enzymes in the sarcoplasm of graft muscle cells is soon followed by death and necrosis of fibers without any host coelomocyte penetration into the grafted tissues. It is reasonable to expect that lysosomal enzymes are involved in cellular defense since under normal conditions a relatively small amount of enzymatic activity is noted. We suggest that autolysis of grafts is initiated by the inhibiting action of host tissues on repressors which normally control the production of lysosomal enzymes in graft cells.

Leukocyte Activity

After 12 days, host coelomocytes not only surround the periphery of grafts but many of them infiltrate the degenerated musculature. Most invading coelomocytes are similar to the macrophages described by many authors in vertebrate graft reactions. They arise from small undifferentiated splanchnic cells, resembling, by many features of their progeny, vertebrate reticular cells. A first and interesting form arising from undifferentiated splanchnic cells is a lymphocytoid cell characterized by a reduced cytoplasmic component rich in free ribosomes. Another form which contains much rough-surfaced endoplasmic reticulum resembles the vertebrate plasma cells. These two types of cells are always found in small numbers in the coelomic cavity. On the other hand, macrophagelike cells can be very numerous, chiefly in various pathological cases: these large cells contain varying amounts of rough-surfaced endoplasmic reticulum, a large number of free ribosomes, and an important Golgi apparatus. Macrophages are implicated in the elimination of grafted tissues by engulfing autolysed cells. Both macrophages and engulfed tissues are then enclosed in brown bodies; these are nodules composed of aggregated coelomic corpuscles and waste substances. Later, brown bodies migrate through the coelomic cavity in the posterior part of the body (see Hostetter and Cooper for diagrams of this process).

Second-Set Anamnestic Response

Similar events are found in the rejection of a second graft, but both cellular synthesis and self-destruction are less important. The grafted tissues are attacked early by leukocytes of the host. Five days after a second graft, a high number of macrophagelike cells occur in the coelom surrounding the graft. We had previously noted that such accumulations of leukocytes occur only ten or twelve days after a first graft. Macrophages invade the transplanted tissues about six days after a second graft. They cling to one another and produce clumps which closely adhere to the transplant cells and finally engulf them. This phenomenon is different from phagocytosis. It is soon followed by the death of both engulfed cells and macrophages. Regeneration by undifferentiated cells of the host begins before degeneration of the graft is completed, leading to the differentiation of a new body wall.

Stimulation of second graft resorption is specific. Xenograft immunity can be transferred by coelomic cells from an immunized worm (Bailey *et al.*, 1971; Valembois, 1971*b*). Therefore, coelomocytes are involved in xenograft immunity. More precisely, coelomocytes involved in graft immunity seem to be macrophages differentiated from small and undifferentiated cells of the splanchnic layer.

COMPARISON BETWEEN THE GRAFT REACTION IN LUMBRICIDS AND SOME OTHER METAZOA

"Induced" Self-Destruction of the Graft

It seems that rejection mechanisms are not only restricted to lumbricids. Data from several authors suggest that these mechanisms are also present in other invertebrate groups. Graft rejection in gorgonians (Theodor, 1970, 1971) involves a mechanism of self-destruction similar to the first step in earthworm graft rejection. The destruction of a grafted explant in gorgonians is expressed by collapse of the tissues. The histopathologic phenomena disappear if the graft is subjected to antibiotic action; this shows the active role played by the graft in mediating its own self-destruction. In the case of grafts performed in mollusca, Cheng and Galloway (1970) described autolytic processes prior to invasion of transplanted tissues by coelomocytes. In the course of studies of colonial fusion in compound ascidians, Freeman (1970) showed that some necrosis also occurs at the contact surface between the two colonies. However, no cellular movements were noted. The incompatibility manifested in xenogeneic parabiosis in amphibian embryos (Gipouloux, 1966) suggests an autolytic process analogous to those described in gorgonians and in lumbricids: A neurula of *Rana esculenta* was fused belly to belly with a neurula of *Rana temporaria*: In this case, only the first embryo was perfectly viable while the second always necrosed and died. This destruction was produced neither by leukocytes nor by antibodies: The young amphibians acquired immune competence only one month after hatching has occurred.

Cellular Immune Reactions

Little is known about the cellular mechanisms underlying graft rejection in vertebrates. The recipient lymphocytes play an important part in the process. Almost certainly, they carry surface recognition sites, and they have a specific cytotoxic effect on allogeneic transplanted cells. On the other hand, macrophages or cell populations rich in macrophages have been associated with the major events in transplantation immunity. It has been suggested that stimulated lymphocytes could transform to macrophages. As already mentioned, antigenic information in earthworms is acquired by small, undifferentiated cells which produce macrophagelike cells that mediate graft destruction. Thus, in both lumbricids and vertebrates, similar processes of rejection are executed by analogous systems of leukocytes. Graft rejection in lumbricids is the only example we have of adaptive immunity in invertebrates. But it is important to point out that uniformity in leukocyte structure and function occurs in most coelomates (Fauré-Fremiet, 1927; Wagge, 1955). Such uniformities suggest similar capabilities for performing specific cellular immune reactions. Failure to obtain this kind of reaction in other coelomate invertebrates could be due mainly to unsolved technical problems (Tripp, 1970).

Phylogenetic Implications

Analogous processes of graft rejection are demonstrable in different groups of metazoa: gorgonians and lumbricids. A specific and anamnestic cellular response is found in lumbricids and in vertebrates. Though our study has emphasized common features in graft responses of different invertebrate groups, the basis of this likeness remains to be elucidated. For instance, it remains to be determined whether the specific response characteristic of lumbricids is related to the vertebrate immune response in a straight phylogenetic line or whether the resemblance in the responses results from convergent evolution. Considering that the Annelida and Vertebrata are not directly related, it seems reasonable to expect that the immunological resemblances may be only the result of convergent evolution. However, we suggest that graft rejection involving self-destruction of transplants could be an archaic mechanism manifested by acoelomates and some coelomates. Only some coelomates having more highly differentiated leukocyte systems are able to show specific cellular immune reactions (Valembois, 1973).

REFERENCES

Bailey, S., Miller, B. J., Cooper, E. L., 1971, Transplantation immunity in Annelids. II. Adoptive transfer of the xenograft reaction, *Immunology 21*:81-86.

Burnet, F. M., 1959, *The Clonal Selection Theory of Acquired Immunity, p. 209*, Cambridge University Press, Cambridge.

Burnet, F. M., 1968, Evolution of the immune process in Invertebrates, *Nature (London) 218*:426-430.

Chapron, C. and Valembois, P., 1967, Infrastructure de la fibre musculaire pariétale des Lombriciens, *J. Microscop. 6*:617-626.

Cheng, T. C. and Galloway, P. C., 1970, Transplantation immunity in Mollusks: the histoincompatibility of *Helisoma duryi normale* with allografts and xenografts, *J. Invertebr. Pathol, 15*:177-192.

Cooper, E. L., 1968, Rejection of xenografts exchange between *Lumbricus terrestris* and *Eisenia foetida, Transplantation 6*:322-337.

Cooper, E. L., 1969, Chronic allograft rejection in *Lumbricus terrestris*, *J. Exp. Zool.* *171*:69-74.

Duprat, P., 1964, Mise en évidence de réactions immunitaires dans les homogreffes de paroi du corps chez le Lombricien *Eisenia foetida typica*, *Comp. Rend. Acad. Sci. Paris* *259*:4177-4180.

Duprat, P., 1967, Étude de la prise et du maintien d'un greffon de paroi du corps chez le Lombricien *Eisenia foetida typica*, *Ann. Inst. Pasteur, 113*:367-88.

Ehrlich, P., 1900, On immunity with special reference to cell life, *Proc. Royal Soc.* *66*:424-448.

Fauré-Fremiet, E., 1927, Les amibocytes des Invertébrés à l'état quiescent et à l'état actif, *Arch. Anat. Microscop. Morphol. Exp 23*:99-173.

Freeman, G., 1970, Transplantation specificity in Echinoderms and lower Chordates, *Transplant. Proc. 2*:236-239.

Gipouloux, J. D., 1966, Observations sur la compatibilité ou l'incompatibilité entre embryons parabiotiques chez les Amphibiens Anoures, *Comp. Rend. Soc. Biol.* *160*:2291-2294.

Hilgard, H. R., 1970, Studies of protein uptake by Echinoderm cells: their possible significance in relation to the phylogeny of immune responses, *Transplant. Proc. 2*:240-242.

Hilgard, H. R. and Phillips, J. H., 1968, Sea urchin response to foreign substances, *Science, 161*:1243-1245.

Hilgard, H. R., Wander, R. H., and Hinds, W. E., 1973, Specific receptors in relation to the evolution of immunity (this symposium).

Jerne, J., 1970, The natural selection theory of antibody formation, *Proc. Nat. Acad. Sci. U.S. 41*:849-857.

Theodor, J., 1970, Distinction between "self" and "not-self" in lower Invertebrates, *Nature* (*London*) *227*:690-692.

Theodor, J., 1971, Reconnaissance du "self" ou reconnaissance des "not-self," *Arch. Zool. Exp. Gen. 112*:113-116.

Tripp, M. R., 1970, Immunity in Mollusca, *Transplant. Proc. 2*:231-232.

Valembois, P., 1963, Recherches sur la nature de la réaction antigreffe chez le Lombricien *Eisenia foetida Sav., Comp. Rend. Acad. Sci., Paris. 257*:3489-3490.

Valembois, P., 1971*a*, Evolution de la musculature d'un xénogreffon de paroi du corps chez un Lombricien. *J. Microscop. 11*:339-352.

Valembois, P., 1971*b*, Rôle des leucocytes dans l'acquisition d'une immunité antigreffe spécifique chez les Lombriciens, *Arch. Zool. Exp Gen. 112*:97-104.

Valembois, P., 1973, Quelques aspects phylogéniques de la réaction d'incompatibilité aux greffes chez les Métazoaires, *Ann. Biol. 12*:1-26.

Wagge, L. E., 1955, Amoebocytes, *Intern. Rev. Cytol. 4*:31-78.

Chapter 11

Graft Rejection and the Regulation
of Length in Hydra viridis

Stanley Shostak

Department of Biology
University of Pittsburgh
Pittsburgh, Pennsylvania

INTRODUCTION

At a recent meeting of comparative immunologists an argument took place about how to conduct research on evolutionary questions. The speaker had said that to trace the origins of the immune system the essential question was, "What characteristics of the primitive organism could give rise to the immune system?" not, "What characteristics of the immune system are found in primitive organisms?" The former question acknowledges the ambiguous antecedents of immunity while the latter question predetermines the answer and limits the potential for research. The moderator reproachfully argued that proceeding without the classical definitions of immunity justifies any sort of research as immunology. He was urged to work on primitive organisms to break down his vertebrate-bound immunologic chauvinism.

The object of comparative immunology is to explore the biological roots of recognition, sensitivity, specificity and anamnesis. My position is a compromise between both sides of the dispute. I pursue answers to the question, "What does a primitive organism do in response to a challenge which a vertebrate would respond to with its immune system? Specifically, how does a *Hydra* respond to grafting, and what are the controls of graft rejection?"

POSITION OF COELENTERATES IN INVERTEBRATE
IMMUNOLOGY RESEARCH

Coelenterates figure in many studies of primitive organisms because their basic radial symmetry places them at the nexus of evolution toward increasing complexity. Campbell and Bidd (1970) and Shostak (1970) reviewed the variety of immunologically relevant research projects on coelenterates which range from the recognition and binding of protein suitable for digestion (Phillips, 1966) and the uptake of symbiotic algae in different species of *Chlorohydra* (Park *et al.*, 1967) to the initiation of budding.

Much of the work capitalizes on the unique feature of the hydrozoans, the ease with which they can be grafted. In particular, the fresh-water hydrozoan, *Hydra,* is virtually capable of being taken apart and put back together again. Because of the cavity that runs throughout the length of the animal, annuli cut out of animals can be skewered on a hair, pushed together, and, after healing between the pieces (about 3 hr), removed from the hair as a reconstituted composite or graft animal. Depending on the number of pieces grafted together, the process from cutting to pushing the pieces together takes between 2 and 15 min. Many grafts can be made and a statistical approach to the response of animals to grafting or graft rejection is feasible.

Heterografts have been successful, if only occasionally, among some species of *Hydra* and even produce chimeric buds (see review by Campbell and Bidd, 1970). Lowell and Burnett (1969) achieved unique xenogeneic intertissue chimeras by combining the outer cell layer (epidermis) from animals of one species, with the inner cell layer (gastrodermis) from animals of another species. A still more provocative development in xenografting is that of Saffitz *et al.* (1972), who transfused hydra of one species depleted of pluripotential interstitial cells with interstitial cells from members of another species. The possibilities for using interstitial cell transfusions in studies of species specificity is only beginning to be explored.

SEPARATION

Under some conditions successful grafts break apart. The process of graft separation begins with a constriction of waist at the graft border. Although at first food passes beyond the waist, within a day or two after its appearance food fails to pass, even though large quantities of food can be present distal to the waist. The graft piece proximal to the waist, therefore, receives no direct nutrition unless buds or an ectopic head are present. The gastrodermis then disappears in the waist. In *Hydra viridis,* where the green algal symbiont lives exclusively within gastrodermal cells, loss of green color in the waist indicates loss of gastrodermal cells. Ultimately, only a strand of epidermal cells connects the two graft pieces. This strand is then broken. The animal's head and foot will attach to the substratum as far apart as the full stretch-length allows. A violent contraction breaks the connecting strand, releasing the graft pieces with an elastic reaction. The time between a waist's first appearance and separation varies between 1 and 3 days. Rarely, a waist disappears and the graft remains intact, but almost all separations are preceded by the formation of a waist.

The histology of graft separation has not been studied, but the identical process of bud detachment has been studied by Tannreuther (1909). Cell movement seems to be chiefly responsible for thinning the attaching strand rather than cell death.

INTRASPECIFIC GRAFTS

Although as a rule, grafts between members of the same species of Hydra are successful, there are exceptions. For instance, some species such as *Hydra pseudologactis* are notoriously hard to graft compared to others such as *Hydra viridis*. There are also conspicuous differences between the ease with which different parts of an animal are grafted. The budding region and upper peduncle are the "stickiest" parts of an animal. Would healing and the formation of graft borders between the grafted pieces occur more rapidly in these regions than elsewhere (Shostak, 1968).

Ectopic structures, mainly heads (ring of tentacles surrounding a mouth with associated tissue) and feet (basal adhesive disk surrounding an aboral pore with associated tissue) can form at the borders between grafted pieces. Feet form on the apical graft piece and heads on the basal graft piece. Results on the frequencies of head and foot regeneration at graft borders has been presented (Shostak, 1972, 1973) and need not be further reviewed here. Heads and feet regenerate as frequently in the vicinities of graft borders that ultimately separate as in vicinities of borders that do not, but separation occurs more rapidly when regenerated structures are present in the vicinity of the waists.

Three general rules can be formulated for success in grafting animals without producing heads and feet or giving way to separations at graft borders: (1) Do not elongate the animals by grafting, i.e., add only as much tissue as is removed. (2) Strictly observe and retain the original polarity of each graft piece in the final graft animal. (3) Graft pieces together so that they reside in the final graft animal in the same positions that they originally occupied. Due caution should also be observed in matching the graft pieces by size and aligning them to meet across as broad a surface as possible. Finally, the duration between wounding and grafting should be as brief as possible and not exceed 15 min. When these rules are observed, no heads, feet, or separations occur, in virtually all cases, even if the head or foot is amputated either before or after grafting (Shostak, 1972).

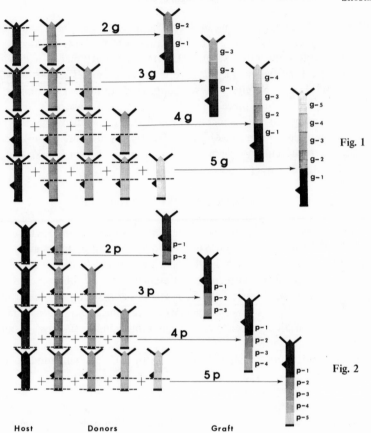

Fig. 1

Fig. 2

Host   Donors   Graft

Figs. 1 and 2. Illustrate the grafting procedures and nomenclature. Each row shows another combination of multiple gastric region grafts (Fig. 1) or multiple peduncle grafts (Fig. 2). The names of each type of graft are given above the arrows connecting the host and donor animals (left) with the graft (right). The normal and untraumatized parts of the animals (such as heads, budding regions, and feet) and the parts not involved in the grafted parts (peduncles in the case of gastric region grafts, or gastric regions in the case of peduncle grafts) are not mentioned in the names. Thus, only the distinguishing features of the graft appear in the name. The number refers to the total number of either gastric regions or peduncles present, not merely to those from donor animals.

The dashed lines passing through the host and donor animals and extending on both sides indicate where the host and donor are cut to provide the parts of each graft. The "graft" columns indicate how the parts are assembled. The animals and their parts are drawn proportionally to the lengths of these animals with a scale of 16:1. The head is represented by two symbolic tentacles lying at right angles from the pointed apical end (hypostome). The budding region is represented by an arrow protruding to the left of each animal. The gastric region is the part of the animal between the head and budding region. The feet of the hydras are symbolized by the bold lines at their lower ends. The peduncle is the part of the animal between the budding region and foot. For identifying the parts of the graft, the letter g is used for gastric region, and p for peduncle. The host is considered the part containing an original budding region and is always the largest part of the graft. The host's gastric region and peduncle are labeled number one (1). The adjacent grafted parts are numbered consecutively. These designations correspond to those used in the Tables.

Acquiring material for studying graft rejection, therefore, requires breaking one or another of these rules. Campbell and Bidd (1970) broke the rule on the retention of polarity and obtained separations between graft pieces that were also regenerating structures at the original point of healing. I broke the rule against elongating because it does not necessarily involve the regeneration of additional structures at the graft border and it can, therefore, be free of interference from the regenerating structures. The experiments discussed here involve elongating *Hydra viridis* by adding multiple gastric regions or peduncles to host animals. The types of grafts and the nomenclature employed are shown in Figs. 1 and 2.

MULTIPLY GRAFTED ANIMALS

The fact that graft pieces separate when they represent additional tissue i.e., more tissue is presented than removed, while similar graft pieces do not separate when additional tissue is not supplied, suggests that *Hydra* possesses a quantitative sense of self. Experimentally elongated animals somehow can measure the amount of tissue available and proceed to reject excess tissue by forming waists and separations. The object of the present research was to illuminate the basis of quantitative self-recognition and the method of self-regulation through graft rejection. The underlying question is, "Is there a quantitative surveillance system operating in *Hydra* which, when triggered, results in graft rejection?"

Doubling the Gastric Region (2g) or Peduncle (2p)

The frequencies of waists and separations and the sums of these frequencies for different types of multiply grafted animals on the second day after grafting are listed in Tables I–III. Frequency refers to the number of times the event occurs at a particular graft border as a function of the number of graft animals in a particular sample. Since waists almost always lead to separations, the sums of the frequencies are the ultimate frequency of separations, in effect, predicting the fate of the waists. These sums are plotted as functions of the distances from the heads and feet of the animals in Fig. 3.

Animals with just one additional segment, i.e., two gastric regions (2g) or two peduncles (2p), always have lower frequencies of waists and separations than graft animals with more segments. The 2g and 2p graft animals are the only ones in which all graft pieces have a terminal structure, the head being on the apical piece and the foot on the basal one. In all other cases, central graft pieces lack terminal structures entirely, having instead graft borders at both ends. The presence of terminal structures is constructive for the formation of patent graft borders.

The results on animals with both two gastric regions and two peduncles (2g2p animals) are in part consistent with a role of terminal structures in graft

Table I. Frequencies of Waists, Separations, and Their
Sums on Animals with Multiple Gastric Region Grafts

Designations	2g	3g	4g	5g
Number of animals	123	73	76	49
g-5 to g-4				
Waists				0.29
Separation				0.06
Sum				0.35
g-4 to g-3				
Waists			0.17	0.20
Separation			0.11	0.04
Sum			0.28	0.24
g-3 to g-2				
Waists		0.25	0.08	0.08
Separation		0.16	0.05	0.02
Sum		0.41	0.13	0.10
g-2 to g-1				
Waists	0.07	0.10	0.05	0.12
Separation	0.03	0.03	0.03	0.04
Sum	0.10	0.13	0.08	0.16

TABLE II. Frequencies of Waists, Separations, and Their
Sums on Animals with Multiple Peduncle Grafts

Designations	2p	3p	4p	5p
Number of animals	48	57	58	50
p-1 to p-2				
Waists	0.02	0.24	0.24	0.42
Separation	0.04	0.38	0.40	0.16
Sum	0.06	0.62	0.64	0.58
p-2 to p-3				
Waists		0.05	0.09	0.08
Separation		0.02	0.16	0.16
Sum		0.07	0.25	0.24
p-3 to p-4				
Waists			0.07	0.16
Separation			0.04	0.10
Sum			0.11	0.26
p-4 to p-5				
Waists				0.02
Separation				0.04
Sum				0.06

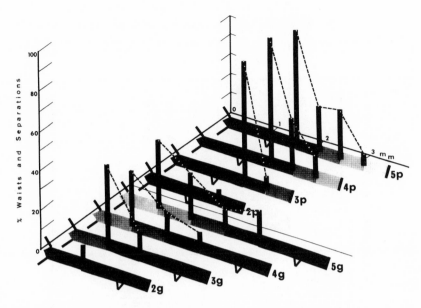

Fig. 3. The frequencies (as percentages) of the sums of waists and separations are shown as functions of distance from the head. The frequencies correspond to those listed in Tables I–II in the rows entitled "Sum." The thick vertical solid bars are proportional to these frequencies. The results for each graft border on animals of the different types are connected by dashed lines. The diagrammatic hydras resemble those in Figs. 1 and 2. The lower half of Fig. 3 corresponds to the grafts illustrated in Fig. 1 of animals with multiple gastric regions. The upper half of Fig. 3 corresponds to the grafts illustrated in Fig. 2 of animals with multiple peduncles. The arrows on the left of each hydra identify the budding region, and thus the host animal. The host's gastric region or peduncle is numbered one (1) in the Tables and Figs. 1 and 2. The grafted segments are indicated by the changing tones. They can be numbered consecutively away from the host segments.

healing. The frequency of waists and separations between the apical gastric region and the central gastric region having only graft borders at its ends are twice the frequency of 2g animals (Table III). The increase in the frequency of separations between the peduncles, however, is nowhere near as large.

Another type of experiment involved the removal, just prior to grafting, of the terminal structures from 2g 2p, and 2g2p animals. The results are presented in Table III. Headless animals with two gastric regions (−H2g) showed a dramatic and statistically significant increase (as shown by Chi square) in both the frequencies of waists and separations. The absence of the terminal foot from animals with two peduncles (2p−F) had no effect. Even more surprising, the removal of the terminal structures from animals with two gastric regions and two peduncles (−H2g2p−F) had no effect on the frequencies of waist and separations.

Table III. Frequencies of Waists, Separations, and Sums on Multiply Grafted Animals with Normal Terminal Structures, Additional, or Missing Ones

Descriptions	3g	2H3g	2g	-H2g	2g2p	-H2g2p-F	2p	2p-F	3p	3p2F
Number of animals	73	72	123	74	55	52	48	48	57	28
g-3 to g-2										
Waists	0.25	0.10								
Separation	0.16	0.31								
Sum	0.41	0.41								
g-2 to g-1										
Waists	0.10	0.04	0.07	0.26	0.15	0.08				
Separation	0.03	0.08	0.03	0.22	0.09	0.12				
Sum	0.13	0.12	0.10	0.48	0.24	0.20				
			$\underbrace{\hspace{2cm}}_{a}$							
p-1 to p-2										
Waists					0.07	0.06	0.02	0.06	0.24	0.22
Separation					0.04	0.06	0.04	0.04	0.38	0.36
Sum					0.11	0.12	0.06	0.10	0.62	0.58
p-2 to p-3										
Waists									0.05	0
Separation									0.02	0
Sum									0.07	0

[a]Probability that difference is due to random error less than 5%

These results can be broadly interpreted in terms of the concept of dominance (Spiegelman, 1945) or of what Child (1941) called physiological competition. Dominance usually refers to the competition of parts of a morphological system for food, but since in *Hydra* food is stored in cells, dominance is competition for cells. The dominant regions of a hydra are the head, budding region, and foot, each of which normally competes for cells. The head and foot ordinarily have priority inasmuch as when there is a dearth of cells, budding is suppressed. On the other hand a well-fed budding animal can lose 80–85% of its cells to developing buds (Campbell, 1967; Shostak and Kankel, 1967; Shostak, 1968). Conceivably, the tension created by physiological competition for cells is both related to successful healing and graft separation.

When the head, budding region, and foot are present on graft animals of normal length or even on animals elongated by the addition of one graft segment, a tension could exist in both directions across the graft border which brings the pieces together and promotes healing. When the head is absent, however, as on headless animals or the central graft pieces in 2g2p animals, this constructive tension would not exist. Possibly the foot and budding region draw cells away from the graft border and prevent adequate healing.

Another possibility also has merit. Following the amputation of a head, a new one begins regenerating immediately. A regenerating head recruits and mobilizes cells for itself more effectively than a normal head. For instance, a regenerating head forms tentacles in two days while normal tentacles undergo turnover in about a week Conceivably the regenerating head competes successfully with the other dominant centers, and it draws cells away from the graft border. Equal and opposite tension across the graft border would be absent as a consequence, and the pieces would fail to heal together adequately and would ultimately separate.

King (1901) and Tardent (1954, 1960) also experimented with elongated animals. Their conclusion that graft separation is a consequence of head regeneration at the graft border is consistent with a role for dominance in separation. When regenerating heads form at a graft border, they could usurp the cells that would otherwise have contributed to healing across the graft border.

Higher Degrees of Multiplicity

A general pattern in the sums of the frequencies of waists and separations can be seen in the results plotted in Fig. 3. Decreasing frequencies occur as functions of increasing distance from the head and decreasing distance from the foot of graft animals of different degrees of multiplicity. The asymmetric pattern does not suggest an effect of dominance, and the fact that the graft borders close to the head are always more vulnerable to separation than other graft borders is inconsistent with a positive effect on healing of the head. Other possibilities are also eliminated. Lines of stress in the multiply grafted animals would have resulted in a parabolic pattern peaking at the central graft borders. Mechanical stress on the borders, therefore, does not explain the observed pattern. Had the distribution of separations been random, the frequencies of separations at different graft borders as a function of distance from the head or foot would have been a straight line with zero slope. The observed pattern, however, is that of a gradient with slopes statistically significantly different from zero. The changing of frequencies of waists, separations, and their sums as a function of distance suggest that an overriding control of graft rejection is due to a diffusion gradient of a material affecting healing.

A model of diffusion gradients in which a diffusible substance is released from a source and used up at a distant sink was suggested by Crick (1970, 1971) and shown to be feasible for multiply grafted animals (Shostak, 1972, 1973) and possibly normal animals (Wolpert *et al.*, 1972). Some of the operational consequences of this model can be tested on the data available here.

The gradients should be linear over the distance between the source and sink if the zone between them is neutral, i.e., neither producing nor using up the diffusible material. There is ambiguity due to the failure to define the source and sink, but the regression of the frequencies of separations does not differ statistically from linearity (Fig. 3). The slopes of the gradients should decrease as the distance between the source and sink increase, if the only factor determining the slope is diffusion through a neutral zone from the source to the sink. In multiply grafted animals, the slopes for the frequencies of separations as a function of distance from the terminal head (Table IV) do, indeed, decrease as the number of grafted pieces increases. The average frequencies of waists and separations between the terminal pieces and the subterminal ones for animals of all lengths should be about the same. If the terminal piece at one end contains the source and at the other end contains the sink, the distance between them should not

Table IV. Average Slopes of the Gradients of Graft Separation

Type of graft	Sum of frequencies of waists and separations per mm from head
3g	−0.28
4g	−0.10
5g	−0.073
3p	−0.79
4p	−0.38
5p	−0.22

affect the frequencies of separations of the end pieces. Once again, the consequences of the Crick model are borne out. On multiply grafted animals of the two types, neither the frequencies found for the apical graft borders nor the frequencies found for the basal graft borders, (Tables I–II) differed statistically significantly.

The experimental results provide, therefore, compelling reasons to conclude that graft rejection in multiply grafted animals is controlled in part by a diffusible material produced at a source and used up at a sink separated from the source by a neutral zone. The control of graft rejection by a diffusible material is in addition to the control by the dominant center. Conflict between the control based on dominance and that based on diffusible material occurs only when the terminal head is amputated. In the absence of the head, the control based on dominant centers predominates and the frequency of graft rejection increases. In multiply grafted animals the rejection of grafts seems to be primarily a function of the action of the diffusible material.

The Diffusion Gradient

The remaining problem is determining whether the head end of the hydras is a source of a promoter of graft rejection and the foot end is the sink, or the foot end is a source of a promoter of graft healing and the head end is the sink. Diffusion gradients of either type of diffusible materials could account for the observed changes equally well since the frequencies of waists and separation decrease as a function of increasing distance from the head or increase as a function of increasing distance from the foot (Fig. 3). The ablation experiments in which the head was amputated suggest that the head plays an active role whereas the amputation of the foot has no significant effect (Table III). However, the role of the head could merely involve dominance rather than diffusion of material. Efforts to specify the source and sink of the diffusible material by adding heads to animals with three gastric regions (2H3g animals), or feet to animals with three peduncles (3p2F), were not illuminating (Table III). The two-headed pieces used in grafting were obtained by Colcemid treatment (Shostak & Tammariello, 1969), and the two-footed pieces were made by surgically splitting the foot of animals and allowing sufficient time for both halves to enlarge to normal size. No significant differences in the frequencies of waists or separations occurred between the two-headed and two-footed animals and their one-headed and one-footed counterparts.

The noteworthy difference between the maximum frequencies of waists, separations, and their sums on animals with multiple gastric region grafts as opposed to animals with multiple peduncle grafts can be classified as a region-specific difference. Perhaps the peduncles are less competent than gastric regions for healing graft pieces together over a long period of time, despite the greater ease with which peduncles stick together initially. Sensitivity to the diffusible material could also be involved. Perhaps the gastric regions are more sensitive to a diffusible material that promotes healing, or perhaps the peduncles are more sensitive to a diffusible material that promotes rejection. The latter possibility has some merit inasmuch as buds normally detach from the parent when in the upper part of the parent's peduncle.

Although the identities of the source and sink remain unknown, as does the identify and function of the diffusible material, there seems little question that a source, sink, neutral zone, and diffusible material which influence healing and graft rejection exists. This conclusion will, no doubt, be greeted enthusiastically by those who have sought to explain pattern formation in systems like hydra in terms of "positional information" (Wolpert, 1968, 1969, 1971). A diffusion gradient could impart to cells "positional information" regarding where they are relative to the ends of the animal. The cell's knowledge about where it should be as opposed to where it is would then trigger it to engage in a healing mode or in a rejection mode of differentiation.

CONCLUDING REMARKS

The *Hydra* has two systems for quantitatively measuring itself, one involving the dominant centers and the other a diffusion gradient of a material affecting healing. The role of dominance in normal animals may be less important except following amputation, but the diffusion gradient could have several normal functions even in the absence of wounding. Given that the animal has been molded by evolution to a maximal adaptive size suitable for coping with currents, nutrition, transpiration, and structural demands, a gradient system would be an exquisite way for the animal to measure up to its maximal adaptive size. "Positional information" could instruct cells to break down the substratum to which cells adhere, for instance, during bud detachment, or not to synthesize new substratum at the points of normal cell attrition and turnover. If throughout the invertebrates qualitative self-recognition within a species is lacking or weak, as shown by allograft rejection, it might be because qualitative self-recognition is not at the root of histocompatibility. Quantitative self-recognition, on the other hand, may be more widespread, and therefore more fundamental.

REFERENCES

Campbell, R. D., 1967, Tissue dynamics of steady state growth in *Hydra littoralis*. II. Patterns of tissue movement, *J. Morph. 121*: 19.

Campbell, R. D. and Bidd, C., 1970, Transplantation in coelenterates, in: *Phylogeny of Transplantation Reactions* (W. H. Hildemann and E. L. Cooper, eds.), Transplantation Proceedings, Vol. II, p. 202.

Child, C. M., 1941, *Patterns and Problems of Development,* University of Chicago Press, Chicago.

Crick, F. H. C., 1970, Diffusion in embryogenesis, *Nature* 225:420.

Crick, F. H. C., 1971, The scale of pattern formation, *Symp. Soc. Exp. Biol.* 25:429.

King, H. D., 1901, Observations and experiments on regeneration in *Hydra viridis, Arch. Entwicklungsmech. Organ.* 13:135.

Lowell, R. D. and Burnett, A. L., 1969, Regeneration of complete hydra from isolated explants, *Biol. Bull.* 137:312.

Park, H. D., Greenblatt, C. L. Mattern, C. R. T., and Meril, C. R., 1967, Some relationships between *Chlorohydra*, its symbionts and some other chlorophyllous forms, *J. Exp. Zool.* 164:141.

Phillips, J. H., 1966, Immunological processes and recognition of foreignness in the invertebrates, in: *Phylogeny of Immunity*, p. 133 (R. T. Smith, P. A. Miescher, and R. A. Good, eds.), University of Florida Press, Gainsville.

Saffitz, J. E., Burnett, A. L., and Lesh, G. E., 1972, Nervous system transplantation in Hydra, *J. Exp. Zool.* 179:215.

Shostak, S., 1968, Growth in *Hydra viridis, J. Exp. Zool.* 169:431.

Shostak, S., 1970, Transplantation in Cnidaria, in: *Phylogeny of Transplantation Reactions* (W. H. Hildemann and E. L. Cooper eds.), Transplantation Proceedings, Vol. II, p. 212.

Shostak, S., 1972, Inhibitory gradients of head and foot regeneration in *Hydra viridis, Develop. Biol.* 28:620.

Shostak, S., 1973, Evidence of morphogenetically significant diffusion gradients in *Hydra viridis* lengthened by grafting, *J. Embryol. Exp. Morphol.* 29:311.

Shostak, S. and Kankel, D. R., 1967, Morphogenetic movements during budding in *Hydra, Develop. Biol.* 15:451.

Shostak, S. and Tammariello, R. V., 1969, Supernumerary heads in *Hydra viridis, Nat. Cancer Inst. Monograph* 31:739.

Spiegelman, S., 1945, Physiological competition as a regulatory mechanism in morphogenesis, *Quart. Rev. Biol.* 20:121.

Tannreuther, G. W., 1909, Budding in *Hydra, Biol. Bull.* 16:210.

Tardent, P. E., 1954, Axiale Verteilungs-Gradienten der interstitiellen Zellen bei *Hydra* und *Tubularia* und ihre Bedeutung fur die Regeneration, *Entwicklungsmech. Organ.* 146:593.

Tardent, P. E., 1960, Principles governing the process of regeneration in hydroids, in: *Developing Cell Systems and Their Control* p. 21 (E. M. Rudnick, ed.), Ronald Press, New York.

Wolpert, L., 1968, The French flag problem: a contribution to the discussion on pattern development and regulation, in: *Towards a Theoretical Biology, I. Prolegomena*, p. 125 (C. H. Waddington, ed.), Edinburgh University Press, Edinburgh, U.K.

Wolpert, L., 1969, Positional information and the spatial pattern of cellular differentiation, *J. Theoret. Biol.* 25:1.

Wolpert, L., 1971, Positional information and pattern formation, in: *Current Topics in Developmental Biology, Vol. 6.,* p. 183 (A. A. Moscona and A. Monroy, eds.), Academic Press, New York.

Wolpert, L., Clarke, M. R. A., and Horbrunch, A., 1972, Positional signaling along *Hydra, Nature, New Biol.* 239:101.

Chapter 12

Tissue Transplantation in
Diverse Marine Invertebrates

W. H. Hildemann,* Trevor G. Dix,† and John D. Collins

School of Biological Sciences
James Cook University of North Queensland
Townsville, Australia

INTRODUCTION

The search for the origins and early mechanisms of immunocompetence among the invertebrates is now well underway. Tissue transplantation is recognized as a sensitive and perhaps universally applicable tool for investigation of immunoresponsiveness. Indeed, only orthotopic tissue transplantation may allow meaningful comparisons of reactivity to potentially immunogenic cells among phylogenetically diverse animals. This is because responses to xenogeneic or exotic macromolecules may be limited by the enzymes available to a species rather than by immunologic potential as such. Moreover, endotoxins inherent in many microbial antigen preparations may have effects ranging from stimulating to fatal, depending on the recipient species. A purified protein such as bovine serum albumin is an excellent, satisfactory, or poor immunogen depending on whether the recipient is a rabbit, goldfish, or mouse, respectively (Vredevoe, 1964, Trump, 1970). Thus the choice of test immunogen rather than the innate immunologic capacity of the recipient may be decisive and thus, results can be misleading.

Although refined surgical techniques have allowed detailed assessment of responses to grafted tissues in all classes of vertebrates, such studies of invertebrates are still in the pioneering phase. Experimental approaches and their

*Present address: Department of Medical Microbiology and Immunology University of California, Los Angeles, California 90024. Aided by NIH research grant AI-07970.
†Present address: Sea Fisheries Division, Department of Agriculture, G.P.O. Box 192B, Hobart 7001, Australia.

shortcomings, as applied to invertebrates, were recently reviewed by Hildemann (1972). The question posed for molluscs by Tripp (1970), "Can successful autografts or allografts be made routinely?" must still have a negative answer for a surprisingly large number of invertebrate groups. A large part of the difficulty hinges on adequate animal care to assure prolonged survival under laboratory conditions. Most marine animals have specialized requirements and a narrow range of tolerance for abnormal conditions. Little is known about anesthetics, infectious agents, or use of antibiotics among invertebrates.

Our recent transplantation studies of corals, bivalve molluscs, and echinoderms indicate the diversity of approaches required among invertebrates. The difficulties encountered in anesthesia, surgical techniques, reactions to injury, and graft scoring are also cited in brief as a guide to others embarking on similar studies.

CORALS

Branching staghorn corals of *Acropora* species found in many bays around Magnetic Island near Townsville, Australia, have been maintained for long periods in running seawater aquariums with microscopic food provided, as in nature, by the constantly renewed seawater. Indeed, such optimal conditions appear essential to keep living corals healthy.

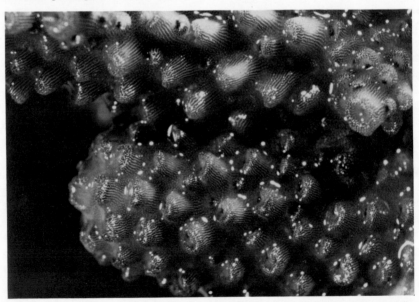

Fig. 1. Compatible lateral fusion of two intracolony branches of living *Acropora* at five weeks after grafting at 25°C. Both soft tissue (coenenchyme) and skeletal tissue fusion occurred and persisted indefinitely.

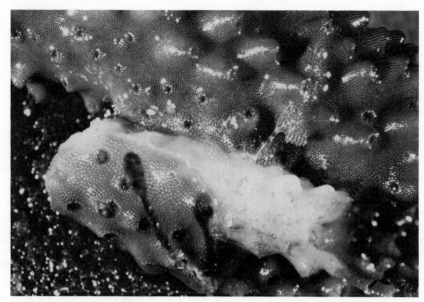

Fig. 2. Incompatible lateral fusion of two xenogeneic branches of living *Acropora* at about five weeks after grafting at 25°C. Branches remain held together by monofilament nylon loop (center), but blanched area of tissue death in contact zone is obvious. Invasion of blanched graft skeletal tissue by dark pigmented recipient coenenchyme is evident.

Quite simple techniques have sufficed to yield viable grafts among staghorn corals, and anesthesia is not required for successful "surgery." A 2–5 cm terminal piece of a staghorn branch is broken off to provide a graft which is simply tied firmly alongside a recipient branch with a single loop of 0.2 mm monofilament nylon. This brings graft and recipient soft tissues (i.e., coenenchyme) into intimate contact as illustrated in Fig. 1. When graft and recipient are derived from the same colony (i.e., branches of the same original clone), one would expect compatibility, since the relationship is that of an autograft or isograft. Indeed, *Acropora* isografts have invariably shown compatible fusion of soft tissue and cementing of skeletal tissue with the recipient in 6–8 days at 25°C. Such fusion persists indefinitely or >300 days (Fig. 1). Often when scuba diving on the Great Barrier Reefs, compatible fusion of separate intracolony branches is observed to have occurred following accidental breakage. In many species, repeated compatible fusion of intracolony branches occurs naturally during normal growth—a process which has the obvious advantage of sustaining the structural integrity of the whole colony against wave action.

Stereomicroscopic observation of fused isografts in the graft–recipient contact zone reveals intact polyps and persistence of pigmented zooanthellae in the coenenchyme, just as found in adjacent normal tissue. The viable integrity of isograft and recipient is also verifiable by a simple direct test. A gentle probing of polyp tentacles induces a withdrawal response (Horridge, 1957) which is instantly transmitted across the graft—recipient interface via the nerve net. This has proved to be a quite sensitive and unequivocal test of functional graft survival. In contrast with isografts, xenografts between *Acropora* species have shown no persistent tissue fusion. Although graft/recipient contact is quickly established, a zone of cell death develops after about a week. This is followed by obvious regression of soft tissues at the interface (Fig. 2). Subsequent overgrowth of the exposed skeleton by either graft or recipient tissue is then typical. Acute or subacute rejection of xenografts, at least in certain species combinations of *Acropora*, appears to be the rule.

Preliminary study of *Acropora* allografts (i.e., intercolony grafts) has revealed moderate incompatibilities. Functional fusion of graft and recipient occurs as rapidly and as completely as with isografts. However, after several to many weeks, incompatibility leading to soft-tissue death in the contact zone has frequently been observed.

The capacity for nonself recognition followed by antagonistic reactions is clearly present even at this early phylogenetic level of the coelenterates. To what extent immunologic components of specificity and memory are involved in allogeneic/xenogeneic rejection remains to be determined. Additional methods to evaluate histological changes at graft sites could be most helpful in scoring the more attenuated or chronic reactions characteristic of allogeneic combinations.

The lack of sharp taxonomic distinctions among *Acropora* species poses some problems in deciding whether certain grafts are allogeneic or xenogeneic. Moreover, if test *Acropora* are taken from the same bay or reef area, one cannot always be sure whether separate colonies may have originated by breakage from the same colony during stormy weather. Although distinctive species of *Acropora* were used for grafting, their identification by name is still uncertain (Collins, in preparation). Many species of diverse corals coexist in close proximity on tropical reefs. The integrity of each species, if not each clonal colony, requires recognition mechanisms to prevent random tissue fusion under natural reef conditions. Both "transplantation" compatibility and incompatibility, then, are regularly seen among hard coral species in nature (Whitefield, 1901) and have a *raison d'etre* readily understood in terms of population genetics and ecology.

PEARL OYSTERS (*Pinctada margaritifera*)

In contrast to the technical ease of hard coral transplantation, our extensive work on pearl oysters has led to numerous difficulties which have only partly been solved. The primary aim was to develop successful orthotopic transplantation techniques. Mantle tissue was selected for several reasons: (a) mantle tissue is most accessible to surgical manipulation, (b) mantle tissue has a texture and organization amenable to microsurgical techniques, (c) the orange versus black color dimorphism of the marginal mantle of individual oysters provides unequivocal indication of viability. Initially, an anesthetic was sought to open the shell and relax the mantle for surgery. Many possible anesthetics reviewed by Kaplan (1969) proved unsuitable, but 0.25% propylene phenoxetol (Nippa Laboratories Ltd., U.K.) in sea water anesthetizes pearl oysters effectively in 10–20 min. Following surgery (10–15 min), animals began to recover several minutes after return to running sea water. No adverse effects were noted.

Mantle pieces including marginal and pallial tissue were removed with fine scissors and forceps from anesthetized pearl oysters. These trapezoidal or rectangular tissue pieces were then sutured into their original position, optimally with 6–0 monofilament nylon (Ethicon Inc., Somerville, N.Y.) affixed to a curved cutting-point needle. A binocular "opti-Visor" magnifier (3X) with adjustable headband proved essential. Many variations in technique were attempted. These included the size and shape of the transplant, number and position of sutures, type of suturing, and application of absorbable gelatin and/or tetracycline wound powder along the graft contact zone.

Regardless of the detailed technique no mantle transplants remained viable and intact longer than about 16 days. Seven trapezoid grafts ($\sim$8 mm $\times$ 4-5 mm)

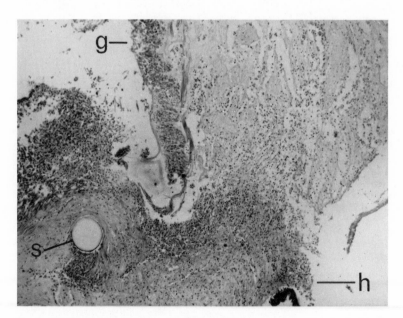

Fig. 3. Histological appearance of weakly-healed but necrosing orthotopic mantle graft in *Pinctada margaritifera* after 5–8 days at 25°C. Note large numbers of hemocytes in contact zone of pale graft (g) and host (h) tissue. (S) indicates position of 6–0 monofilament nylon suture.

examined at 1, 2, 5, 8, 16 and 23 days postoperation illustrate the pattern which was usually observed All grafts appeared fully viable and neatly in place at day 2. Although all were still in place at days 5 and 8, three exhibited signs of necrosis at day 5; by day 8 only one graft appeared viable. After 16 days only two grafts remained intact, and by day 23 none remained. Histological sections at various times after operation indicated that the graft often fused or healed, at least weakly (Fig. 3), although necrosis and graft loss subsequently ensued. The reasons for these losses are unclear. Early technical losses attributable to pulling out of sutures by the strong mantle muscles were prevented in several ways. Transplants were made smaller (~6 X 3-5 mm) with little inclusion of soft pallial tissue. Extra 6-0 sutures were inserted to give up to three on each of the three contact sides or margins of the graft in the tougher part of the marginal mantle. In still other specimens a loop suture was inserted to join host tissue lateral to the transplant; this served to reduce muscle tension on the transplant sutures.

The pearl oyster mantle, particularly the inner pallial epithelium, is quite vulnerable to visible damage from forceps pressure and needle holes. Every effort was made to minimize such physical trauma during transplantation, but some damage to grafts was unavoidable and may have been at least partly responsible for graft loss. Although pearl oysters were kept in nonsterile running sea water or actually in the sea postoperatively, bacterial or protozoan invasion of grafts was rarely detectable. Bacterial invasion was found only in grafts at stages of advanced necrosis.

Recent studies (Dix, in preparation) indicate that sutured incisions, through the mantle edge and also in the visceral mass of the pearl oyster, are capable of rapid healing with firm union of wound surfaces. Suturing is an effective means of maintaining ectopic mantle grafts in the visceral mass. Experiments to assess cellular reactions to such autografts, allografts, and xenografts are underway. Modified operative procedures may yet allow successful orthotopic mantle grafts. In our view, comparative evaluation of transplantation reactivity and immunity among different animal species requires orthotopic grafting, since heterotopic grafting necessarily involves placement of tissues in an abnormal microenvironment. Previous workers have often broken the shell lip or have made holes in the shell to perform surgery on bivalve molluscs (Des Voigne and Sparkes, 1968, 1969; Pauley and Sparkes, 1967; Ruddell, 1971). Apart from the physiological stress entailed, this approach stimulates a cellular shell repair response which could complicate reactions to nearby transplants. However, this or other radical approaches may prove essential whenever natural opening of the shell under anesthesia provides insufficient access to facilitate orthotopic grafting.

ECHINODERMS

One colorful representative of each of two disparate classes has recently been studied in considerable detail (Hildemann and Dix, 1972). The sea cucumber, *Cucumaria tricolor,* (Class Holothuroidea) and the horned sea star, *Protorea-ster nodosus,* (Class Asteroidea) are both found on the Barrier Reefs and else-where in the tropical Indo-Pacific. The integumentary pigmentation patterns of each species facilitated transplantation of skin of one color into an area of contrasting coloration. Operative procedures were evolved with difficulty after numerous trial-and-error experiments, although both species survived very well under laboratory conditions in running sea water at ambient temperatures of 21°–27°C. Propylene phenoxetol, as described for pearl oysters, was superior as an anesthetic in producing quiescence and relaxation in both sea cucumbers and sea stars. No adverse effects were noted.

Successful attachment of orthotopic *Protoreaster* skin grafts was rarely a-chieved until conventional suturing was abandoned in favor of simply winding 6–0 monofilament nylon repeatedly and firmly around a recipient's arm directly over the graft. The pigmented skin overlying the hard endoskeleton was cut free as 5–6 mm² × 1 mm thick grafts which were individually fitted to beds along the dorso-lateral surface of one of the five arms in an area of contrasting color-ation. Initial graft fusion and subsequent healing within 2–3 days appeared to be aided by dusting of the contact zone with absorbable gelatin powder and tetra-cycline wound powder. Under these conditions, autografts remained fully viable by all criteria indefinitely, whereas initial allografts consistently showed chronic rejection with survival times of 153 to 177 days in a small series.

After extensive experimentation with operative techniques in *Cucumaria,* the following method was adopted. Integumentary grafts, 8–10 mm² × 2–3 mm thick, were excised with scalpels and loosely sutured in individual open fitting beds at each of the four corners with 6–0 monofilament nylon affixed to a curved cutting-point needle. Light dusting of the graft–recipient contact zone with wound powder and gelatin powder led to formation of a sealing gel after reaction with local plasma exudate. Technical success was achieved if animals refrained from excessive body distension or contortion within the first 2 days, and firm healing occurred within 4 days. With increased body distension, even grafts with numerous, loose-fitting sutures deep in the leathery integument can be torn out and lost. Unfortunately, such responses to repeat or second-set grafts usually occurred as if the animals were quite determined to remove any renewed source of irritation. Sixteen animals received single, first-set allografts plus a concurrent control autograft which remained fully viable. All allografts exhibit-ed slow rejection at 21°–27°C with survival times of about 129 to 185 days. Three successfully accomplished second-set grafts, made while initial allograft rejection was still in progress, all showed accelerated rejection at 28–50 days.

Donor pigment cells served as viability markers for repeated stereomicro-scopic scoring *in vivo* of both *Cucumaria* and *Protoreaster.* Chronic allograft rejection in both species was progressively indicated by superficial, cloudy hy-perplasia along the graft–recipient contact zone, by donor pigment destruction, and by invasive replacement of graft tissue. Zero survival end points were based on eventual disappearance of distinctive donor pigmentation. Biopsies of autografts and allografts were also removed at various times or stages of rejection for histological evaluation. Leukocytes of multiple types, including macrophages, small lymphocytes (hemocytes), and eosinophilic granulocytes, infiltrated echinoderm skin allografts in process of rejection. Illustrations of sequential transplantation reactions in echinoderms may be found elsewhere (Hildemann and Dix, 1972).

DISCUSSION AND CONCLUSIONS

Characteristically slow allograft rejection has previously been reported with varying degrees of conviction among invertebrates in certain coelenterates (Campbell and Bibb, 1970; Hauenschild, 1956; Theodor, 1970), annelids (Cooper, 1970; Duprat, 1970), and tunicates (Freeman, 1970). Certain molluscs appear able to distinguish between autografts, allografts, and xenografts (Cheng, 1970; Cheng and Galloway, 1970; Tripp, 1970), but the specificity of observed rejection reactions is not yet clear. Although annelid worms develop short-lived immunologic memory with considerable specificity toward transplantation antigens, the existence and characteristics of memory have scarcely been investigated in other invertebrates. The *Cucumaria* studies summarized here suggest the existence of specific immunologic responsiveness at the echinoderm level of phylogeny (Bruslé, 1967; Ghiradella, 1965). The immunologic potentialities of echinoderms invite more detailed study because this group is ancestrally close to the vertebrates.

At the primitive phylogenetic level of coelenterates, recognition of foreignness or incompatibility mechanisms to prevent indefinite xenogeneic or allogeneic tissue fusion already appear well developed. The *Acropora* coral studies reported here augment earlier work with other classes of coelenterates revealing impressive, though perhaps limited, capacity for "nonself" recognition. The molecular basis of this capacity is unknown and may not even depend on immunologic mechanisms. Antagonistic interspecific reactions among scleractinian corals which are brought or come into contact with each other, have been interpreted as "aggressive interactions" (Lang, 1971) or even reciprocal cannibalism, but such reactions may be limited to the larger polyps of mussid-type corals. At several intermediate levels of invertebrate phylogeny, typified by our still inconclusive pearl oyster studies, decisive evidence from orthotopic tissue transplantation experiments is still lacking mainly because of difficulties in achieving adequate animal care and operative techniques (cf. Anderson, 1971; Triplett *et al.*, 1958; Tripp, 1970).

Very simple experimental techniques may suffice with certain species, as in the coral and sea star studies just cited. In colonial tunicates, mere surface contact between the outer cellular tunics appears to be a sufficient test of compatibility. Necrosis at the contact surface between two incompatible colonies of various species has been repeatedly observed (Oka and Watanabe, 1960; Mukai, 1967; Freeman, 1970). Isogeneic pieces from the same colony always fuse to share a common vascular system, whereas random colonies are rarely compatible.

An essential requirement, then, is that control autografts or isografts, using a given technique in a given species, are regularly successful. Otherwise, the fate of similar allografts or xenografts may be meaningless. In contrast with familiar laboratory mammals, the current pioneering stage of work with marine invertebrates demands that attention be given to effects of anesthetics, need for sterile techniques and influence of antibiotics, and adequacy of food sources.

Despite many information gaps, a quite new post-Metchnikoff conception of invertebrate potentialities is emerging as follows: Essential cellular immunocompetence evolved among certain metazoan invertebrates well before the additional vertebrate capacity to produce immunoglobulin antibodies. Capacity for recognition of and reaction to foreign tissue evolved still earlier and is now demonstrable even toward allografts in coelenterates. Cell surface recognition units and perhaps even primordial immunoglobulins may yet be found in "advanced invertebrates" (i.e., echinoderms and tunicates) possessing diverse types of leukocytes, including small lymphocytelike cells.

ACKNOWLEDGMENTS

We thank Mr. Ian Croll and the staff of the Marine Gardens, Magnetic Island for generous support and assistance. We also thank Professor C. Burdon-Jones and the staff of the School of Biological Sciences, James Cook University for substantial logistical support.

REFERENCES

Anderson, R. S., 1971, Cellular responses to foreign bodies in the tunicate *Molgula manhattensis, Biol. Bull. 141*:91-98.

Bruslé, J., 1967, Homogreffes et hétérogreffes réciproques du tégument et ses gonades chez *Asterina gibbosa* et *Asterina pancerii, Cahiers Biol. Marine 8*:417-420.

Campbell, R. D. and Bibb. C., 1970, Transplantation in coelenterates, *Transplant. Proc. 2*:202-211.

Cheng, T. C., 1970, Immunity in Mollusca with special reference to reactions to transplants, *Transplant. Proc. 2*:226-230.

Cheng, T. C. and Galloway, P. C., 1970, Transplantation immunity in molluscs: the histoincompatibility of *Helisoma duryi normale* with allografts and xenografts, *J. Invertebr. Pathol. 15*:177-192.

Cooper, E. L., 1970, Transplantation immunity in helminths and annelids, *Transplant. Proc. 2*:216-221.

Des Voigne, D. M. and Sparks, A. K., 1968, The process of wound healing in the Pacific oyster, *Crassostrea gigas, J. Invertebr. Pathol. 12*:53-65.

Des Voigne, D. M. and Sparks, A. K., 1969, The reaction of the Pacific oyster, *Crassostrea gigas*, to homologous tissue transplants, *J. Invertebr. Pathol. 14*:293-300.

Duprat, P. C., 1970, Specificity of allograft reaction in *Eisenia foetida, Transplant. Proc. 2*:222-225.

Freeman, G., 1970, Transplantation specificity in echinoderms and lower chordates, *Transplant. Proc. 2*:236-239.

Ghiradella, H. T., 1965, The reaction of two starfishes. *Patiria miniata* and *Asterias forbesi*, to foreign tissue in the coelom, *Biol. Bull. 128*:77-89.

Hauenschild, C., 1956, Über die Vererbung einer Gewebverträglichkeits-Eigenschaft bei dem Hydroidpolypen, *Hydractinia echinata, Z. Naturforsch. 11*:132-138.

Hildemann, W. H., 1972, Phylogeny of transplantation reactivity, in: *The Transplantation Antigens*, Academic Press, New York, pp. 3-73.

Hildemann, W. H. and Dix, T. G., 1972, Transplantation reactions of tropical Australian echinoderms, *Transplantation 15*:624-633.

Horridge, G. A., 1957, The coordination of the protective reaction of coral polyps, *Phil. Trans. Roy. Soc.* (London) *240*:495-529.

Kaplan, H. M., 1969, Anesthesia in invertebrates, *Federation Proc. 28*:1557-1569.

Lang, J., 1971, Interspecific agression by schleractinian corals. I. The rediscovery of *Scolymia cubensis, Bull. Marine Sci. 21*:952-959.

Mukai, H., 1967, Experimental alteration of fusibility in compound ascidians, *Sci. Rep Tokyo Kyoiku Daigaku B. 13*:51-73.

Oka, H. and Watanabe, H., 1960, Problems of colony specificity in compound ascidians, *Bull. Biol. Asamushi 10*:153.

Pauley, G. B. and Sparks, A. K., 1967, Observations on experimental wound repair in the adductor muscle and Leydig cells of the oyster, *Crassostrea gigas, J. Invertebr. Pathol. 12*:52-65.

Ruddell, C. L., 1971, Elucidation of the nature and function of the granular oyster amebocytes through histochemical studies of normal and traumatized oyster tissues, *Histochemie 26*:98-112.

Theodor, J. L., 1970, Distinction between "self" and "not-self" in lower invertebrates, *Nature 227*:690-692.

Triplett, E. L., Cushing, J. E., and Durall, G. L., 1958, Observations on some immune reactions of the sipunculid worm, *Dendrostomum zostericolum, Am. Naturalist 92*:287-293.

Tripp, M. R., 1970, Immunity in Mollusca, *Transplant. Proc. 2*:231-232.

Trump, G. N., 1970, Goldfish immunoglobulins and antibodies to bovine serum albumin, *J. Immunol. 104*:1267-1275.

Vredevoe, D. L., 1964, The production and transfer of immune reactions to bovine serum albumin in isogeneic and allogeneic mice. I. Transfer of antibody formation, *J. Immunol. 92*:709-716.

Whitfield, R. P., 1901, Notice of a remarkable case of combination between two different genera of living corals, *Bull. Am. Museum Nat. Hist. 14*:221-222.

Chapter 13

Specific Receptors in Relation to
the Evolution of Immunity

Henry R. Hilgard, Robert H. Wander, and William E. Hinds

Division of Natural Sciences
University of California
Santa Cruz, California

INTRODUCTION

The principal concepts of immunology, developed during the past hundred years, have their origins in experimental studies carried out mostly in the warm-blooded vertebrates. Hence, when one searches broadly among the phyla for the evolutionary origins of immunity, one naturally tends to search for an immune system which has the characteristics of the familiar vertebrate immune system. These characteristics are recognition of nonself, specificity, and memory (alteration of response due to prior contact with antigen). In our view, all metazoan immune systems are characterized at least by specificity and by recognition of nonself. Although there is increasing evidence that cellular immune memory does occur in some annelids (Cooper, 1969; Chateaureynaud-Duprat, 1970) and in some echinoderms (Hildemann and Dix, 1972), the lower metazoans in general seem to lack memory (Good and Papermaster, 1964; Teague and Friou, 1964; Chadwick, 1967; Cushing, 1967; Feng, 1967).

Let us consider for a moment the properties of an invertebrate humoral immune system — one which lacks memory. We can visualize the following model: immunocompetent cells synthesize specific receptors (analogous to antibodies) and carry these receptors on their surfaces. When an immunocompetent cell encounters an antigen for which it possesses the complementary receptor, a receptor—antigen complex is formed. This complex serves as the signal for the synthesis of receptor molecules to replace those which have already complexed with antigen. As long as there is free antigen to combine with receptors, there is rapid synthesis of new receptor molecules. After all of the antigen has been complexed, the system returns to its original state: the same number of cells producing receptors at the same rate as they were before the encounter with antigen. It would be very difficult for a vertebrate immunologist to detect such an immune system (Burnet, 1968; Hilgard, 1970). There is no immune memory, so there is no accelerated antigen clearance following immunization; there is no production of receptors beyond those needed to complex with antigen, so there are no circulating antibodies (overproduced receptors) to detect. Nonetheless, there is recognition of nonself and there is specificity.

SPECIFIC UPTAKE OF PROTEIN BY SEA URCHIN COELOMOCYTES

Our own investigations have been designed to detect specificity in systems which seemed to lack the memory component. We have been looking for evidence that specific receptors are involved in the processes by which cells take up proteins and amino acids. Much of our work has involved the responses of the sea urchin, *Strongylocentrotus purpuratus,* to the proteins bovine serum albumin (BSA), human serum albumin (HSA), and chicken serum albumin (CSA). The method which we used has been reported elsewhere (Hilgard *et al.,* 1967; Hilgard and Phillips, 1968). The plan of attack in these experiments was as follows: we placed sea urchin coelomocytes, *in vitro,* in an artificial sea water environment containing varying amounts of C^{14}-labeled protein with or without added unlabeled protein. The concentration of labeled protein was carefully selected to be high enough so that it would saturate the cellular uptake mechanism. Then, working at the saturation level for the labeled protein, we asked the following question: would one kind of protein (CSA, for example) which was not labeled interfere with the uptake of a different protein (BSA, for example) which was labeled? We reasoned that if there are separate receptors and separate uptake mechanisms for BSA and CSA, then there should be no inhibition of BSA uptake by CSA. If the same receptor is used for the uptake of both proteins, then we would expect the uptake of BSA-C^{14} to be reduced, because the CSA would occupy some of the pertinent receptors.

The results of experiments employing labeled BSA are shown in Figs. 1a and 1b. Note that there is very little increase in uptake when the concentration of BSA-C^{14} is raised from 20 μg/ml (Fig. 1a) to 80 μg/ml (Fig. 1b). Thus cellular uptake of BSA is nearly saturated at 20 μg/ml. It is also clear that at saturation the uptake of BSA-C^{14} is inhibited only by addition of unlabeled BSA and not by unlabeled CSA or HSA, suggesting that there are separate receptors involved in the uptake of these various proteins. However, these results are also compatible with the possibility that there is only a single receptor which has a greater affinity for BSA than for HSA or CSA. In order to validate this last possibility, we also studied the uptake of CSA-C^{14}. Fig. 2a shows the uptake of CSA-C^{14}

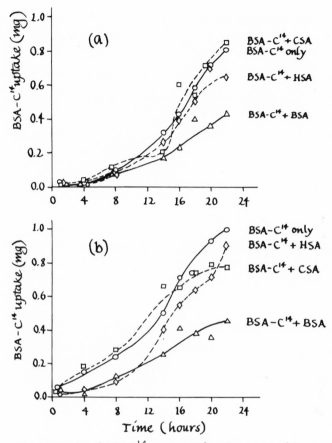

Fig. 1. Uptake of BSA-C[14] by 5 × 10[5] coelomocytes of *S. purpuratus* cultured *in vitro*. The concentrations of BSA-C[14] were 20 μg/ml (Fig. 1*a*) or 80 μg/ml (Fig. 1*b*). Some cultures contained only cells and BSA-C[14] (○); to other cultures unlabeled BSA (△), HSA (◇), or CSA (□) were added. The concentration of each unlabeled protein was the same as the concentration of the BSA-C[14] to which it was added: 20 μg/ml (Fig. 1*a*) or 80 μg/ml (Fig. 1*b*).

from solutions containing 80 μg/ml of CSA-C[14]. To some of the solutions were added 80 μg/ml of the unlabeled proteins BSA, HSA, or CSA. Unlabeled CSA, but not BSA or HSA, inhibited the uptake of CSA-C[14]. Similar results were obtained at 160 μg/ml of CSA-C[14] (Fig. 2*b*). These results rule out the possibility that there is a single receptor which has a greater affinity for BSA than for CSA, and are consistent instead with the hypothesis that sea urchin coelomocytes possess some receptors which combine relatively specifically with BSA and some which combine relatively specifically with CSA.

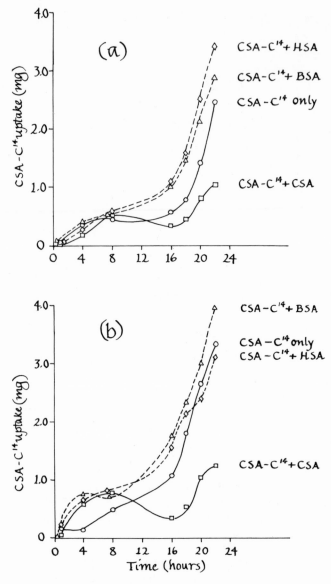

Fig. 2. Uptake of CSA-C^{14} by 5 × 10^5 coelomocytes of *S. purpuratus* cultured *in vitro*. The concentrations of CSA-C^{14} were either 80 μg/ml (Fig. 2*a*) or 160 μg/ml (Fig. 2*b*). Some cultures contained only cells and CSA-C^{14} (○); to other cultures unlabeled BSA (△), HSA (◇), or CSA (□) were added. The concentration of each unlabeled protein was the same as the concentration of the CSA-C^{14} to which it was added: 80 μg/ml (Fig. 2*a*) or 160 μg/ml (Fig. 2*b*).

SELECTIVE UPTAKE OF AMINO ACIDS BY AMOEBAE

We recently studied an uptake process (endocytosis) of ^{3}H-labeled L-amino acids in *Amoeba proteus*. We wished to know if this process also involved specific receptors. It is already known (a) that the amino acids arginine (arg), glutamic acid (glu), and lysine (lys) are endocytotically taken in by *A. proteus* with the inducing optimum being around pH 8 (Chapman-Andresen, 1964), and (b) that an important component of the induction of endocytosis is binding of the molecules to the cell membrane (Chapman-Andresen, 1965). We felt that specific receptors might be involved in the binding and subsequent transport of amino acids into the cell, and, hence, we did a series of uptake studies to shed light on this question of specificity.

Many of the techniques we used in these amoebae studies are modifications of Schumaker's procedures (Schumaker, 1958). All amino acid uptake studies were carried out at pH 8.0 and 23°C, and uptake was determined by the amount of ^{3}H-labeled amino acid which became associated with the cells. We exposed amoebae uniformly to solutions containing labeled amino acid for 30 min, since the maximum period of endocytosis usually lasts from 20 to 30 min under these conditions and is followed by several hours of rest even though the amoebae remain in an excess of inducing solution (Chapman-Andresen, 1964, 1965). After the 30-min period amoebae were washed in unlabeled amino acid solutions of the identical composition, molarity, and pH as the original solutions containing labeled amino acids. Amoebae were then transferred into glass vials for scintillation counting. In preliminary studies we determined the toxic concentrations for each amino acid; toxicity was indicated by bursting of cells during the 30-min period of exposure to various concentrations of amino acids. Arginine and lysine were toxic above $2.0 \times 10^{-2} M$, but glutamic acid was nontoxic even at its maximum solubility in water ($5.0 \times 10^{-2} M$).

Using labeled amino acid tracers to monitor total uptake, we measured the uptake of arginine, lysine, and glutamic acid per 100 amoebae over a wide molarity range (Fig. 3). In the region above $1.1 \times 10^{-3} M$ for arginine, small increases in the molarity of the arginine resulted in marked increases in its uptake. Utilizing this steep part of the uptake curve as a guide for concentration, we set up experiments to determine how the uptake of labeled arginine would be affected by the presence of glutamic acid. Fig. 4 shows the uptake of labeled arginine when the total molar concentration was raised above $1.0 \times 10^{-3} M$ with unlabeled arginine or unlabeled glutamic acid. In each case, the amount of labeled arginine present in the inducing solution was kept constant. Increasing the molarity with unlabeled arginine caused the uptake of the labeled arginine to increase considerably, as expected in this molarity range; however, the uptake of labeled arginine was not affected when the molarity was increased with unlabeled glutamic acid. Our interpretation of these results is that separate receptor

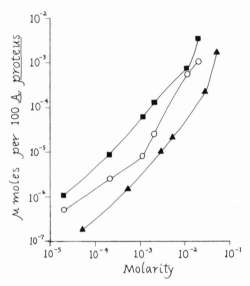

Fig. 3. Uptake of arginine (○), lysine (■), and glu
tamic acid (▲) per 100 *A. proteus* over a wide molar
ity range.

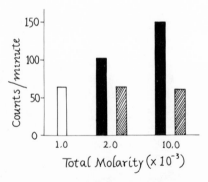

Fig. 4. Uptake of ³H-labeled arginine per 100
A. proteus in the presence of unlabeled arginine
or glutamic acid. Molarity was increased above
the basic $1.0 \times 10^{-3}M$ arginine (□) by adding
unlabeled arginine (■) or unlabeled glutamic
acid (▨). The amount added was either 1.0×10^{-3} (for final total molarity of $2.0 \times 10^{-3}M$)
or $9.0 \times 10^{-3}M$ (for final total molarity of 10.0
$\times 10^{-3}M$). Each uptake value represents the
mean of three studies.

molecules are involved in the binding and subsequent transport of these molecules into the cell. Hence, unlabeled arginine affects ^{3}H-arginine uptake but unlabeled glutamic acid does not. In any case, although these findings are preliminary, they are compatible with the hypothesis that specific processes are involved in the endocytotic uptake of amino acids.

EVOLUTIONARY IMPLICATIONS

These investigations, then, of the uptake of proteins by sea urchin coelomocytes, and of the uptake of amino acids by amoebae, suggest that specificity (or at least selectivity) is associated with these uptake processes. This is not surprising, since specific cell receptor molecules seem to be involved in other biological processes as well — processes such as hormonal triggering (Gorski et al., 1969) and cellular recognition during metazoan embryonic development (Lilien 1969). Therefore, it is tempting to speculate that the vast vocabulary of vertebrate receptors (antibodies), apparently present in even the most primitive vertebrate species (Hildemann and Thoenes, 1969; Hildemann, 1970), may have evolved gradually from a vocabulary of receptors already possessed by an invertebrate ancestor (Burnet, 1968, 1971). In fact, the receptors of all metazoans, vertebrates, and invertebrates alike may have evolved from surface receptors such as those associated with the binding of proteins (Chapman-Andresen, 1965) and amino acids to the cell membranes of amoebae. Ultimately, of course, it will be necessary to isolate and purify cell-surface receptors in order to determine evolutionary relationships with certainty.

Assuming the existence of immune systems characterized only by recognition of nonself and by specificity, would there be any selective advantage to adding on a memory system? Perhaps so, particularly for an organism with a long lifespan, because immune memory provides a mechanism whereby specific responses can be adjusted to reflect the individual experience of the organism. Furthermore, immune memory might be of advantage to a species which produced only a small number of offspring, because such a species cannot easily rely on the mechanisms of mutation and selection to meet environmental challenges. Hence, the capacity of the organism to modify its responses on the basis of experience would be of selective advantage. An immune system with recognition and specificity could hypothetically evolve a memory system in either of two quite simple ways. Cells which carry receptors might proliferate after contact with antigen, or cells might permanently step up their synthesis of surface receptors after contact with antigen. Perhaps events such as these played a role in the evolution of immune memory.

ACKNOWLEDGMENTS

These investigations were supported in part by Grant AI 05098-06 from the National Institutes of Health, U.S.P.H.S., and in part by Contract

N00014-69-A-0200-7003 from the Office of Naval Research, and were carried out during the tenure of an established investigatorship of the American Heart Association awarded to H.R.H.

REFERENCES

Burnet, F. M., 1968, Evolution of the immune process in vertebrates, *Nature 218*:426-430.
Burnet, F. M., 1971, 'Self-recognition' in clonal marine forms and flowering plants in relation to the evolution of immunity, *Nature 232*:230-235.
Chadwick, J. S., 1967, Serological responses of insects, *Federation Proc. 26*:1675-1679.
Chapman-Andresen, C., 1964, Measurement of material uptake by cells: pinocytosis, in: *Methods in Cell Physiology, Vol. 1,* pp. 277-304 (D. W. Prescott ed.), Academic Press, New York.
Chapman-Andresen, C., 1965, The induction of pinocytosis in amoebae, *Arch. Biol. (Liège) 76*:189-207.
Chateaureynaud-Duprat, P., 1970, Specificity of allograft reaction in *Eisenia foetida, Transplant. Proc. 2:222-225.*
Cooper, E. L., 1969, Specific tissue graft rejection in earthworms, *Science 166*:1414-1415.
Cushing, J. E., 1967, Invertebrates, immunology, and evolution, *Federation Proc. 26*:1666-1670.
Feng, S. Y., 1967, Responses of molluscs to foreign bodies with special reference to the oyster, *Federation Proc. 26*:1685-1692.
Good, R. A. and Papermaster, B. W., 1964, Ontogeny and phylogeny of adaptive immunity, *Adv. Immunol. 4*:1-115.
Gorski, J., Shuamala, G., and Toft, D., 1969, Interrelationships of nuclear and cytoplasmic estrogen receptors, in: *Current Topics in Developmental Biology, Vol. 4,* pp. 149-167 (A. A. Moscona and A. Monroy, eds.), Academic Press, New York.
Hildemann, W. H., 1970, Transplantation immunity in fishes: Agnatha, chondrichthyes, and Osteichthyes, *Transplant. Proc. 2*:253-259.
Hildemann, W. H. and Dix, T. G., 1972, Transplantation reactions of tropical Australian Echinoderms, *Transplantation 15*:624-633.
Hildemann, W. H. and Thoenes, G. H., 1969, Immunological responses of Pacific hagfish. I. Skin transplantation immunity. *Transplantation 7*:506-521.
Hilgard, H. R., 1970, Studies of protein uptake by Echinoderm cells: their possible significance in relation to the phylogeny of immune responses, *Transplant. Proc. 2*:240-242.
Hilgard, H. R., Hinds, W. E., and Phillips, J. H., 1967, The specificity of uptake of foreign proteins by coelomocytes of the purple sea urchin, *Comp. Biochem. Physiol. 23*:815-824.
Hilgard, H. R. and Phillips, J. H., 1968, Sea urchin response to foreign substances, *Science 161*:1243-1245.
Lilien, J. E., 1969, Towards a molecular explanation for specific cell adhesion, in: *Current Topics in Developmental Biology, Vol. 4,* pp. 169-195 (A. A. Moscona and A. Monroy, eds.), Academic Press, New York.
Schumaker, V. N., 1958, Uptake of protein from solution by *Amoeba proteus, Exp. Cell Res. 15*:314-331.
Teague, P. O. and Friou, G. J., 1964, Lack of immunological responses by an invertebrate, *Comp. Biochem. Physiol.12*:471-478.

Chapter 14

Recognition of Foreignness in the Fresh-Water Crayfish, Parachaeraps bicarinatus

C. J. Tyson, D. McKay,* and C. R. Jenkin

Department of Microbiology
University of Adelaide
Adelaide, South Australia

INTRODUCTION

In the vertebrates, recognition of foreignness by phagocytic cells is mediated by interaction of specific immunoglobulins with foreign material. As a result of this interaction, the foreign material–antibody complex adheres to the membranes of phagocytic cells and is engulfed. These specific recognition factors (immunoglobulins) may be present in the serum or adsorbed to the surface of the cell. The number of molecules of immunoglobulin required per foreign particle to bring about this recognition varies according to the immunoglobulin class and the size of the particle. However, the recognition of bacteria by peritoneal macrophages from the mouse requires only a few hundred molecules of antibody per bacterial cell (Rowley and Turner, 1966; Jackson et al., 1968).

The phagocytic cells from invertebrates are just as capable as those from vertebrates in distinguishing self from foreignness, yet we know very little regarding the mechanism involved. We studied this mechanism using cells from the fresh-water crayfish (Parachaeraps bicarinatus), and the findings we wish to present indicate that the recognition of particles such as erythrocytes and bacteria involves the interaction of these particles with recognition factors either free in the hemolymph or associated with cell membranes.

The fresh-water crayfish (Parachaeraps bicarinatus) is widely distributed throughout South Australia, particularly in the Murray River and associated

---

*Present address: National Biological Standards Laboratory Canberra, A.C.T.

lakes. Animals weighing from 35 g–400 g may be obtained in large numbers throughout the year. The animals are easily maintained under laboratory conditions for many months or even years, and the fact that 20% of their weight is hemolymph containing from $2-5 \times 10^6$ cells/ml makes them ideal animals for studies on cellular recognition and other immune phenomena (McKay and Jenkin, 1969).

PREPARATION OF HEMOCYTE MONOLAYERS

Since our method of preparing monolayers of hemocytes has been modified over the past two years, it might be pertinent to outline the method before discussing the results of our studies on the factors involved in the recognition of foreignness (McKay *et al.*, 1969; McKay and Jenkin,1970; Tyson and Jenkin, unpublished observations). Crayfish were injected via the ventral sinus with 2 ml of 0.25% cysteine hydrochloride in physiological saline containing 10 units of heparin/ml at pH 6.2. After a period of three minutes the animals were bled from the ventral sinus using a 10-ml syringe and 19-gauge needle. The syringe contained 1 ml of ice cold 0.25% cysteine hydrochloride and 10 units* of preservative-free heparin/ml. The cysteine hydrochloride prevents hemolymph clotting without damaging the cells. We have recently found that while heparin had no effect on the clotting mechanism, it prevented cell clumping, which, had been one of the problems in the past. The contents of the syringe, after removing the needle, were gently squirted into an ice cold tube and centrifuged at 50 g for 10 min at 4°C. Following centrifugation the cells were resuspended in ice cold Van Harreveld's medium at pH 7.2 (Van Harreveld, 1936) containing 10 units* of heparin/ml and were washed several times by centrifugation, depending on the needs of the experiment. Following washing, the cells were added to tissue culture tubes at 4°C and were allowed to settle onto the glass. Plastic petri dishes may also be used. The cells were allowed to settle for an hour at 4°C, then were brought into the laboratory and allowed to reach room temperature. Under these conditions, the cells rapidly spread to form complete monolayers.

RECOGNITION OF ERYTHROCYTES BY CRAYFISH HEMOCYTES

The crayfish, like many other invertebrate species, has agglutinins in its hemolymph which show specificity for erythrocytes from different vertebrate species (McKay *et al.*, 1969). Vertebrates also have similar hemagglutinins in their serum. These vertebrate hemagglutinins are immunoglobulins and function as opsonins for their specific red cells. It was therefore of some interest to determine if these hemagglutinins in the crayfish would function in an analogous fashion to the vertebrate hemagglutinins. Sheep erythrocytes and human blood group B erythrocytes were treated with hemolymph (as outlined in Table I) and

*Units refers to international units per mililiter.

Table I. Specificity of Opsonic Activity of Normal Crayfish
(*Parachaeraps bicarinatus*) Hemolymph

Test erythrocytes	Hemolymph used to sensitize red blood cells	Phagocytosis	
		% hemocytes phagocytosing red blood cells	Red blood cells per 1000 hemocytes
Sheep	Saline	0.8	12
Sheep	Normal crayfish hemolymph	12.0	210
Sheep	Crayfish hemolymph adsorbed with sheep red blood cells	2.0	35
Sheep	Crayfish hemolymph adsorbed with human red blood cells	6.4	125
Human B	Saline	2.5	25
Human B	Normal crayfish hemolymph	19.0	365
Human B	Crayfish hemolymph adsorbed with sheep red blood cells	13.0	265
Human B	Crayfish hemolymph adsorbed with human red blood cells	0.9	9

were added to monolayers of crayfish hemocytes such that the ratio of erythrocytes to hemocytes was of the order of 10:1. The data given in Table I indicate that phagocytosis of erythrocytes by crayfish hemocytes is dependent on the red cell having been pretreated with hemolymph. Adsorption experiments also showed that there is some specificity in the opsonic activity of the serum (McKay and Jenkin, 1970). Since the adsorption of serum with one type of erythrocyte not only removed the hemagglutinin, but also the opsonin to that erythrocyte, it is not unreasonable to argue that the hemagglutinin and opsonin were identical materials. Further support for this is found in the facts that the hemagglutinating activity of hemolymph from various individuals paralleled the opsonic activity and that in purification studies, the opsonic activity was always found in that fraction which had the hemagglutinating activity.

In vertebrates, a monophyletic group of animals, antibodies will function as opsonins across class barriers. Thus antibodies from the shark (*Emissola antartica*) and lizard (*Tiliqua rugosa*) will enhance the phagocytosis of bacteria and erythrocytes by mouse peritoneal macrophages. The invertebrates are a polyphyletic group, and it was of some interest to see if the hemagglutinins present in the hemolymph of individuals from different phyla would function as recognition factors for hemocytes from the crayfish. Studies by other workers have shown that in the molluscs, phagocytosis of erythrocytes is dependent on a factor in the hemolymph (Tripp, 1966; Stuart, 1968; Prowse and Tait, 1969). The data given in Table II indicate that hemolymph or serum from animals outside of the phylum Arthropoda, while possessing hemagglutinating activity

162   Tyson, McKay, and Jenkin

Table II. Phagocytosis by Crayfish Hemocytes of Red Blood Cells
Sensitized with Hemolymph from Various Species of Invertebrates

| | | | Phagocytosis | |
Red blood cells	Hemolymph used to sensitize red blood cells	Titer[a]	% Hemocytes showing phagocytosis	Red blood cells per 1000 hemocytes
Sheep	Saline	–	0.8	9
Sheep	Crayfish (*Parachaeraps bicarinatus*)	1/32	13.0	180
Sheep	Reef crab (*Ozius truncatus*)	1/32	12.5	220
Sheep	Snail (*Helix aspersa*)	1/64	0.7	7.0
Sheep	Rabbit antisheep R.B.C. antibody	1/32	0.0	0.0
Mouse	Crayfish (*Parachaeraps bicarinatus*)	1/128	8.0	140
Mouse	Swan Mussel (*Velesunio ambiguus*)	1/128	0.0	0.0
Sheep	Salter (*Porcellio laevis*)	1/2	0.5	5.1

[a]Agglutinin titer of the hemolymph used to sensitize red cells for phagocytosis. All cells opsonized with two agglutinating doses.

against sheep or mouse erythrocytes, will not enhance the phagocytosis of these cells by crayfish hemocytes.

RATE OF ELIMINATION OF BACTERIA FROM THE CIRCULATION OF THE CRAYFISH

In the vertebrates, if one injects a known concentration of bacteria intravenously, they are cleared from the circulation at an exponential rate by the phagocytic cells of the liver and spleen. The clearance rate, denoted by the phagocytic index K, varies with the strain of bacteria and is related to the titer of circulating antibody (Benacerraf et al., 1959; Jenkin, 1964). The results of

Table III. Rate of Elimination (K) of Various Strains of Bacteria
from the Circulation of the Crayfish (*Parachaeraps bicarinatus*)

| Strain of bacteria | Phagocytic index K for concentration of bacteria injected | | | |
	5×10^7	1×10^8	5×10^8	1×10^9
Salmonella typhimurium C5	0.03	0.03	0.03	0.03
Salmonella abortus equi	0.11	0.12	0.15	0.20
Staphyloccus aureus	0.14	0.18	0.15	0.11
Escherichia coli 086	0.22	0.16	0.19	0.21
Pseudomonas strain C.P.	0.09	0.08	0.08	0.10

similar experiments in the crayfish show that different strains of bacteria were eliminated from the circulation at different rates (Table III). These experimental results are merely suggestive by analogy with the system in vertebrates that factors in the hemolymph may be necessary for the phagocytosis of bacteria. More conclusive data were obtained by the following *in vivo* and *in vitro* experiments.

FACTORS INVOLVED IN THE REMOVAL OF BACTERIA FROM THE CIRCULATION OF THE CRAYFISH

If in vertebrates that have just eliminated a primary dose of bacteria from the circulation, a second similar dose of bacteria is injected, the latter is removed much more slowly, and one refers to the animal as having been blockaded by the first dose. However, if the second dose is pretreated (opsonized) with specific antibody, the rate of clearance may be returned to normal. This type of experiment is a very sensitive assay for antibody. Similar experiments to these were performed in the crayfish and the results are given in Table IV. It is clear that reversal of blockade may be effected by pretreating the second dose of bacteria with hemolymph. Prior adsorption of the hemolymph used for opsonization of the second dose with the specific strain of bacteria prevents the reversal of blockade. Further, if the primary dose of bacteria is pretreated with hemolymph prior to injection, thus preventing removal of recognition factors when injected, the animal is not blockaded and the second dose is cleared at normal rates. Similar results were obtained using other strains of bacteria.

Table IV. The Clearance of Bacteria from the Circulation of Normal and Blockaded Crayfish

Treatment of animals	Challenge organism	Phagocytic index
None	*Salmonella abortus equi*	0.15
Salmonella abortus equi	*Salmonella abortus equi*	0.035
Salmonella abortus equi	*Salmonella abortus equi* pretreated with normal hemolymph	0.15
Salmonella abortus equi	*Salmonella abortus equi* pretreated with hemolymph adsorbed with *Salmonella abortus equi*	0.035
Salmonella abortus equi pretreated with normal serum	*Salmonella abortus equi*	0.11

IN VITRO STUDIES ON THE PHAGOCYTOSIS OF BACTERIA BY CRAYFISH HEMOCYTES

Monolayers of crayfish hemocytes were prepared as above, and various strains of bacteria were added to these cultures before and after treatment with hemolymph. The results of these experiments showed that bacteria were ingested and killed by the phagocytic cells irrespective of whether they had been pretreated with hemolymph. These findings suggested that the phagocytic cells had either recognition receptors as an integral part of the membrane or had adsorbed to their surfaces the recognition factors found in the hemolymph. In order to decide between these two possibilities, the following experiments were done. Monolayers of crayfish hemocytes were treated at room temperature for a period of 2 hr with 0.005% trypsin. Prior experiments had established that this concentration of trypsin had no effect on the viability of the cells as judged by trypan blue exclusion. Following trypsin treatment, the monolayers were washed several times with tissue culture medium and bacteria added to them before and after opsonisation with hemolymph. In this particular series of experiments, the percentage of unopsonized bacteria phagocytosed was significantly reduced by trypsin treatment (Table V) compared with that observed using untreated cells. These experiments suggested that the trypsin labile recognition factor on the surface of the cells was similar to the recognition factor in the hemolymph. Further experiments supported this view. Trypsin-treated cells maintained in tissue culture medium for periods varying from 4 to 24 hr failed to regain their capacity to phagocytose unopsonized bacteria. However, if such cells were incubated in the medium in the presence of hemolymph, this capacity was restored. One could argue that because of the more nutritional medium, the

Table V. Phagocytosis of Opsonized and Unopsonized Bacteria by Hemocytes from the Crayfish (*Parachaeraps bicarinatus*) before and after Trypsin Treatment

	Percentage phagocytosis of bacteria in 60 min[a]		
Strain of bacteria	Trypsin treated cells		Normal cells
	Opsonized	Unopsonized	Unopsonized
Salmonella abortus equi	52	11	59
Escherichia coli 086	43	16	38
Salmonella typhimurium	53	35	58
Pseudomonas strain C.P.	43	17	70

[a]These values are the average of three separate experiments. The variation among experiments was not greater than 8%.

**Table VI. Phagocytosis of Unopsonized *Salmonella abortus equi*
by Trypsin-Treated Hemocytes before
and after Exposure to Hemolymph**

Cells	Percentage phagocytosis in 60 min[a]
No hemolymph	19
Incubated with hemolymph	50
Incubated with hemolymph previously absorbed with *S. abortus equi*	18

[a]These values are the average of three separate experiments. The variation among experiments was not greater than 5%.

cells were able to resynthesize these membrane-associated recognition factors. This appears to be an unlikely explanation since this capacity was not restored when hemolymph that had been previously adsorbed with bacteria was added to the culture medium (Table VI). Thus, these *in vitro* data indicate that the recognition of bacteria by phagocytic cells is mediated by factors which may be associated either with the cell membrane, as cytophylic antibody is in the vertebrates, or free in the hemolymph. These preliminary experiments also suggest that the membrane-bound recognition factors are similar to those in the hemolymph. At present, the specificity and nature of these recognition factors is being investigated.

At first, these data might appear to conflict with the observations on the recognition and uptake of erythrocytes by crayfish hemocytes where it was shown that phagocytosis or binding of the red cell to the membrane did not take place unless the erythrocyte had been pretreated with hemolymph. Results of similar experiments in the vertebrates have shown that the amount of antibody required to facilitate the uptake of erythrocytes by phagocytes is much greater than that required for bacteria, due to the difference in surface area between the two particles. It is possible, therefore, that the concentration of these molecules on the membrane is not sufficient to bind the red cell but is sufficient to bind bacteria. The interesting experiments of Scott (1971) with hemocytes from the cockroach show that recognition of erythrocytes by these cells appears to be independent of factors in the hemolymph. However, the capacity to recognize erythrocytes was destroyed by treating the cells with trypsin. It seems not improbable that the crayfish and cockroach have similar recognition mechanisms, but in the case of the cockroach, the recognition factors have a much higher affinity for cell membranes and so very few of these molecules appear free in the hemolymph, the concentration being sufficient to enhance adhesion and ingestion of erythrocytes by trypsin treated hemocytes.

In conclusion, the recognition of foreignness by hemocytes of the crayfish (*Parachaeraps bicarinatus*) appears to be mediated by recognition factors which are either free in the hemolymph or associated with the membranes of the cells. These factors function in a way similar to the antibodies of vertebrates.

REFERENCES

Benacerraf, B., Sebestyan, M. N., and Schlossman S., 1959, A quantitative study of the kinetics of blood clearance of P^{32} labeled *Escherichia coli* and Staphylococcus by the reticulo-endothelial system, *J. Exp. Med.* 110:27-33.

Jackson, G. D. F., Rowley, D., and Jenkin, C. R., 1968, Further studies with artificial antigens and immunity mouse typhoid. I. Use of O-acetylated galactans in the purification of specific antibody against Antigen 5, *Immunology* 15:789-798.

Jenkin, C. R., 1964, The immunological basis for the carrier state in mouse typhoid, in: *Bacterial Endotoxins*, pp. 263-274, Quinn and Boden Co. Inc., Rahway, New Jersey.

McKay, D. and Jenkin, C. R., 1969, Immunity in the invertebrates. II. Adaptive immunity in the crayfish (*Parachaeraps bicarinatus*), *Immunology* 17:127-137.

McKay, D. and Jenkin, C. R., 1970, Immunity in the invertebrates. The role of serum factors in phagocytosis of erythrocytes by hemocytes of the fresh-water crayfish (*Parachaeraps bicarinatus*), *Australian J. Exp. Biol Med. Sci* 48:139-150.

Prowse, R. H. and Tait, N. N., 1969, *In vitro* phagocytosis by amoebocytes from the hemolymph of *Helix aspersa* (Müller). I. Evidence for opsonic factor(s) in serum, *Immunology* 17:437-443.

Rowley, D. and Turner, K. J., 1966, Number of molecules of antibody required to promote phagocytosis of one bacterium, *Nature (London)* 210:496-498.

Scott, M. T., 1971, Recognition of foreignness in invertebrates. II. *In vitro* studies of cockroach phagocytic hemocytes, *Immunology* 21:817-828.

Stuart, A. E., 1968, The reticulo-endothelial apparatus of the lesser octopus (*Eledone cirrosa*), *J. Pathol. Bacteriol.* 96:401-412.

Tripp, M. R., 1966, Hemagglutinin in the blood of the oyster (*Crassostrea virginica*), *J. Invertebr. Pathol.* 8:478-484.

Van Harreveld, A., 1936, A physiological solution for fresh-water crustaceans, *Proc. Soc. Exp. Biol. Med.* 34:428-432.

Chapter 15

Insect Immunity to Parasitic Nematodes

George O. Poinar, Jr.

Division of Entomology and Parasitology
University of California
Berkeley, California

INTRODUCTION

Immune or defense reactions by insects to parasitic nematodes was discussed by Salt (1963) and later reviewed by Poinar (1969). No attempt will be made here to discuss the works already cited by these authors. The purpose of this paper is to present some original findings on this subject, review the different types of immune responses produced by insects to nematodes, and to discuss current literature in the field. The definitions of immune responses in insects as related to host escape, cellular responses, melanization, and humoral responses are similar to those presented earlier (Poinar, 1969).

SIMPLE ENCAPSULATION

The term encapsulation is defined as the accumulation of host cells (usually hemocytes) around a parasite, resulting in the formation of a capsule. Other terms are sometimes confused with encapsulation. These are phagocytosis—when an individual cell engulfs or encloses foreign material, and encystment—when a parasite produces a membrane or cyst around itself. Simple encapsulation represents an accumulation of host cells around a parasite without any secondary melanization reactions. This type of encapsulation appears in Fig. 1. Here an adult male of *Mesodiplogaster lheritieri* occurs within a hemocytic capsule from *Galleria* larvae. The nematodes were injected into the body cavity of last instar larvae of *Galleria mellonella* L. Numerous layers of blood cells surrounded the nematode and each other to form an egg-shaped capsule. Although

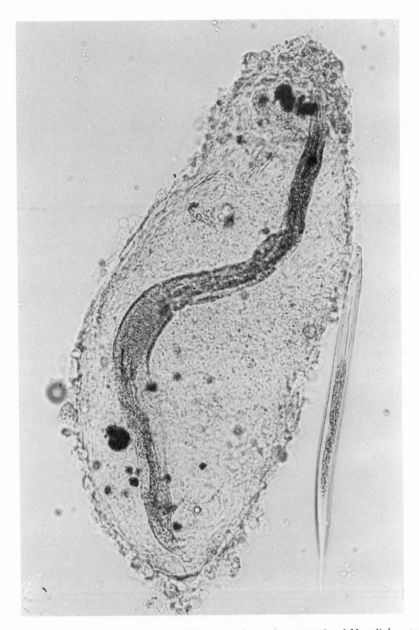

Fig. 1. An example of simple encapsulation around a male nematode of *Mesodiplogaster lheritieri*. Note the dauer stage of the same species to the right, which was removed from the same host, but did not elicit an immune response (magnification 220X).

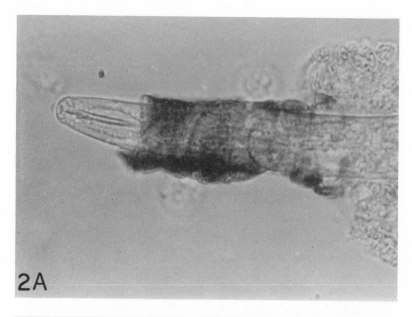

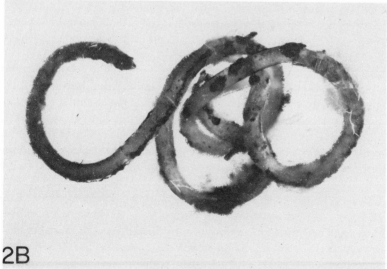

Fig. 2. Examples of melanotic encapsulation. *a*. The infective stage juvenile of *Filipjevimermis leipsandra* removed from the body cavity of a *Diabrotica* beetle larva. Note the collar of melanized blood cells around the anterior part of the nematode (magnification 230X). b. A specimen of *Hexamermis arvalis* (?) removed from the body cavity of an adult alfalfa weevil, *Hypera postica*. Note the melanotic areas on the cuticle of the nematode (magnification 25X).

a few melanotic areas are present, there is no general melanization as it occurs in a melanotic capsule. The smaller nematode next to the capsule is a dauer stage of the same species and was also removed from the same *Galleria* larva. It is interesting that although both had been introduced at the same time, the dauer stage elicited no host response, but the adult male did. The dauer is enclosed in a lipophilic second-stage cuticle which may not attract blood cells. Another case resembling simple encapsulation was reported by Nelmes and Hussain (1972) with the tylenchid nematode, *Contortylenchus* sp. in the bark beetle, *Ips sexdentatus* (Burn). The multilayered capsules were found attached to various host tissues.

MELANOTIC ENCAPSULATION

In contrast to simple encapsulation, melanotic encapsulation occurs when the surrounding blood cells produce a dark pigment, generally referred to as melanin, around the body of the parasite. A typical case of melanotic encapsulation was demonstrated by Poinar *et al.* (1968) as an immune response of *Diabrotica* beetles against invading juveniles of the mermithid, *Filipjevimermis leipsandra* (Fig. 2*a*). Host hemocytes were lysed after making contact with the parasite, and within 6–8 hr after initial entry, an inner layer of melanin had formed around the nematode. The remains of the original hemocytes were just exterior to this layer with a layer of necrotic, partially melanized cells (Fig. 4*b*).

Similar host reactions were reported by Nappi and Stoffolano (1971) and Stoffolano and Streams (1971) for dipterous hosts to the nematode *Heterotylenchus autumnalis* Nickle. The immune responses of *Musca domestica* L., *Orthellia caesarion* (Mg.), and *Ravinia l'herminieri* R.-D. involved the formation of melanotic capsules around the developing gamogenetic female nematodes. The authors recorded an initial aggregation and fusion of hemocytes to form a multinucleate syncytium while melanin was deposited on the nematode. Additional hemocytes adhered to the periphery of the capsule, forming a thick, syncytial mass.

Occasionally, developing females of *Praecocilenchus rhaphidophorus* Poinar, removed from the hemocoel of their normal host, *Rhynchophorus bilineatus* (Montr.), exhibited melanotic encapsulation. The immune response began with the deposition of hemocytes on the cuticle of the nematode. These hemocytes became pigmented (Fig. 3*a*), and eventually the entire nematode was encased in a melanotic capsule.

Mature juvenile mermithids may also elicit a response in their host. A specimen of *Hexamermis,* possibly *arvalis* Poinar and Gyrisco, removed from an adult alfalfa weevil, exhibited a response similar to melanotic encapsulation. Large masses of melanized hemocytes formed an irregular layer over the nematode's cuticle (Fig. 2*b*).

HUMORAL MELANIZATION

Although earlier studies suggested that such a phenomenon as humoral melanization existed, it was only confirmed recently by ultrastructural studies. In culicids (mosquitoes), chironomids (midges), and probably other groups, circulating blood cells are rare, and at least some species can melanize invading parasites by means of components in the noncellular portion of the blood.

In studying the immune response of *Culex pipiens* L. larvae to *Neoaplectana carpocapsae*, Poinar and Leutenegger (1971) showed that a homogeneous deposit quickly surrounded the nematode in just one hour after it had entered the host (Fig. 3*b*). Pigment granules began to form within this deposit, eventually enlarged, and coalesced to form a layer of melanin around the parasite (Fig. 4*a*).

The whole process of melanization was accomplished without the direct presence or action of blood cells, and the original deposit was attributed to components in the noncellular portion of the hemolymph that coagulated on the nematode's surface. This type of melanization clearly differs from the common cellular type.

What appeared to be a similar type of response was reported by Petersen *et al.* (1969) in larvae of *Aedes triseriatus* (Say) attacked by the mermithid, *Reesimermis nielseni* T. and G. Such lethal host reactions could definitely limit the use of this nematode in biological control programs of mosquitoes. The same rapid melanization reactions were also observed in *Anopheles sinensis* Wiedemann against the same mermithid nematode (Mitchell *et al.*, 1972).

Although rarely occurring against parasites in their "natural hosts," humoral melanization may be a fairly common response when parasites invade "foreign" hosts. I observed that when infective stage juveniles of the blackfly mermithid, *Gastromermis viridis* Welch, invaded larvae of *Culex pipiens* L., they were quickly melanized and killed.

In working with *Chironomus* larvae, Götz (1969) also reported humoral melanization against juveniles of the mermithid, *Hydromermis contorta* (Köhn). A pigmented substance, presumably melanin, was deposited directly on the surface of the nematode without the participation of blood cells. The same response was elicited if the nematodes entered hosts or were placed in a drop of chironomid blood *in vitro*.

INTRACELLULAR MELANIZATION

Very little is known about the intracellular responses of insects to nematodes since most entomogenous nematodes rarely enter individual host cells. However, microfilariae commonly initiate their development within cells of their intermediate host and, under some circumstances, may elicit a cell response which could curtail further growth. Dead melanized microfilariae of *Dirofilaria*

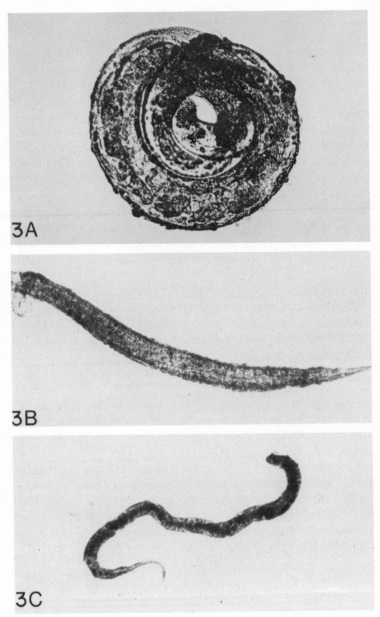

Fig. 3. *a.* A case of melanotic encapsulation of a female of the tylenchid nematode, *Praecocilenchus rhapidophorus* removed from the body cavity of the adult weevil, *Rhynchophorus bilineatus* (magnification 220×). *b.* An example of humoral melanization of the dauer stage of *Neoaplectana carpocapsae* removed from the body cavity of a *Culex pipiens* larva (magnification 260×). *c.* A case of intracellular melanization of a microfilaria of *Dirofilaria immitis* removed from a Malpighian tubule cell of an adult *Aedes aegypti* (magnification 350×).

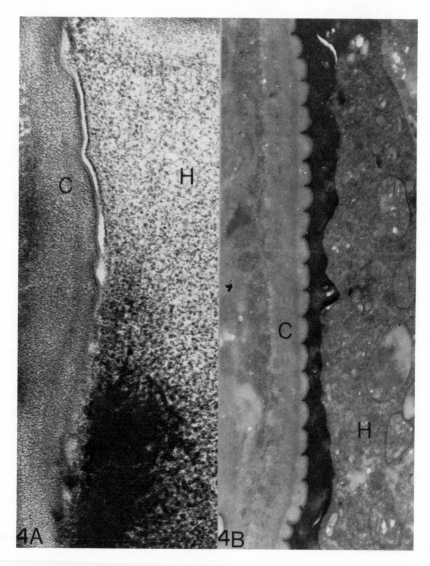

Fig. 4. Ultrastructural view of two different types of melanization. *a.* Humoral melanization of *Neoaplectana carpocapsae* in *Culex pipiens.* Note the homogeneous granular deposit (H) adhering to the nematode's cuticle (C). The granules darken and coalesce, as shown in the bottom of the figure (magnification 70,000×). *b.* Hemocytic melanization forming a melanotic capsule around *Filipjevimermis leipsandra* in *Diabrotica* sp. Note the layer of lysed and necrotic hemocytes (H) overlying a layer of melanin adjacent to the nematode's cuticle (C) (magnification 15,000×).

immitis (Leidy) were found within the Malpighian tubule cells of *Aedes aegypti* (Fig. 3*c*) by Dr. P. McGreevy. These microfilariae were covered with a deposit, presumably melanin, and, generally, the physical nature of the response resembled that of humoral melanization. Whether intracellular melanization proceeds in a fashion similar to extracellular melanization is a challenging goal for future investigators.

TISSUE RESPONSES

Evidence indicates that tissues other than the blood also can react to the presence of nematode parasites. Soon after the spirurid nematode, *Abbreviata caucasica* v. Linstow entered the epithelial cells of the colon wall in the roach, *Blatella germanica* L., the surrounding host cells became a syncytial giant cell. Large polychromatic epithelial cell nuclei occurred throughout the giant cell and the nematodes moved freely within the cytoplasmic matrix. After reaching the

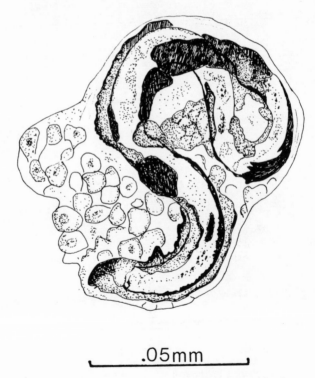

.05mm

Fig. 5. A melanized juvenile of *Abbreviata caucasica* in an atrophied capsule removed from the ileum of the posterior intestine of *Blatella germanica*.

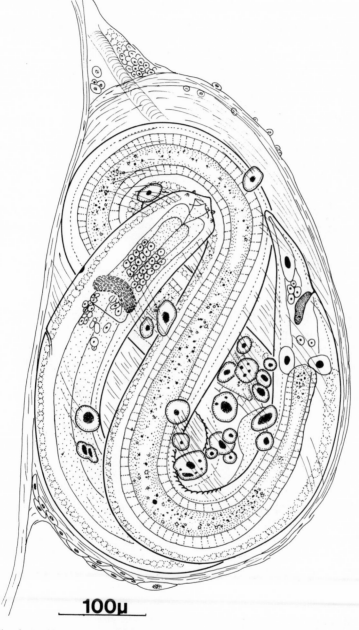

Fig. 6. A third stage juvenile of *Abbreviata caucasica* resting in a giant cell attached to the colon wall of *Blatella germanica*. Note the associated polychromatic epithelial cell nuclei.

third stage, the nematode remained in a quiescent state within the vacuolated giant cell (Fig. 6). In the early stages of development, the giant cell was surrounded by blood cells responding to the disruption; however, they rarely made contact with the parasite. In the ileum portion of the gut where the epithelial cells apparently did not always respond to the parasite, the surrounding blood cells then encapsulated and melanized the nematode (Fig. 5). Thus, when the protecting giant cell is not formed, the nematodes are more likely to be encapsulated and destroyed.

In addition to a response by the intestinal epithelium, Schacher and Kahlil (1968) cite evidence of an immune response against the filarial nematode, *Foleyella philistinae* Schacher and Khalil by the fat body cells of *Culex pipiens molestus*. The authors recorded the appearance of dark pigment granules in the fat body adjacent to the developing nematode and noted that these granules were deposited in and on the head and rectum of the parasites. Since the authors also show host hemocytes adhering to the nematode within the fat body, it is conceivable that some of the pigment could have originated from the blood cells.

CONCLUSION

In conclusion, we note that in addition to simple and melanotic encapsulation, humoral melanization occurs against nematodes in at least two insect families, and intracellular and tissue responses may also be more common than supposed earlier. Not only the physical location, but also the chemical pathways of melanin formation require further investigation. Moreover the basic question of how hosts recognize foreign invaders, even under a layer of their own hemocytes, remains unanswered.

Concerning unanswered questions, we come to another category of immune responses where we know very little indeed. This category has been called humoral immunity and defined as including those factors in the noncellular portion of the blood that have an adverse effect on the parasite (Poinar, 1969). The response may be expressed only by an abnormal growth pattern which may eventually result in death. The hemolymph may lack an essential factor required by the parasite or contain inhibitory substances that prevent its development.

In studying the development of *Brugia* spp. in *Aedes aegypti*, Beckett and MacDonald (1971) found abnormal nematodes that exhibited degenerative changes, i.e., a general thickening, nuclear pycnosis, cell hypertrophy, vacuolation, and other changes. There was very little evidence of melanization, and it was apparent that humoral factors were responsible for these abnormal conditions. The identification of these factors is still another challenging goal for future investigators of insect immunity to internal parasites.

SUMMARY

The present account discusses insect immunity to parasitic nematodes. A case of simple encapsulation of the nematode, *Mesodiplogaster lheritieri* in *Galleria mellonella* larvae and melanotic encapsulation of *Praecocilenchus rhaphidophorus* and *Hexamermis arvalis* (?), in their weevil hosts, *Rhynchophorus bilineatus* and *Hypera postica,* respectively, are presented. Another case of intracellular melanization is recorded in *Dirofilaria immitis* which was removed from a Malpighian tubule cell of *Aedes aegypti,* and a response of the intestinal cells of *Blatella germanica* against the developing juveniles of *Abbreviata caucasica* is discussed. Studies on the chemical pathways of melanin formation, the various types of tissue capable of immune responses, host recognition of foreign parasites, and the identification of factors in the noncellular portion of the blood responsible for humoral immunity, are challenging goals for the future.

REFERENCES

Beckett, E. B. and MacDonald, W. W., 1971, The survival and development of subperiodic *Brugia malayi* and *B. pahangi* larvae in a selected strain of *Aedes aegypti, Trans. Roy. Soc. Trop. Med. Hyg. 65*:339-346.

Götz, P., 1969, Die Einkapselung von Parasiten in der Hämolymphe von *Chironomus − Larven (Diptera), Zool. Anz., Suppl. 33*:610-617.

Mitchell, C. J., Chen, P. S., and Chapman, H. C., 1972, Exploratory trials utilizing a mermithid nematode as a control agent for *Culex* mosquitoes in Taiwan (China), WHO/ VBC/72.*410*:1-10.

Nappi, A. J. and Stoffolano, Jr., J. G., 1971, *Heterotylenchus autumnalis* hemocytic reactions and capsule formation in the host, *Musca domestica, Exp. Parasitol. 29*:116-125.

Nelmes, A. J. and Hussain, W. I., 1972, The response of the bark boring beetle, *Ips sexdentatus* infected by a nematode parasite, *Contortylenchus* sp., *11th Intern. Symp. Nematol. Reading, Abstr.* p.48.

Petersen, J. J., Chapman, H. C., and Willis, O. R., 1969, Fifteen species of mosquitoes as potential hosts of a mermithid nematode *Romanomermis* sp., *Mosquito News 29*:198-201.

Poinar, Jr., G. O., 1969, Arthropod immunity to worms, in: *Immunity to Parasitic Animals, Vol. 1,* p. 173, (G. Jackson, R. Herman, and I. Singer, eds.), Appleton-Century Crofts, New York.

Poinar, Jr., G. O. and Hess, R., 1974, An ultrastructural study of the response of *Blatella germanica*(Orthoptera: Blattidae) to the nematode *Abbreviata caucasica* (Spirurida: Physalopteridae), *J. Ultrastruct. Res.* (in press).

Poinar, Jr., G. O. and Leutenegger, R., 1971, Ultrastructural investigation of the melanization process in *Culex pipiens* (Culicidae) in response to a nematode, *J. Ultrastruct. Res. 36*:149-158.

Poinar, Jr., G. O., Leutenegger, R. and Götz, P., 1968, Ultrastructure of the formation of a melanotic capsule in *Diabrotica* (Coleoptera) in response to a parasitic nematode (Mermithidae), *J. Ultrastruct. Res. 25*:293-306.

Salt, G., 1963, The defense reactions of insects to metazoan parasites, *Parasitology 53*:527-642.

Schacher, J. F. and Khalil, G. M., 1968, Development of *Foleyella philistinae* Schacher and Khalil, 1967 (Nematoda: Filarioidea) in *Culex pipiens molestus* with notes on pathology in the arthropod, *J. Parasitol. 54*:869-878.

Stoffolano, Jr., J. G. and Streams, F. A., 1971, Host reactions of *Musca domestica, Orthellia caesarion,* and *Ravinia l'herminieri* to the nematode *Heterotylenchus autumnalis, Parasitology 63*:195-211.

Chapter 16

Control Mechanisms of
Leafhopper Endosymbiosis

Werner Schwemmler

Institut für Biologie II
Lehrstuhl für Mikrobiologie
Universität Freiburg
Freiburg i. Br., B.R.D.

INTRODUCTION

As for many insects, the existence of the small leafhopper *Euscelis plebejus* F. (Homoptera, Hemiptera), depends on intracellular symbionts. Two types of symbionts can be distinguished: the *a*- and the *t*-symbionts (Müller, 1949). In a preliminary classification, they were placed as "protoplastoids" between viruses and mycoplasma (Schwemmler, 1971). The *a*- and *t*-symbionts occur in two morphologically different stages: an intracellular, larger, optically transparent, noninfectious, vegetative, and proliferative stage, and an extracellular, smaller, optically denser, infectious stage transmitted to the next generation (Körner, 1969; Schwemmler, 1974).

The transmission process involves the insertion of the infectious symbionts between the egg envelope and the egg where they form the symbiont ball (Figs. 1, 2*a*). During embryogenesis, the *a*-infectious symbionts are incorporated into polyploid host cells which are designated as a_1-mycetocytes. The a_1-mycetocytes disintegrate at a later stage and the free infectious *a*-symbionts now infect binucleated, polyploid host cells, the a_2-mycetocytes. Only at this stage are the infectious *t*-symbionts incorporated into polyploid host cells, the *t*-mycetocytes. Both the a_2- and *t*-mycetocytes containing the vegetative stages of the *a*- and *t*-symbionts combine to form a common organ, the primary mycetome (Fig. 1). The primary mycetome later becomes divided and forms the two lateral mycetomes. Each lateral mycetome consists of a peripherally located, syncytial *a*-mycetome and a centrally located *t*-mycetome. The *a*- and *t*-mycetomes are separated by an epithelium free of symbionts. During the five larval instars, no significant changes in the two lateral mycetomes can be detected. In the adult female, cells of ovarian origin become incorporated into the a-mycetome. These cells form a special structure, called the infectious mount, in which the vegetative a-symbionts are incorporated and develop into the a-infectious stage (Schwemmler, 1973a). In regions where the t-mycetome comes in contact with the ovary, infectious t-symbionts develop in migratory t-mycetocytes. During the infectious process, both infectious stages a and t are released into the hemolymph and are subsequently incorporated into specialized follicle cells, the wedge cells, and from there they enter the egg (Körner, 1969). Those symbionts which remain in the wedge cells are lysed, thus completing the symbiontic cycle.

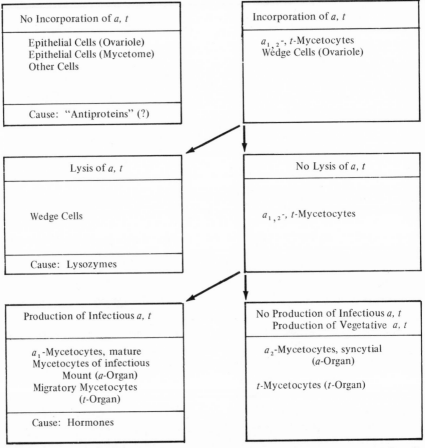

Diagram 1. Classification of the different cells in the endosymbiontic system of *Euscelis plebejus* F. according to the possible distributions of "antiproteins," lysozymes, and hormones.

Depending on their behavior toward the a- and t-symbionts, the host cells which participate in the symbiontic cycle can be distinguished as follows (Diagram 1):

1. Cells which do not incorporate symbionts, such as the epithelial cells of ovarioles and the epithelial cells of the mycetomes;
2. Cells which incorporate symbionts, such as the wedge cells and the mycetocytes, the former incorporating both a- and t-symbionts, the latter selectively incorporating a- or t-symbionts. Furthermore, cells which incorporate symbionts (2) can be subdivided as follows:

   a. Cells which after a certain time lyse the incorporated symbionts, such as the wedge cells;
   b. Cells which do not lyse but integrate the incorporated symbionts, such as the mycetocytes. Finally, the mycetocytes (b) themselves are subdivided into: (i) Mycetocytes which produce infectious symbionts, such as the mature a_1-mycetocytes, the a-mycetocytes of the infectious mount, and the migratory t-mycetocytes; (ii) Mycetocytes which exclusively produce vegetative symbionts, such as the young a_1-mycetocytes, the a_2-mycetocytes, and the t-mycetocytes.

LYSOZYME CONTENT

This investigation is an attempt to understand the causal relations between symbionts and host cells. The control mechanisms underlying leafhopper endosymbiosis were investigated by immunological techniques. In order to analyze the incorporation specificity of symbionts into wedge cells and mycetocytes, female *Euscelis* larvae and adults were fed 0.1% tetracycline dissolved in a natural or synthetic diet (Schwemmler, 1972; Schwemmler *et al.,* 1973). Tetracycline inhibits the translation step in protein synthesis (Schlegel, 1969). Embryos derived from treated females contained t-mycetocytes infected with both t- and a-symbionts (Figs. 4, 5, 6). Infection of epithelial cells of both ovarioles and mycetomes with a-symbionts was observed by light microscopy, but not yet verified by electron microscopy.

The results indicate that a specific protein mechanism ("antiprotein") exists in the plasma or in the membranes of t-mycetocytes and epithelial cells of both the ovarioles and the mycetomes which inhibits specific incorporation of the a-symbionts. A parallel mechanism which inhibits specifically the incorporation of t-symbionts may exist in a-mycetocytes as well as in epithelial cells of ovarioles and mycetomes. At present, a suitable antibiotic is not known which specifically inhibits this mechanism. The distribution of a- and t-specific "antiproteins" in host cells would explain why symbionts are specially incorporated by host cells and how passage of symbionts from the mycetome to the oocytes is regulated.

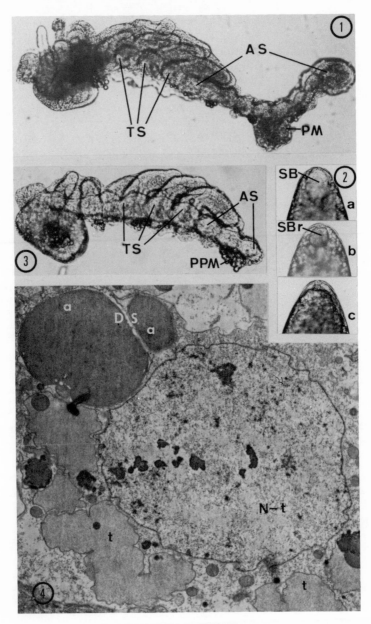

Fig. 1. Embryo of *E. plebejus* F., of age 6 days (100×).

Fig. 2. *a*. Abdominal egg pole with symbiont ball. (100×) *b*. Abdominal egg pole with reduced symbiont ball (treatment with lysozyme). (100×) *c*. Abdominal egg pole without symbiont ball (treatment with tetracycline). (100×).

Fig. 3. "Head-embryo" of age 6 days with reduced abdomen from the egg in Fig. 2*b*. (100×).

Fig. 4. Double infection of *t*-mycetocyte with *t*- and *a*-symbionts (treatment with tetracycline) (7500×).

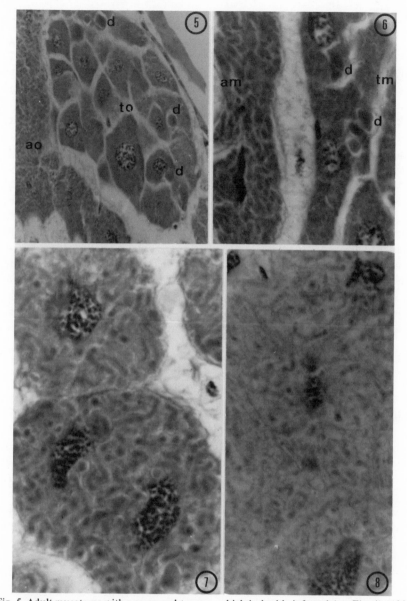

Fig. 5. Adult mycetome with a-organ and t-organ, which is double infected (see Fig. 4) (420X).

Fig. 6. a-Mycetocytes and t-mycetocyte with double infections (see Fig. 4) (1050X).

Fig. 7. a-Mycetocytes in which the a-symbionts are partially lysed (tetracycline) (1050X).

Fig. 8. a-Mycetocytes, completely lacking symbionts (tetracycline) (1050X).

Abbreviations for Figs. 1−8: a = a-symbiont, am = a-mycetocyte, ao = a-organ, AS = abdominal segments, d = double infection, DS = division of an a-symbiont, N-t = nucleolus of t-mycetocyte, (P)PM = (symbiont-free) primary mycetome, SB (r) = symbiont ball (reduced), t = t-symbiont, tm = t-mycetocyte, to = t-organ, TS = thoracic segments.

Several investigations have been reported regarding lysis specificity of wedge cells and mycetocytes. Malke (1964a,b), Ehrhardt (1966), and Hinde (1971) analyzed lysozyme content in cells and hemolymph of insects and observed the lytic effect on intracellular symbionts. Lysozyme lyses the 1.4 glycosidic bond of aminoacetylpolysaccharides of muramic acid in cell walls of prokaryotes and prokaryotic symbionts (Schlegel, 1969). The temporal and local distribution and effects of lysozyme on the endosymbiontic complex of *Euscelis* have been investigated by *in vivo* and *in vitro* methods (Schwemmler, 1972; Schwemmler *et al.*, 1973). The lysozyme content of ovarioles, eggs, and mycetomes or portions of them was determined by a "plaque test" (Ceriotti, 1964; Mohrig and Messner, 1968). The sheath cells of both the ovarioles and the mycetomes, as well as the oocytes themselves, show high lysozyme activity, which is comparable to the lysozyme activity of the hemolymph during egg infection (see below). The symbiont balls and the mycetocytes of the embryo, larva, and adult exhibit no lysozyme activity. This indicates that no host cells with permanent symbionts, such as the mycetocytes, possess detectable amounts of lysozyme. In contrast, all cells with no incorporated symbionts, such as the epithelial cells and the oocytes, possess large amounts of lysozyme. The wedge cells, which lyse the remaining symbionts within a week, possess intermediary amounts of lysozyme.

THE PROCESS OF ENDOSYMBIOSIS

The lysozyme content of hemolymph from newly hatched female *Euscelis* adults corresponds to an intermediate value of 200 ± 100 μg/ml, which is within the range observed for other insect hemolymphs (Mohrig and Messner, 1967). During egg infection by the symbionts, lysozyme concentration in female hemolymph increases up to 5 times the normal concentration. However, it never reaches the extreme value of approximately 10,000 μg/ml (50 times the normal concentration) measured for insects following microbial infection (Mohrig and Messner, 1967). Generally, the increase of lysozyme concentration in infected insect hemolymph induces lysis of microbes. Similarly, increased lysozyme content of *Euscelis* female hemolymph during egg infection serves to destroy those symbionts not incorporated by wedge cells within a week. If the lysozyme content of hemolymph is increased artificially 50–10,000-fold (10,000–2,000,000 μg/ml) of the normal content either by injection of lysozyme (1–2% dissolved in 0.5% NaCl in distilled water) or by feeding 0.1% lysozyme in a synthetic diet, the symbionts are lysed (Schwemmler *et al.*, 1973). The degree of lysis is different in vegetative and infectious symbionts. The vegetative symbionts of mycetocytes become lysed only partially and preferentially in developing embryonic and larval mycetomes (Fig. 7). When high doses of lysozyme are applied, *a*- and *t*-mycetocytes completely lacking symbionts may appear (compare also with Fig. 8). However, these remain intact and become reinfected by symbionts of undamaged, neighboring mycetocytes when lysozyme application is interrupted. Thus, mycetocytes free of symbionts cannot be detected a week after lysozyme application. Likewise, mycetocytes cultured *in vitro* are freed of their symbionts by application of 0.01–1% lysozyme, survive, and are sensitive to reinfection (Schwemmler *et al.,* 1971). In contrast to vegetative symbionts, the infectious stages are lysed in the hemolymph at lower doses of lysozyme. Thus, egg infection is partially or completely interrupted and resulting eggs have reduced (Fig. 2*b*) or lack the symbiont ball. Eggs without a symbiont ball develop exclusively into embryos lacking an abdomen. Such embryos have been designated as "head-embryos" (Fig. 3) (Schwemmler *et al.,* 1973). Application of tetracycline also produces eggs free of symbionts (Fig. 2*c*) and therefore results in "head-embryos" or symbiont-free mycetocytes (Figs. 7, 8). In contrast to the vegetative symbionts which possess three membranes, the infectious symbionts possess only two and are far more sensitive to the lytic effect of lysozyme, especially so since the exterior membrane of infectious symbionts possesses a lysozyme-sensitive cell wall complex.

The infectious symbionts develop only during certain stages of host growth. Perhaps this specificity is controlled by the host developmental stage and it cannot be influenced by exogenous factors (Schwartz, 1932). Since the production of infectious symbionts begins just before egg maturation (approximately 2 days after the hatching of female adults), it is possible that this process is coordinated with changes in sexual hormones of the host. This assumption is supported by the observation that the infectious "mount," where the *a*-infectious stages are differentiated, is formed by immigration of the ovary cells, and that the migratory *t*-mycetocytes, which produce the *t*-infectious stages, originate in contact with the ovary. Addition of a preparation extracted from mature female gonads correspondingly results in the *in vitro* production and release of infectious symbionts in mycetocyte cultures (Schwemmler, 1972; 1973*a*; 1974). Coordination with the hormone system ensures that infectious symbionts are produced only at predetermined host developmental stages, namely, a short time before maturation. Possibly, synthesis in mature a_1-mycetocytes is controlled by the hormone pool released during oogenesis.

CONCLUSIONS

In conclusion, the specificity of incorporation of the symbiontic cell complex is caused by *a*- and/or *t*-specific "antiproteins," but lysis specificity results from the action of antimicrobial lysozyme. Specificity of infectious symbiont production is determined by the host's sexual hormone system (Diagram 1). Diagram 2 shows the probable distribution of "antiprotein," lysozymes, and sexual hormones in different cell types participating in the symbiontic complex. According to this diagram, epithelial cells of both the ovarioles and the myce-

Diagram 2. Preliminary model of the endosymbiotic control mechanism in *E. plebejus* F. according to the possible extra- or intracellular distributions of lysozymes, hormones, and "antiproteins."

$a_{1,2}$-M = $a_{1,2}$-mycetocyte
E = epithelial cell
I = infectious mount cell
K = wedge cell
O = oocyte
S = symbiont ball
t-M = t-mycetocyte
W = migratory cell
$A_{a,t}$ = "antiproteins" (prohibiting incorporation of a and t)
$a_{i,v}$ = a-symbiont: infectious, vegetative stage
H = hormones (inducing production of a_i and t_i)
L+,$^\pm$,– = lysozymes: much, little, none (effecting lysis of a_i, t_i)
$t_{i,v}$ = t-symbiont: infectious, vegetative stage

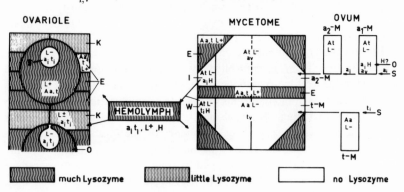

tomes contain a- and t-specific "antiproteins," a high concentration of lysozyme, and possess no relationship with the hormonal system of the host. Wedge cells possess neither a- nor t-specific "antiprotein," have a low concentration of lysozyme, but are free from control by sexual hormones. The t-mycetocytes have an a-specific "antiprotein," a correlation with the host hormone system in the migratory t-mycetocytes, but no detectable activity of lysozyme. The a-mycetocytes show a t-specific "antiprotein," a correlation with the host hormone system in the a_1-mycetocytes as in the a-mycetocytes of the infectious mount, but no detectable lysozyme activity. The extracellular hemolymph system contains high lysozome activity during egg infection and production of sexual hormones. The symbiont balls are free of lysozyme but not controlled by hormones. Many questions are left unanswered: For example, the mechanism of hormonal regulation and release of the infectious symbionts is not known. These and other questions such as the relationship of lysozyme to insect immunity must be solved by further systematic experiments. The model of control mechanism of leafhopper endosymbiosis represents a first attempt only to evaluate this schematically presented data.

REFERENCES

Ceriotti, G., 1964, Quantitative determination of lysozyme, *Atti III. Symp. Intern. Lisozima Fleming, Milano,* Ser 1:22-23.

Ehrhardt, P., 1966, Die Wirkung von Lysozyminjektionen auf Aphiden und deren Symbionten, *Z. Vergleich. Physiol. 53*:130-141.

Hinde, R., 1971, The control of the mycetome symbiotes of the aphids *Brevicoryne brassicae, Myzus persicae,* and *Macrosiphum rosae, J. Insect Physiol. 17*(9):1791-1800.

Körner, H., 1969, Die embryonale Entwicklung der symbiontenführenden Organe von *Euscelis plebejus* (Homop., Cicad.), *Oecologia (Berlin) 2*:319-346.

Malke, H., 1964*a*, Wirkung von Lysozym auf die Symbionten der Blattiden, *Z. allgem. Mikrobiol. 4*:88-91.

Malke, H., 1964*b*, Production of aposymbiotic cockroaches by means of lysozyme, *Nature 204*:1223-1224.

Mohrig, W. and Messner, B., 1967, Lysozym im humoralen Abwehrmechanismus spezifisch und unspezifisch immunisierter Insektenlarven, *Biol. Rundschau 5*(4):181-183.

Mohrig, W. and Messner, B., 1968, Immunreaktionen bei Insekten. I. Lysozym als grundlegender antibakterieller Faktor im humoralen Abwehrmechanismus der Insekten. *Biol. Zb. 87*:439-470.

Müller, H. J., 1949, Zur Systematik und Phylogenie der Zikadenendosymbiose. *Biol. Zb. 68*:343-368.

Schlegel, H., 1969, *Allgemeine Mikrobiologie. Georg Thieme Verlag, Stuttgart.*

Schwartz, W., 1932, Neue Untersuchungen über die Pilzsymbiose der Schildläuse (Lecaniinen), *Arch. Mikrobiol. 3*:446-472.

Schwemmler, W., 1971, Intracellular symbionts: a new type of primitive prokaryotes, *Cytobiologie 3*(3):427-429.

Schwemmler, W., 1972, *In vivo* und *vitro* Analysen zur Struktur, Funktion und Evolution der Endosymbiose von *Euscelis plebejus* F. (Hemip. Homop., Cicad.), Dissertation, Universität Freiburg (Bibliothek).

Schwemmler, W., 1973*a*, Beitrag zur Analyse des Endosymbiosezyklus von *Euscelis plebejus* F. (Hemip., Homop., Cicad.) mittels *in vitro* Beobachtung, *Biol. Zb. 92*:6, 749-772.

Schwemmler, W., 1973*b*, *In vitro* Vermehrung intrazellulärer Zikaden-Symbionten und Reinfektion asymbiontischer Mycetocyten-Kulturen, *Cytobios 8*:63-73.

Schwemmler, W., Quiot, J.-M., and Amargier, A., 1971, Etude de la symbiose intracellulaire sur cultures organotypiques et cellulaires de l'homoptère *Euscelis plebejus* F. (Cicad.) en milieux à fractions standard, *Ann. Soc. Entr. Fr. 7*(2):423-438.

Schwemmler, W., Duthoit, J.-L., Kuhl, G., and Vago, C., 1973, Sprengung der Endosymbiose von *Euscelis plebejus* F. und Ernährung asymbiontischer Tiere mit synthetischer Diät (Hemiptera, Cicadidae), *Z. Morphol. Oekol. Tiere 74*:297-322.

Schwemmler, W., 1974, Studies on the fine structure of leafhopper intracellular symbionts during their reproductive cycles (Hemiptera, Deltocephalidae). *Appl. Entomol. Zool.,* in press.

Chapter 17

Cellular and Noncellular Recognition of and Reactions to Fungi in Crayfish

Torgny Unestam and Lars Nyhlén

Institute of Physiological Botany
University of Uppsala
Uppsala, Swedden

INTRODUCTION

According to current literature, the fungi are of minor importance as parasites on vertebrates where bacteria dominate completely. Schäperclaus (1954) in his book on fish diseases lists many more bacterioses than mycoses. In many invertebrate groups, however, the situation is different. Fungi "compete" successfully with bacteria in insects (Steinhaus, 1963) and according to the recent bibliographies on diseases of invertebrates other than insects (Johnson, 1968; Johnson and Chapman, 1969), far more work is listed on fungal than on bacterial parasites of different host groups.

The reasons for these differences are not known. There is no ground to believe that mycoses should be more interesting to scientists or more apparent in one group of animals than in another. It must be questioned whether the vertebrates have evolved a better protection mechanism than other animals. It may be that the vertebrate immunoglobulin system is more effective against fungi or that the vertebrates have evolved some additional (unknown) defense resisting fungal invasion.

Certainly, fungi have unique properties which make them different from other organisms. The ability to translocate intracellular material over long distances, to penetrate mechanically through rigid barriers, and to react chemotropically are some of the more obvious specialties of a hypha. The composition of its cell wall is also different from that of other organisms.

When invading animals such as crayfish, the fungus first has to penetrate the chitinous cuticle or the intestinal wall which is also chitinous in parts. To grow further, it must pass the epidermal cell layer before it reaches the hemolymph (blood) and other tissues. On its way, the hypha will probably cause physical or chemical disturbance which will give rise to reactions in the host tissue; the hypha will be recognized. Some reactions may be of a general nature while some may be more fungal-specific. Basically the same reaction could occur in many tissues, but tissue-specific responses must also exist. Finally, some of the observed reactions, if not all, may be part of a defense system.

REACTIONS IN THE HEMOLYMPH

In the hemolymph of some planktonic crustaceans, phagocytosis of yeast cells and spores seems to be very effective (Metschnikoff, 1884; Pixell-Goodrich, 1928), but in crayfish no such activity against fungi has been found with certainty (Unestam and Weiss, 1970; Unestam and Nylund, 1972). Live bacterial and protozoan parasites were not phagocytized in *Astacus astacus* and the crab, *Carcinus maenas*, respectively (Cuenot, 1895; Poisson, 1930), but dead parasites were phagocytized.

Hyphae of the crayfish plague fungus, *Aphanomyces astaci*, and some other Phycomycetes penetrating into the abdominal hemolymph of the European crayfish, *Astacus astacus*, or the American, *Pacifastacus leniusculus*, were always

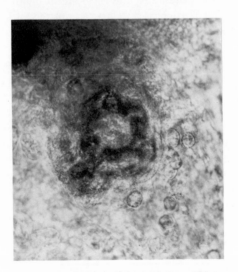

Fig. 1. A conidium of *Entomophthora coronata* encapsulated *in vivo* by hemocytes and melanized on its surface in *Pacifastacus leniusculus* hemocoel. × 260.

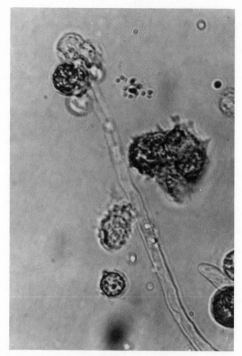

Fig. 2. Crayfish blood cells in an artificial blood
stream sticking to a hypha of *Aphanomyces astaci*.
× 520.

soon encapsulated by hemocytes, as long as the animals were otherwise healthy
(Unestam and Weiss, 1970). Artificially injected spores of different fungi were
similarly encapsulated (Fig. 1). Our recent (unpublished) work has shown that
Australian and New Guinean crayfish exhibit the same type of reactions.

In an artificial blood stream, the immediate events following the first contact between crayfish blood and hyphae, which finally gave rise to encapsulation, were studied (Unestam and Nylund, 1972). Very brief chance contact with
a hypha, or with cell extensions from blood cells or a blood-cell clump on the
hypha, caused cells to stop and adhere (Fig. 2). The clump of blood cells thus
agglomerated on the hypha and became more densely packed due to forces
between the cells inside the clump. As cells became attached to a cell clump,
many soon disintegrated and released their contents of granules and other organelles.

Our recent work with a number of Basidiomycetes, Ascomycetes, Zygo-
mycetes and Oomycetes showed that all tested fungal cells are encapsulated in

Table I. Reactions on the Hyphal Wall of a Number of Fungi (Cells Killed
in Boiling Water) after Addition of Hemolymph of the Crayfish
Pacifastacus leniusculus

Fungi	Cell walls containing	Hemocytes trapped[a]	Light-refracting particles attach[a]	Melanin formation[a]
Oomycetes	Cellulose			
Aphanomyces astaci		+	+	+
A. stellatus		+	+	+
Saprolegnia sp.		+	+	+
Zygomycetes	Chitin			
Entomophthora apiculata		+	+	+
Phycomyces blakesleeanus		+	0	0
Ascomycetes	Chitin			
Ophiostoma multiannulatum		+	+	+
Saccharomyces cerevisiae		+	+	+
Basidiomycetes	Chitin			
Armillaria mellea		+	0	0
Stereum purpureum		+	0	0
Fomes tomentosus		+	0	0
Algae				
Vaucheria dichotoma	Cellulose	+	0	0
Cotton fibers	Cellulose	+	0	0
Nylon fibers		+	0	0

[a]Reaction seen (+); no reaction (0).

the same way (Table I). The same was true for cotton and nylon fibers. The
recognition by blood cells of the hyphal surface as *not-self* seems, therefore, to
be instantaneous and very nonspecific (cf. Salt, 1970) and does not involve any
important chemotactic factor (Unestam and Nylund, 1972).

The sticking of blood cells to the hyphal surface was very reminiscent of the
first phase of clot formation in the hermit crab (Bang, 1967), a process strongly
inhibited by 0.01 M N-ethyl maleimide (NEM). Thus, NEM (final concentration
about 0.01 M), added to the artificial blood stream of *Astacus astacus* blood,
completely inhibited the sticking and clumping of blood cells on the hyphae
and, consequently, also encapsulation.

In vivo, soon after blood cells clumping onto injected spores or hyphae of
the crayfish plague fungus occurred, a light-refracting layer was always formed on

parts of the hyphal surface; within a few hours this layer became yellow, and later brown, due to melanin formation. Melanin formation was especially strong in crayfish resistant to the crayfish plague, e.g., *Pacifastacus leniusculus* (Unestam and Weiss, 1970). After introduction by injection into the abdominal hemocoel, other fungi were also melanized in the same way in *Astacus* or *Pacifastacus* (Fig. 1). Events were the same in some Australian crayfish into which the crayfish plague fungus was injected (unpublished).

Granules of the granular hemocytes in these two crayfish were filled with thin tubules (apparent in the electron microscope). They also contained polyphenoloxidase (Unestam and Nylund, 1972). During cell clumping on the hyphae or after mixing fresh blood with a buffer or sucrose solution, these granules were released, sometimes without complete disintegration of blood cells (Fig. 3), and budded off smaller particles which spread in the hemolymph (plasma) or diluted blood.

After removing the cells by centrifugation, such plasma gave rise to light-refracting particles or zones of particles (as *in vivo*) on the cell wall when added to an *Aphanomyces* mycelium (Fig. 4) or a suspension of encysted zoospores. No melanin in or around this light-refracting material was formed, however, unless dihydroxyphenylalanine (DOPA) was supplied as substrate for pigment formation, or whole blood was added together with or instead of plasma (Fig. 5). The light-refracting material, therefore, contained the melanin-forming enzyme, a polyphenoloxidase (PPO), which was specifically activated by close contact with the cell wall. By heating blood or plasma (55°C, 30 min), the fixation capacity of the particles was destroyed, but the enzyme was activated. The

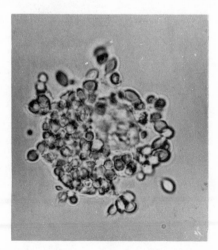

Fig. 3. Release of granules from a granular crayfish hemocyte. × 1200.

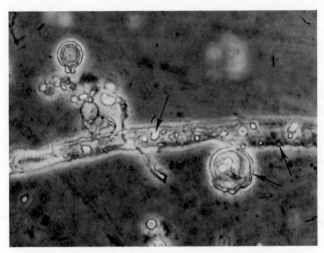

Fig. 4. Light-refracting particles and zones (arrows) on hyphae
and spores of *Aphanomyces astaci*. Phase contrast. ×600.

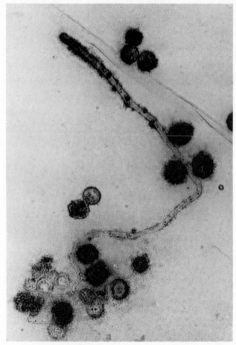

Fig. 5. Melanin formed on the surface of encysted
zoospores and on a hyphal tip of *Aphanomyces
astaci* after addition of crayfish plasma and 0.04%
DOPA. ×420.

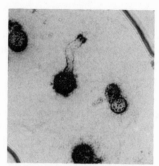

Fig. 6. Melanin on an empty zoospore cyst wall. Note especially that the opening is surrounded by a zone of melanin. ×500.

hemocytes must also have caused the release of the natural substrate. Our recent (unpublished) experiments have shown that this particle-bound enzyme is o-diphenol specific and that the intensity of the melanin formation on the fungal wall is proportional to the number of hemocytes present. When melanized in this way, the growth of the hyphal tip is often disturbed or inhibited and branching is abnormal. The process of particle (refracting zone) fixation and enzyme activation occurs equally well on the walls of killed (boiled) *Aphanomyces* cells or empty cell walls (Unestam and Nylund, 1972).

In recent work, we found that these processes have a great deal of specificity, since they occur to the greatest extent on hyphal tips, zoospore walls, and empty cyst walls, especially at the edge of cyst openings (Figs. 5 and 6). The zoospore wall surface of the Oomycetes seems to be very different in composition from that of the hypha (Tokunaga and Bartnicki-Garcia, 1971) and so is most probably the hyphal tip. Our attempts to inhibit the fixation (recognition) process has, up to now, been successful only when the wall was pretreated with formalin and then with albumin. Possibly, free amino groups of the cell wall surface were involved in the receptor site. Preheating or pretreatment with a number of enzymes was not effective in inhibition.

The described processes were also examined in a number of other fungal groups, in an alga, and in some fibers (Table I). Refracting zones and melanization occurred only in some of the tested fungi, but no good correlation with taxonomic position or cell wall content of chitin or cellulose could be found. When melanization occurred normally, hyphal tips were most heavily affected. Cellulose fibers or nylon did not fix or activate the particulate polyphenol oxidase.

The examined noncellular recognition processes apparently have a much greater specificity than recognition by blood cells, but whether they are part of an undescribed immuno-system remains to be determined. A gradually darkening secretion (thought to be "chitinous") on yeast cells, trapped by hemocytes in the planktonic crustacean *Gammarus* spp. (Pixell-Goodrich, 1928), makes a comparison very interesting. Similar events have been observed in insects (Salt, 1970; Poinar *et al.*, 1968; Götz, 1969). A report of an electron-dense sheath surrounding phagocytized hyphae of *Aspergillus* in fowl chicks (Campbell, 1970) should also be mentioned here. In the electron microscope the light-refracting, PPO-containing layer on the hyphal wall apparently contains mostly particles and balls composed of thin tubules (Fig. 7) of the size found in the hemocyte granules (Unestam and Nylund, 1972).

REACTIONS IN INNER ORGANS

Reactions to the presence of fungal cells in inner organs are almost unknown in crayfish. The crayfish plague fungus is normally found only in the integument and to a limited extent in the hemolymph of its host, *Astacus astacus* (Nybelin, 1936; Schäperclaus, 1935). Hyphae, very scarcely penetrating

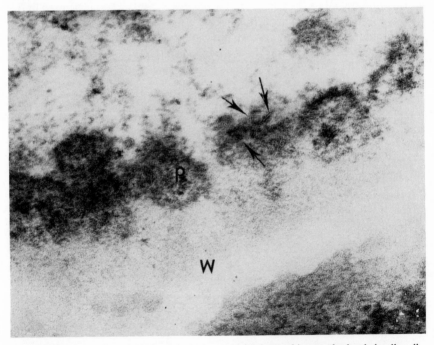

Fig. 7. Electron micrograph of particulate material (p) attaching to the hyphal cell wall (W) of *Aphanomyces*. The material has become partly electron dense with DOPA. Note the thin tubules (arrows) in the particles. Glutaraldehyde-osmium. ×120,000.

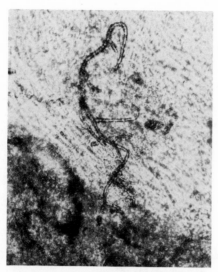

Fig. 8. Melanized hyphae of the crayfish plague fungus in the abdominal muscle of live *Astacus astacus.* ×140.

muscular tissues, or zoospores, experimentally injected into such tissues, always become heavily melanized in *Astacus astacus* and *Pacifastacus leniusculus,* and further growth is strongly inhibited (Unestam and Nylund, 1972) (Fig. 8). Collard (1966) studied a parasite, *Thallassomyces californiensis* (possibly a fungus), on a shrimp, but, although the parasite penetrated deep into the eye stalk and into the optic nerve, the brain, and the ventral nerve cord, there was no visible histological damage or reaction in the host.

REACTIONS IN THE INTEGUMENT

During natural infection, the crayfish plague fungus is mostly found in the soft integumental parts of its host. In fact, resistance to the disease in *Astacus astacus* was much higher when spores were injected into the hemocoel (LD^{50}: 2 × 10^4 zoospores/crayfish) than when the spores were added to the aquarium water (LD^{50}: 30 spores/ml) (Unestam and Weiss, 1970).

Hyphae growing in the inner layers of the cuticle (close to the epidermis) or in the epidermis usually became heavily melanized (Unestam and Weiss, 1970; and unpublished results) (Figs. 9 and 10). Further out in the soft cuticle this reaction was much weaker, or no reaction at all was seen around the hyphae which looked healthy and branched normally. In the outer soft cuticle, especial-

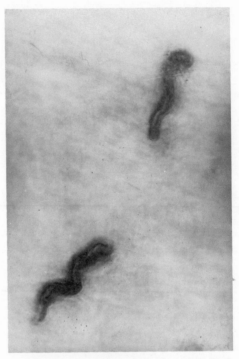

Fig. 9. Heavily melanized hyphae of *Aphanomyces* penetrating the inner layer of the soft, intersegmental membrane of a live *Pacifastacus leniusculus.* × 250.

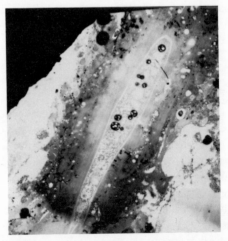

Fig. 10. Electron micrograph of a melanized hypha in the inner layer of an intersegmental membrane of a live *Astacus astacus.* Note the thick, double layer of lining on the cell wall. Glutaraldehyde-osmium, Pb-citrate. × 3000.

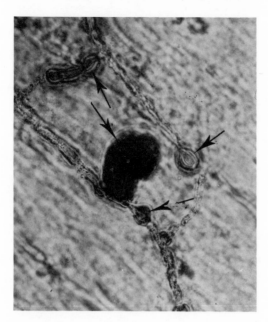

Fig. 11. Hyphae of the crayfish plague fungus growing close to the epicuticle in the intersegmental membrane of a live *Astacus astacus*. Light-refracting, more or less melanized material (arrows) attaches to the hyphal wall. × 320.

ly very close to the epicuticle, localized formation of light-refracting and, later, melanized zones on the hyphae were observed (Fig. 11). Pigment formation was enhanced by placing the cut portion in 0.04% DOPA solution and the process, as a whole, was surprisingly similar to that in hyphae encapsulated by blood cells. The limitation of these areas or spots suggests that the enzyme-containing material was "mobilized" only in certain areas for some unknown reason, or that the material was unequally distributed. Whether the substrate for melanin formation is always available everywhere in this layer of the cuticle or must be mobilized by the presence of the hypha, as in the hemolymph, is, however, not known.

By cutting out parts of soft cuticle (epidermis taken away) of *Astacus,* partly "peeling" off the epicuticle, placing it in a humid chamber (15 or 20°C), and adding a drop of zoospore suspension on the "peeled" surface, the events could be studied continually under the microscope. In a few hours, the light-refracting zones and weak melanization could be observed on the spore walls. (Where the epicuticle remained intact, added spores were not affected, however.) Therefore, all necessary components for these reactions on the hyphal wall were present, and the process proceeded normally without the presence of epicuticle and epidermis and without contact with the live animal. Melanization was

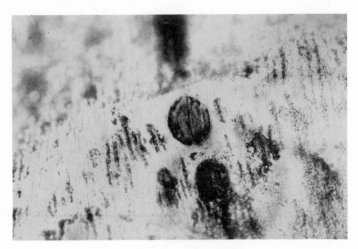

Fig. 12. A brown spot of melanin below the epicuticle in an intersegmental membrane of a live *Astacus astacus.* X 130.

strongly inhibited by KCN and diethyldithiocarbamate. It is interesting to note that in intact healthy crayfish, small, round, brown spots are always found here and there in the soft cuticle but only immediately below the epicuticle (Fig. 12). It could well be that these spots are signs of unsuccessful surface attacks by some fungus (or other microorganism), or that they are spontaneous "outbreaks" of the latent melanization mechanism present in this layer. Certainly, merely pricking the intact surface with a needle gives brown spots within a few days. But only the _border_ of a "peeled" area in a live crayfish (= the edge of the intact epicuticle) soon becomes brown from melanin, not to any greater extent than the "peeled" surface where the added spores become specifically melanized. Thus, nonspecific melanization in the wounded cuticle surface is probably in some way different from the more specific reactions on the fungal wall surface.

All the events described for the cuticle of the European crayfish, *Astacus astacus,* are also found in the American, *Pacifastacus leniusculus* (more resistant to the crayfish plague). But there is one great difference. In natural attacks in *Pacifastacus,* the hyphae are always much more melanized, usually almost black. In some Australian crayfish (susceptible), the processes were also basically the same as those in *Astacus astacus,* summarized in Fig. 13.

Entomophthora apiculata, the insect parasite, was able to penetrate the cuticle of *Astacus* and *Pasifastacus* from inside after experimental injection of conidia into the hemocoel (Unestam and Weiss, 1970). In the inner cuticle, the melanization around the hyphae was heavy, and often very wide, brown zones

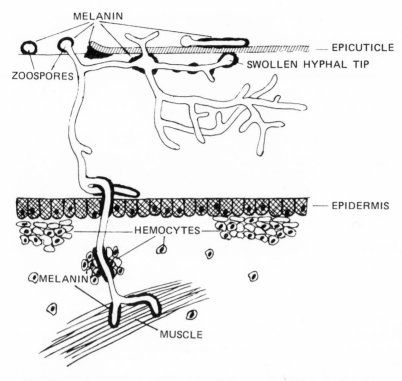

Fig. 13. A diagram summarizing some of the reactions against the invading *Aphanomyces astaci* in *Astacus astacus*.

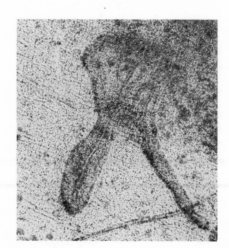

Fig. 14. Hyphae of *Entomophthora apiculata* penetrating the inner layer of an intersegmental membrane of *Pacifastacus leniusculus*. Note the wide reaction zone around the hypha. × 65.

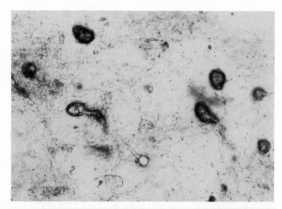

Fig. 15. Swelling hyphal tips (some melanized) of *Aphano-myces astaci* just about to penetrate out through the epi-cuticle of an abdominal, intersegmental membrane of *Astacus astacus.* × 180.

were found around a hypha (Fig. 14). Perhaps exudates from the hypha rather than the hyphal wall was the triggering factor here.

Before hyphae penetrated out through the intact epicuticle, the tip always swelled abnormally (Unestam and Weiss, 1970), both in intact animals (Fig. 15) and in cuticle kept *in vitro*. Often, but not always, these swollen tips were melanized on the surface. In cut, heated cuticle (100°C, 10 min) no such swelling was seen (unpublished). Whether this reaction was due to an insuscepti-bility factor (Read, 1970) or was due to a reaction in the cuticle toward the hyphal tip is not known.

Phenolic tanning and pigmentation in the cuticle of *Austropotamobius* (Astacus) *pallipes* and other Crustacea were studied by Dennell (1947) and in the crab, *Carcinus maenas,* by Krishnan (1951). Tanning and pigment-forming phenol oxidase is present in the calcified or hardening cuticle and the epicuticle, at least during some periods of the molt—intermolt cycle, and may be supplied from the epidermis or from the tegumental glands. In the soft cuticle of crayfish, there are, however, few or no such glands and, normally, very little pigmenta-tion. Perhaps the cell-wall-activated enzyme in such cuticle is very stable and is deposited in the outer cuticle together with it, or that the cuticular plasma canals function throughout the intermolt cycle and transport fresh enzyme from the cells inside the cuticle. The substrate [probably a phenolic amino acid supplied from the hemolymph (Krishnan, 1951)] may not, in our case, have to be kept apart from this enzyme since activation is needed.

Heavy hemocyte accumulation on the inner surface of the epidermis was often seen when the cuticle of *Astacus astacus* was heavily penetrated by the plague fungus (unpublished results). The same response was also found after a few hours inside "peeled" (epicuticle removed) areas of the soft cuticle of crayfish kept in water (15°C) and was probably a result of a "signal" transferred through the cuticle to the epidermal cells, which became "sticky."

In the "burn spot" diseases, caused by some Fungi Imperfecti in *Astacus* spp., *Orconectes limosus*, and the crab, *Eriocheir sinensis* (Mann and Pieplow, 1938; Mann, 1940), hyphae penetrated mainly the calcified portions of the exoskeleton. Brown pigment (probably melanin) was always formed around the penetrating hyphae and the similarities with the reactions toward *Aphanomyces* and *Entomophthora* in the soft crayfish cuticle are striking.

Surprisingly, we have also found that Aphanomyces hyphae may be layered upon by melanin when outside but in contact with the epicuticle (Fig. 16). This was found both in intact American and Australian crayfish about a week after addition of a great number of zoospores to the aquarium water. No visible influence on the epicuticle or cuticle underneath the hypha was seen in the electron microscope (Fig. 17), but the PPO-containing epicuticle may be involved. The nature of this noncellular "recognition" of a hypha is not known.

Penetration of the intact exoskeleton in live crayfish is probably a capacity given to few microorganisms outside the Fungi. The responses upon such pene-

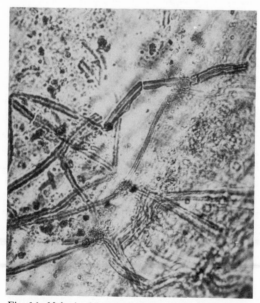

Fig. 16. Melanized hyphae on the surface of an intersegmental membrane of *Pacifastacus leniusculus.* × 260.

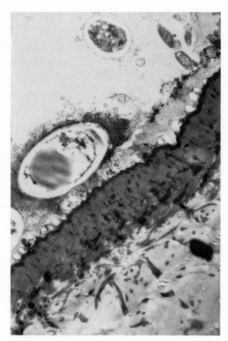

Fig. 17. Electron micrograph of a sectioned
hypha on the surface of an intersegmental
membrane of *Astacopsis gouldi* from Tas-
mania. Glutaraldehyde-osmium. Uranyl acetate. × 8000.

tration, therefore, becomes more or less "specific" to parasitic hyphae. These
responses in the crayfish are summarized in Fig. 13. The crucial events or factors
determining the resistance level in crayfish toward the crayfish plague fungus
may also be located within the cuticle (Unestam and Weiss, 1970).

FINAL REMARKS

    Melanin formation does not necessarily have to constitute the defense pro-
cess against fungi in crayfish but could be a "by-product" of such processes, as it
is in plants. Melanin and resistance toward parasites in insects has been discussed
several times (e.g., Salt, 1963; Chadwick, 1966; Taylor, 1969; Poinar *et al.*,
1968; Pye and Yendol, 1972). The reciprocal genetic adaptation of certain parasites and insects (Salt, 1970), a protozoan and crayfish (Unestam, unpublished observations), and *Thallassomyces* and shrimp (Collard, 1966) includes
lack of hemocyte and other host recognition of the parasite surface as "not-
self." Lack of recognition of a relatively harmless, but unavoidable parasite, may

be beneficial to both host and parasite. On the other extreme, in fungal parasites living in the cuticle of crayfish, for instance, a much heavier host response (melanin formation, *etc.*) is seen in the compatible (usual) host–parasite relationship (like *Pacifastacus–Aphanomyces*) than in the noncompatible one (like *Astacus–Aphanomyces*) where *Astacus* is oversusceptible (Unestam, 1969). The limitation (by inhibition) of the unavoidable attack by *Aphanomyces* in *Pacifastacus* is, of course, in the long run, beneficial to both.

REFERENCES

Bang, F. B., 1967, Blood clot formation in the antenna of the hermit crab, *Pagurus longicarpus, Biol. Bull. 133*:456-457.

Campbell, C. K., 1970, Electron microscopy of aspergillosis in fowl chicks, *Sabouraudia 8*:133-140.

Chadwick, J. S., 1966, The occurrence of polyphenoloxidase in the hemocytes of actively immunized larvae of the greater wax moth, *Galleria mellonella, J. Invertebr. Pathol. 8*:126-127.

Collard, S. B., 1966, *Thallassomyces californiensis* sp.n., a parasite of the nervous system of a shrimp, *Pasiphae emarginata* Rathbun, *Koninkl. Ned. Akad. Wetenschap., Proc. Ser. C 69*:37-49.

Cuenot, L., 1895, Études physiologiques sur les Crustacés Décapodes, *Arch. Biol. (Liege) 8*:245-303.

Dennell, R., 1947, The occurrence and significance of phenolic hardening in the newly formed cuticle of Crustacea Decapoda, *Proc. Roy. Soc. (London) B 134*:485-503.

Götz, P., 1969, Die Einkapslung von Parasiten in der Hämolymphe von *Chironomus*-Larven (Diptera), *Zool. Anz., Suppl. 33*:610-617.

Johnson, P. T., 1968, *An Annotated Bibliography of Pathology in Invertebrates Other than Insects,* Burgess Publishing Co., Minneapolis.

Johnson, P. T. and Chapman, F. A., 1969, *An Annotated Bibliography of Pathology in Invertebrates Other than Insects, Misc. Publ. No. 1,* Center of Pathobiology, University of California, Irvine, California.

Krishnan, G., 1951, Phenolic tanning and pigmentation of the cuticle in *Carcinus maenas, Quart. J. Microscop. Sci. 92*:333-342.

Mann, H., 1940, Die Brandfleckenkrankheit beim Sumpfkrebs (*Potamobius leptodactylus* Eschh), *Z. Parasitenk. 11*:430-432.

Mann, H. and Pieplow, U., 1938, Die Brandfleckenkrankheit bei Krebsen und ihre Erreger, *Z. Fischerei 36*:225-240.

Metschnikoff, E., 1884, Über eine Sprosspilzkrankheit der Daphnien. Beitrag zur Lehre über den Kampf der Phagocyten gegen Krankheitserreger, *Virchows Arch. Pathol. Anat. Physiol. Klin. Med. 96*:177-195.

Nybelin, O., 1936, Untersuchungen über die Ursache der in Schweden Gegenwärtig vorkommenden Krebspest, *Rep. Inst. Fresh-water Res. Drottningholm 9*:3-29.

Pixell-Goodrich, H., 1928, Reactions of *Gammarus* to injury and disease, with notes on some microsporidial and fungoid diseases, *Quart. J. Microscop. Sci. 72*:325-353.

Poinar, Jr., G. O., Leutenegger, R., and Götz, P., 1968, Ultrastructure of the formation of a melanotic capsule in *Diabrotica* (Coleoptera) in response to a parasitic nematode (Mermithidae), *J. Ultrastruct. Res. 25*:293-306.

Poisson, R., 1930, Observations sur *Anophrys sarcophaga* Cohn (A. maggii Cattaneo), *Bull. Biol. (France, Belgique) 64*:288-331.

Pye, A. P. and Yendol, W. G., 1972, Hemocytes containing polyphenoloxidase in *Galleria* larvae after injection of bacteria, *J. Invertebr. Pathol. 19*:166-170.

Read, C. P., 1970, *Parasitism and Symbiology. An Introductory Text,* Ronald Press Co., New York.

Salt, G., 1963, The *Defense* reactions of insects to metazoan parasites, *Parasitology* 53:527-642.

Salt, G., 1970, *The Cellular Defence Reactions of Insects,* Cambridge University Press, London.

Schäperclaus, W., 1935, Die Ursache der pestartigen Krebssterben, *Z. Fischerei 33:*343-366.

Schäperclaus, W., 1954, *Fischkrankheiten,* Akademie-Verlag, Berlin.

Steinhaus, E. A. (ed.), 1963, *Insect Pathology, An Advanced Treatise, Vol. 2,* Academic Press, New York and London.

Taylor, R. L., 1969, A suggested role for the polyphenol—phenoloxidase system in invertebrate immunity, *J. Invertebr. Pathol. 14:*427-428.

Tokunaga, J. and Bartnicki-Garcia, S., 1971, Structure and differentiation of the cell wall of *Phytophthora palmivora:* Cysts, hyphae and sporangia, *Arch. Mikrobiol. 79:*293-310.

Unestam, T., 1969, On the adaptation of *Aphanomyces astaci* as a parasite, *Physiol. Plantarum 22:*221-235.

Unestam, T. and Nylund, J. E., 1972, Blood reactions *in vitro* in crayfish against a fungal parasite, *Aphanomyces astaci, J. Invertebr. Pathol. 19:*94-106.

Unestam, T. and Weiss, D. W., 1970, The host—parasite relationship between fresh-water crayfish and the crayfish disease fungus *Aphanomyces astaci:* Responses to infection by a susceptible and a resistant species, *J. Gen. Microbiol. 60:*77-90.

Chapter 18

Insect Hemocytes and the Problem of Host Recognition of Foreignness

A. J. Nappi

Biological Sciences
State University of New York
Oswego, New York

INTRODUCTION

If cellular and humoral immune reactions of vertebrate species were used as evaluative criteria, insects would not be considered immunocompetent. Immunologic specificity, as defined by antigen—antibody complementarity, and immunologic memory, as measured by anamnestic responses or second-set allograft rejections, are not characterisitc of insect immunity (Good and Papermaster, 1964; Saunders, 1970). However, even in the absence of these and other "deficiencies," cellular and humoral immune reactions of insects are excellent homeostatic adaptations that effectively discern and combat foreignness and abnormal or effete host tissues. Against those foreign organisms too large to be phagocytized, the principal cellular reaction of insects is encapsulation. Typically, the initial reaction is characterized by aggregation of host blood cells or hemocytes to form a capsule around a parasite, and the deposition of melanin on or very near the outer surface of the parasite (c.f. Salt, 1963, 1970; Poinar, 1969; Shapiro, 1969). Against various microbial parasites, some insects produce humoral substances (antibacterial, bactericidal, lytic, etc.) that provide some degree of immunity. Unfortunately, the origin of these substances is unknown. Moreover, except for nonspecificity and lack of similarity to vertebrate antibodies (immunoglobulins), little is known of their chemical nature (Briggs, 1958, 1964; Stephens, 1959, 1962*a,b*, 1963*a—d*; Stephens and Marshall, 1962; Chadwick, 1967; Hink and Briggs, 1968, 1969; Chadwick and Vilk, 1969; Boman *et al.*, 1972).

It is significant that in insects, as in many other invertebrates, transplantation experiments can be performed with very little difficulty (cf. Caspari, 1933; Ephrussi and Beadle, 1935, 1936; Howland *et al.*, 1937; Vogt, 1940, 1942; Kambysellis, 1968, 1970). This situation contrasts markedly with numerous examples of tissue and organ incompatibility in vertebrates which result from immune reactions characterized by specificity and anamnesis (Eichwald, 1963). In insects, the few intraspecific transplant failures reported have usually been attributed to technical or procedural errors.

Unfortunately, we know very little about compatibility involving insect tissue and organ transplantations. For reasons which may best be described as heuristic or historical, this compatibility has generally been attributed solely to the absence of circulating antibodies, an idea first proposed for some lepidopterous insects by Bernheimer *et al.* (1952). However, absence of antibody alone does not account for the encapsulation of certain implants, and the various degrees of intra- and interspecific incompatibility manifested by a grafted host. If we dismiss the few intraspecific insect transplant failures that result from technical difficulties, we should also question what effects such experiments have on the ability of a host to elicit an immune response or repeated responses. This question fails from the classic immunologic standpoint since virtually any inert object of appropriate size introduced into the hemocoele of an insect elicits a hemocytic reaction (Salt, 1970). But how are insect hemocytes stimulated to react against inert objects? If discrimination is based upon contact phenomena, then surface properties are important considerations.

A prerequisite to any significant understanding of cell-mediated immunities is the knowledge of origin and function(s) of immunologically responsive cells and of the mechanisms which regulate their activities during development and under different pathological conditions. Without such information, little more than descriptive accounts can be given of transplantation reactions and host—parasite relations. Thus, fundamental questions concerning the kinetics and interactions of host cells cannot be stated in sufficiently concrete terms to invite experimentation or even analysis.

In spite of extensive literature, the mechanisms underlying the cellular immune reactions of insects have never been clearly established. This situation is not entirely incongruous in view of the dearth of information about blood cells of even a few insects (cf. Wigglesworth, 1959; Jones, 1962, 1964, 1970). Moreover, only recently have attempts been made to rigorously analyze the immune state of insects and the cytological problems involved (Salt, 1970).

HEMOCYTES AND THE PROBLEM OF RECOGNITION
OF FOREIGNNESS

The first investigator to clearly focus attention on the problem of how insect hemocytes discern and combat foreignness was Salt (1956, 1960, 1963,

1965, 1966, 1970). After careful consideration of the available evidence, he proposed that cellular immune reactions of insects were initiated by accidental contact of host hemocytes with foreign organisms rather than specific attraction of these cells from a distance (Salt, 1970). This hypothesis was based primarily on observations of encapsulation as a localized phenomenon. Salt noted that with certain intraspecific organ transplants blood cells aggregated only around the cut ends of attached tracheae and nerves and on those portions of the organs where the surfaces had been broken. Even parasites that normally were not encapsulated provoked hemocytic reactions at or very near the sites of perforations in their integument. Moreover, hemocytes were not repelled at a distance by surfaces which they did not encapsulate, for these cells settled on parasites without any visible evidence of a reaction. Salt believed that if hemocytes had responded to chemotactic stimuli they would have adhered to the surrounding, unaltered surfaces as well. Since there was no general encapsulation, it was assumed that the stimulus which initiated the localized hemocytic reaction had no apparent effect on blood cells circulating in the hemocoele. He further proposed that the success of organ transplants in insects was due to the surface properties of the connective tissues which surround the implants. Salt maintained that the surface properties of intraspecific implants were essentially similar to those of the host and, thus, less likely to provoke hemocytic reactions than the connective tissues of implants from different species or genera (Salt, 1970). As additional evidence, Salt (1970) pointed out that when parasites which normally are encapsulated are implanted into regions of the host body out of the main circulation of blood (i.e., the narrow spaces between the integumentary muscles and epidermis, and the cavity of a femur), hemocytic reactions are lacking or are less vigorous than when the parasites are implanted into the thoracic or abdominal hemocoele.

The observations cited above to support the idea that encapsulation reactions result from fortuitous contacts of blood cells with foreign bodies can be interpreted in two ways with respect to mediation by chemotactic stimuli. The localized aggregation of hemocytes around damaged surfaces and not on nearby unaltered surfaces suggests a directional movement of blood cells in response to the development of a gradient in concentration of a substance(s) released from wounds. In some insects, damaged tissues release substances ("injury factors") which cause the mobilization of hemocytes into the circulation, the deposition of blood cells at the site of the wound, and the formation of membranes by hemocytes which seal the injury (Harvey and Williams, 1961; Wyatt and Linzen, 1965). Because hemocytes settle on the surfaces of parasites that are not encapsulated, Salt (1970) suggested that the cells are not repelled at a distance. But why do the hemocytes fail to adhere to parasites? The idea that insect blood cells fail to react against connective tissues of intraspecific organ implants because of similar or compatible surface properties may be creditable. However, the suggestion that surface properties of all successful entomophilic parasites of different phyla are so similar to host surfaces that they do not provoke a hemocytic response is not entirely valid. Encapsulation and melanization are only visible manifestations of insect cellular immune reactions against internal metazoan parasites. That a parasite develops within a host which shows none of these reactions does not prove that blood cells failed to recognize the parasite as foreign. According to Kitano (1969a), live eggs of the parasite, *Apanteles glomeratus*, whose surfaces are chemically altered, are not encapsulated by hemocytes of its host, *Pierisrapae crucivora*, but dead eggs with unaltered surfaces are encapsulated. An alternate proposal suggests that the success of a parasite is dependent on its ability to produce a substance which directly or indirectly inhibits the hemocytic reaction of the host (Schneider, 1950; Streams and Greenberg, 1969). Indeed, comparative and quantitative hemocytological data indicate that some parasites do suppress the immune reactions of their insect hosts (Walker, 1959; Nappi and Streams, 1969; Kitano, 1969a,b).

In the absence of information of the normal distribution and number of circulating hemocytes, no satisfactory proposal can be given to account for the failure of some parasites to be encapsulated in host body areas removed from the main flow of blood. If under normal conditions hemocytes do not enter certain areas of the body, the presence of even a few blood cells attached or near implanted parasites would be difficult to explain on the basis of contact stimuli.

That many inert objects implanted into the hemocoele of an insect provoke hemocytic reactions is generally regarded as good evidence that blood cells discriminate by means of contact stimuli. Salt (1970) points out that the diffusion of a chemical stimulus can occur when parasites and organ implants are encapsulated, but not when inert objects are encapsulated by many layers of hemocytes. However, it is puzzling how inert objects introduced into the hemocoel avoid even partial coating by substances released from injured integumental and visceral tissues and, thus, stimulate hemocytic reactions.

Recent studies on the distribution and quantitative changes in hemocytes of parasitized insects provide some evidence that chemotactic stimuli are involved in encapsulation reactions (Nappi and Stoffolano, 1971, 1972a,b). In larvae of *Musca domestica* and *Orthellia caesarion*, as in many other dipterous larvae, the majority of hemocytes are accumulated in the posterior segments of the body (Figs. 1, 2). Very few circulating hemocytes are found until pupation, at which time hemocytes in the posterior regions disperse into the hemocoele. However, when larvae are infected with the nematode, *Heterotylenchus autumnalis*, large numbers of hemocytes enter the circulation and can encapsulate parasites in various regions of the body. The reactions involve deposition of melanin around nematodes and aggregation and fusion of hemocytes to form syncytial capsules around the parasites (Figs. 3–7). Differential hemocyte counts from infected larvae show a decrease in the percentages of oenocytoids. Normally, these relatively large hemocytes disappear from the hemolymph only at the time of pupation. Although total hemocyte counts were not made, it was evident from histological examinations that the number of hemocytes in infected larvae was greater than in noninfected larvae. These data suggest that some stimulus in infected larvae, acting on the hemocytes or on the mechanism(s) controlling their activity, causes them to move out of the posterior areas prematurely and to encapsulate the parasites (Nappi and Stoffolano, 1972b).

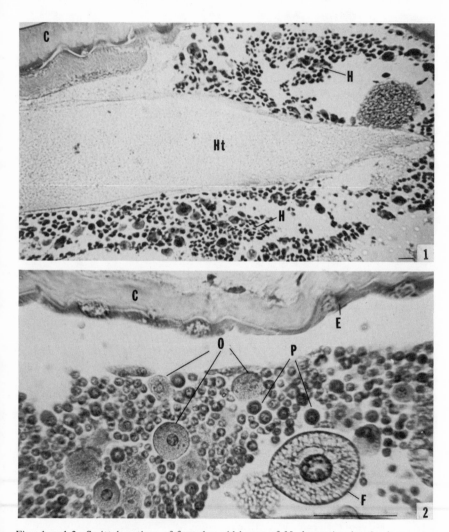

Figs. 1 and 2. Sagittal sections of four day old larvae of *M. domestica* showing hemocytes (H) accumulated within the posterior hemocoele. Ht, heart; C, dorsal cuticle; O, oenocytoids: P, plasmatocytes. Bars = 50 μm.

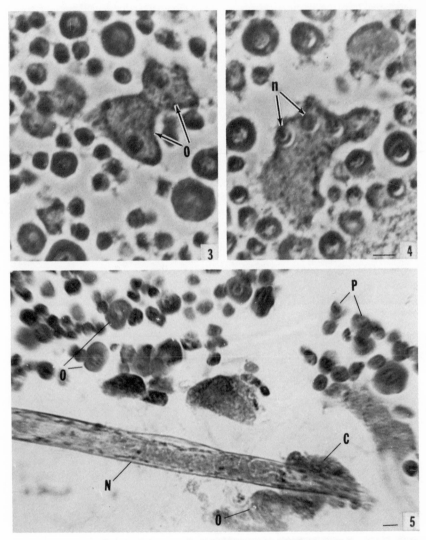

Figs. 3, 4, and 5. Early stages in the encapsulation and melanization of the nematode *H. autumnalis* (N) in larvae of the host *M. domestica*. Note the fusion of oenocytoids (O) and hemocytes adhering to the cuticle of the nematode to form a capsule (C). P, plasmatocytes; n, nuclei of hemocytes. Bars = 10 μm.

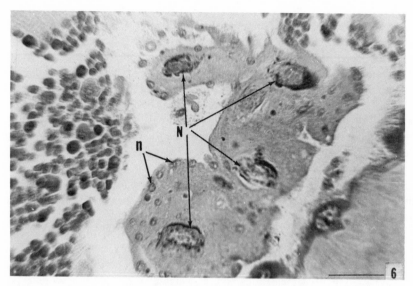

Fig. 6. The nematode *H. autumnalis* (N), seen in transverse section, encapsulated and melanized in a larva of *M. domestica* three days after infection. n, nuclei of hemocytes. Bar = 0.5 μm.

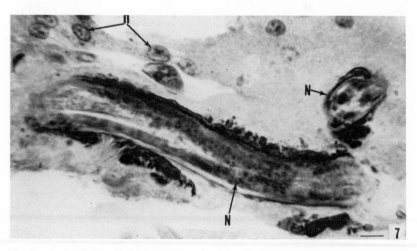

Fig. 7. Longitudinal section of heavily melanized and encapsulated *H. autumnalis* in a larva of *M. domestica* three days after infection. Bar = 10 μm.

Significant changes also occur in the hemocytes of *Drosophila* larvae infected by the solitary, endophagous parasites (parasitoids), *Pseudeucoila bochei* and *P. mellipes* (Walker, 1959; Nappi and Streams, 1969; Nappi, 1970). In larvae of different host species, the parasites are encapsulated and melanized by hemocytes very soon after infection (Figs. 8, 9). The encapsulated and melanized eggs of *Pseudeucoila* are retained within the hemocoele of the host throughout its development with no apparent adverse effect on the fly (Figs. 10–13). In noninfected larvae of *Drosophila melanogaster,* two basic types of hemocytes are found throughout most of larval life: plasmatocytes and crystal cells (Rizki, 1957*a*). Crystal cells (oenocytoids) are readily distinguished from the more numerous plasmatocytes by the presence of cytoplasmic crystals that contain substrate(s) for polyphenoloxidase activity (Rizki and Rizki, 1959). During development, the plasmatocytes gradually enlarge and differentiate into extremely flat, disk-shaped cells known as lamellocytes. At pupation, the crystal cells disappear, and the hemocyte population consists mostly of lamellocytes and plasmatocytes in various stages of differentiation (Rizki, 1957*a*; Nappi and Streams, 1969).

The hemocytic changes that occur in parasitized larvae of *D. melanogaster* include an increase in total numbers of cells, a precocious mass transformation of plasmatocytes to lamellocytes, and a decrease in the percentage of crystal cells (Walker, 1959; Nappi and Streams, 1969). The lamellocytes aggregate around a parasite and adhere to its surface to form a capsule, and the crystal cells lyse and release phenolic substances responsible for the melanization of the capsule. The presence of abnormally large numbers of lamellocytes free in the hemolymph of parasitized larvae during the early stages of infection, even before there is any visible evidence of encapsulation and melanization, suggests that at least some of the hemocytes are stimulated to react without making direct contact with the parasites (Nappi, 1973*b*).

POSSIBLE MECHANISM OF HEMOCYTE ACTIVATION

The hemocytic changes that accompany the encapsulation and melanization of parasites in larvae of *D. melanogaster, M. domestica,* and *O. caesarion* closely resemble those changes that occur in noninfected larvae at the time of pupation (Walker, 1959; Nappi and Streams, 1969; Nappi and Stoffolano, 1971, 1972*b*).

Fig. 8. Dead egg of *P. bochei* removed from a larva of *D. algonquin* 24 hr after infection. Note the melanin (M) deposited on the chorion, especially in the region of the egg stalk (S). Bar = 20 μm.

Fig. 9. Partially encapsulated and melanized egg of *P. bochei* removed from a larva of *D. affinis* 40 hr after infection. Bar = 10 μm.

Fig. 10. Dorsal view of parasitized larva of *D. algonquin* with an encapsulated and melanized egg (E) of *P. bochei.* Bar = 0.5 mm.

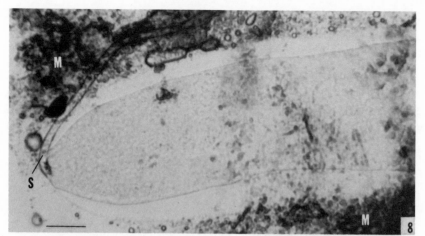

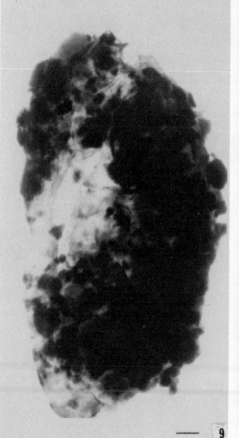

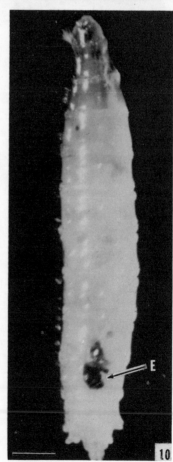

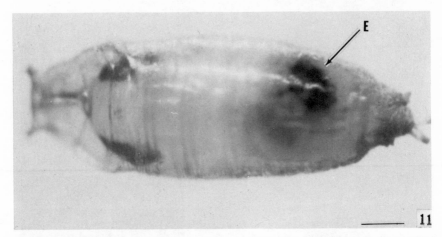

Fig. 11. Four day old parasitized *Drosophila* pupa containing an encapsulated and melanized egg (E) of *P. bochei*. Bar = 0.5 mm.

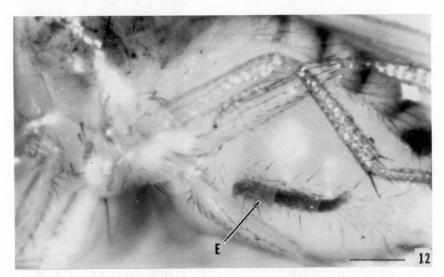

Fig. 12. Encapsulated and melanized egg (E) of *P. mellipes* within the abdomen of an adult *D. melanogaster*. Bar = 0.5 mm.

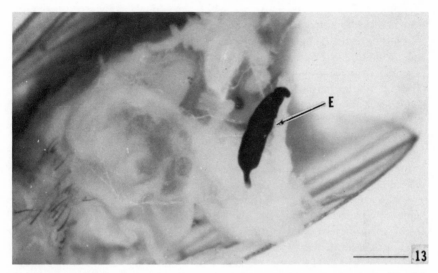

Fig. 13. Specimen shown in Fig. 12 dissected to show the encapsulated egg (E) of *P. mellipes*. Bar = 0.5 mm.

Collectively, these changes include cellular proliferation and differentiation, mobilization of hemocytes, and lysis of certain types of hemocytes. These observations suggest that normal hemocyte activity is regulated by the neuroendocrine system, and that cellular immune reactions of parasitized larvae result from a hormonal imbalance (Nappi, 1973a,b). In infected larvae, hemocytes single out only parasites around which they aggregate, deposit pigment, and form capsules. In noninfected larvae undergoing puparium formation, hemocytes move out of areas where they are normally found and aggregate around metamorphosing and degenerating tissues. In some species where hemocytes have been carefully studied during pupation, there is some evidence that blood cells actively participate in the breakdown of connective tissues covering certain larval structures (Shrivastava and Richards, 1965; Pipa and Woolever, 1965), and in the processing and transporting of material to developing adult tissues (c.f. Whitten, 1964, 1968, 1969; Crossley, 1964, 1965, 1968).

If the neuroendocrine system is involved in immune reactions, what is the origin and nature of the initial stimulus, and what is the sequence of events which this stimulus sets in motion? Since hormones have a widespread effect, why are only the hemocytes affected? Also, how are the hemocytic reactions localized and terminated? Some of these questions were raised, but unsuccessfully answered, in a previous paper (Nappi, 1973b). Without supportive experimental evidence the following account does little to improve upon the situation. However, the problem of how the immune reactions of insects become activated warrants investigation, and a proposal which accommodates some of the observations and can be tested may be helpful.

Although the details of the developmental processes accompanying molting and metamorphosis in the Diptera are far from being completely understood, primary endocrine events involve changes in concentrations of juvenile hormone (JH) and molting hormone or ecdysone (MH). The combined action of MH and a high titer of JH produces a larval molt, and a decrease in the concentration of JH results in a pupal molt. The transformation from pupal to adult stage occurs in the absence of JH. The activities of the endocrine glands throughout development are controlled by the "activation hormone" ("brain hormone") which, in some insects, is known to be produced by the neurosecretory cells of the pars intercerebralis of the brain (Wigglesworth, 1970).

Since the pupal stage is triggered by a low titer of JH, the precocious hemocytic changes in parasitized larvae of *D. melanogaster, M. domestica,* and *O. caesarion* may be due to a decrease in the concentration of this hormone, or to an increase in the amount of MH. Perhaps hemocytes are the most responsive or sensitive host cells to small changes in hormone titers. Recent *in vitro* studies of hemocytes to MH indicate that this hormone markedly affects cell mobility and membrane activity (Judy, 1969; Judy and Gilbert, 1970). According to Judy and Marks (1971), the concentration of circulating hemocytes in the lepidopteran, *Manduca sexta,* may depend directly on MH titer. However, the overall effect of JH is to prevent precocious maturation (Herman, 1968). Some of the known long-term effects of removing the corpora allata, which secrete this hormone, include the accumulation and proliferation of hemocytes, and the encapsulation of certain pathologically changed fat body cells (Novák, 1966). Presumably, JH interacts with the genetic machinery to either promote the differentiation of immature characters, or suppress expression of adult characters latent within the cells (c.f. Wigglesworth, 1970).

The fact that hemocytes specifically single out parasites suggests that the initial stimulus may be a substance released from either the parasites, or the few hemocytes in the circulation when they accidentally make contact with foreign organisms. If a gradient in concentration of the stimulus substance is established, this may provide for the directional movement of hemocytes and the localization of cellular immune responses. However, it is also possible that the stimulus results from the lack of a host metabolite that is rapidly utilized by either the parasite or the hemocytes in contact with the parasite (negative gradient). In any event, the stimulus may act directly on the brain–endocrine complex to affect the production of hormone(s). The hormonal imbalance changes the permeability of the cell membrane of hemocytes to certain metabolites and brings about the premature differentiation and migration of these cells. At or near the surface of the parasite, certain hemocytes lyse and release substances that cause melanization of parasites and aggregation and adhesion of additional hemocytes to form melanotic capsules. The development of a heavily melanized, impervious, and inert capsule would prevent the stimulus from affecting the neuroendocrine system, and the hemocytic reactions would cease (Nappi, 1973b).

It is of interest that the precocious transformation of hemocytes which attends parasite encapsulation and melanization in *D. melanogaster* also occurs in certain mutant strains during the formation of melanotic lesions or "tumors" of the caudal fat body (Rizki, 1957b). Moreover, when tumorous larvae are ligated so that the brain and endocrine gland (ring gland in Diptera) are excluded from hemocytes in the posterior regions, the number of melanotic lesions decreases (Rizki, 1960, 1962). When normal larvae are similarly ligated, there is an early appearance of lamellocytes without pathological effects. If an endocrine gland is implanted into the posterior region of a nontumorous larva, the hemocyte population is normalized.

These results led Rizki (1960) to suggest that hemocytic changes in tumorous larvae result from a hormonal imbalance associated with some physiological abnormality of the endocrine gland. However, since only the caudal fat body is encapsulated and melanized, the hemocytes must also be responding to a stimulus from this tissue which apparently develops asynchronously in tumorous larvae (Rizki, 1957b). Since successful ligation prevents the exchange of material in both directions, perhaps encapsulation and melanization reactions in tumorous larvae occur only after the neuroendocrine center receives a stimulus from the caudal fat cells, and not necessarily because of an abnormal endocrine gland. This may also explain why Burdette (1954) found an increase in tumor frequency in ligated larvae of *D. melanogaster*. Unfortunately, it remains difficult to prove that hemocytic changes in ligated larvae are caused by a hormonal imbalance, and not secondary manifestations to hormone deprivation (Rizki, 1962). However, investigations of nutrient balance in *Drosophila* suggest that melanization of tumors is under hormonal control (Sang and Burnet, 1963) and that an increase in tumor frequency results from a decrease in titers of MH (Sang, 1969). In other insects, extirpation of the corpora allata results in proliferation of hemocytes and formation of tumors (Pflugfelder, 1948).

Regardless of whether cellular immune mechanisms of *D. melanogaster* respond to internal metazoan parasites or to a disruption in synchronous growth and differentiation of host tissues, hemocytic changes in both cases are similar, and the reactions serve to localize and prevent successful establishment of foreign or abnormal cells. What little evidence there is suggests that at least three developmental processes are involved: an upset in the synthesis and release of hormones, hemocyte differentiation in response to hormonal changes, and the mobilization and directional movement of hemocytes in response to chemotactic stimuli. This proposal does not dispute the importance of contact stimuli in the discriminative reactions of hemocytes during capsule formation or in initiating the immune response. It does suggest that chemotaxis is an essential component of the hemocytic reactions of insects. During normal development, the hemocytes may be responding to substances diffusing from metamorphosing and degenerating tissues. If this is true, what characteristics do these tissues have in common with abnormal tissues and parasites which are encapsulated by hemocytes?

It is conceivable that certain parasites and intact intraspecific organ implants are not encapsulated and melanized because they can effectively utilize or manipulate the internal milieu of the host and develop synchronously with host tissues. A considerable number of successful implantation experiments have been performed in *Drosophila* larvae with imaginal discs. These tissues retain an embryonic characteric during larval development but differentiate in the adult stage. However, when certain mutant imaginal discs are implanted into wild-type larvae, these abnormally growing tissues stimulate an intense hemocytic reaction, and are invaded by hemocytes. Unlike wild-type imaginal discs, these mutant discs fail to differentiate in response to hormonal changes at the time of metamorphosis (Gateff and Schneiderman, 1969). The specific recessive gene responsible for the mutation affects other tissues, including the prothoracic gland cells of the ring gland which secrete MH (Hadorn, 1938; Aggarwal and King, 1969). It is also important that the failure of some interspecific ovarian transplants to develop in *Drosophila* has been attributed to a species specificity of hormone necessary for the maturation of the ova (Monod and Poulson, 1937; Vogt, 1940). According to Kambysallis (1970), various expressions of incompatibility in interspecific transplants may be associated with the degree of diversity in the nutritional and/or hormonal milieu of the host. Presumably, when the internal environment of the host is comparable to that of the donor, host reactions do not interfere and the implanted ovaries utilize this environment and reach the stage of complete maturation of the eggs.

CONCLUDING STATEMENT

Our present inability to answer fundamental questions about the kinetics and interactions of insect blood cells is due to a dearth of comparative and quantitative studies of hemocytes during infection (Nappi, 1973*b*). Furthermore, investigations are lacking concerning the surface contact relations of hemocytes and the stimuli that cause these cells to aggregate and form capsules around foreign organisms (Salt, 1970). The problem is further complicated by little information on the functions of specific blood cells, the mechanisms which regulate their differentiation, and their varied activities at different stages during development. Although we know that insect metamorphosis is under hormonal control, we do not understand how hormones interact with cells at the molecular level to initiate those complex physiological and biochemical changes associated with differentiation (Gorell *et al.*, 1972).

If, as a basis of future experimentation, we accept the proposal that a hormonal imbalance causes hemocytic changes leading to encapsulation and melanization of parasites, it may eventually prove valuable if we give some consideration to various genetic aspects of the formation of melanotic tumors and to environmental factors which influence tumor incidence. Experimental transplantations of diverse melanotic tumors into larvae of different genetic strains may provide numerous opportunities for investigating not only the developmental capacities and mode of formation of melanotic lesions, but also the mechanism of activation or inactivation of cellular responses. While it may be of interest to some insect pathologists to search for vertebratelike immunoglobulins and to demonstrate transplantation immunity in such experiments, others may wish to give some consideration to the possible adaptive significance of immune reactions which lack immunologic specificity and anamnesis.

REFERENCES

Aggarwal, S. K. and King, R. C., 1969, A comparative study of the ring glands from wild-type and *1(2)gl* mutant *Drosophila melanogaster, J. Morphol. 129*:171-200.

Bernheimer, A. W., Caspari, E., and Kaiser, A. D., 1952, Studies on antibody formation in caterpillars, *J. Exp. Zool. 119*:23-35.

Boman, H. G., Nilsson, I., and Rasmuson, B., 1972, Inducible antibacterial defense systems in *Drosophila, Nature 237*:232-235.

Briggs, J. D., 1958, Humoral immunity in lepidopterous larvae, *J. Exp. Zool. 138*:155-188.

Briggs, J. D., 1964, Immunological responses, in: *The Physiology of Insecta, Vol. 3*, pp. 259-283 (M. Rockstein, ed.), Academic Press, New York.

Burdette, W. J., 1954, Effect of ligation of *Drosophila* larvae on tumor incidence, *Cancer Res. 14*:780-784.

Caspari, E., 1933, Über die Wirkung eines pleiotropen Gens bei der Mehlmotte *Ephestia kühneilla* Zeller, *Arch. Entwicklungsmech. Organ. 130*:353-381.

Chadwick, J. S., 1967, Serological responses of insects, *Federation Proc. 26*:1675-1679.

Chadwick, J. S. and Vilk, E., 1969, Endotoxins from several bacterial species as immunizing agents against *Pseudomonas aeruginosa* in *Galleria mellonella, J. Invertebr. Pathol. 13*:410-415.

Crossley, A. C., 1964, An experimental analysis of the origins and physiology of hemocytes in the blue blow-fly, *Calliphora erythrocephala, J. Exp. Zool. 157*:375-398.

Crossley, A. C., 1965, Transformations in the abdominal muscle of the blue blow-fly, *Calliphora erythrocephala* (Meig.), during metamorphosis, *J. Embryol. Exp. Morphol. 14*:89-110.

Crossley, A. C., 1968, The fine structure and metabolism of breakdown of larval intersegmental muscles in the blow-fly, *Calliphora erythrocephala, J. Insect Physiol. 14*:1389-1407.

Eichwald, E. J., 1963, Tissue transplantation, *Advan. Biol. Med. Phys. 9*:94-205.

Ephrussi, B. and Beadle, G. W., 1935, La transplantation des ovaries chez la drosophile, *Bull. Biol. (France, Belgium) 69*:492-502.

Ephrussi, B. and Beadle, G. W., 1936, A technique of transplantation for *Drosophila, Am. Naturalist 70*:218-226.

Gateff, E. and Schneiderman, H. A., 1969, Neoplasms in mutant and cultured wild-type tissues of *Drosophila, Nat. Cancer Inst. Monograph 31*:365-397.

Good, R. A. and Papermaster, B. W., 1964, Ontogeny and phylogeny of adaptive immunity, *Adv. Immunology 4*:1-115.

Gorell, T. A., Gilbert, L. I., and Siddal, J. B., 1972, Studies on hormone recognition by arthropod target tissues, *Am. Zool.* *12*:347-356.

Hadorn, E., 1938, Die Degeneration der Imaginalscheiben bei latalen Drosophila Larven der Mutante "lethal giant," *Rev. Suisse Zool.* *45*:425-429.

Harvey, W. R. and Williams, C. M., 1961, The injury metabolism of the *Cecropia* silkworm, I. Biological amplification of the effects of localized injury, *J. Insect Physiol.* *7*:81-99.

Herman, W. S., 1968, Control of hormone production in insects, in: *Metamorphosis: A Problem in Developmental Biology,* pp. 107-141 (W. Etkin and L. Gilbert, eds.), Appleton-Century-Crofts, New York.

Hink, W. F. and Briggs, J. D., 1968, Bactericidal factors in hemolymph from normal and immune wax moth larvae, *Galleria mellonella, J. Insect Physiol.* *14*:1025-1034.

Hink, W. F. and Briggs, J. D., 1969, Immune responses of ligatured *Galleria mellonella* larvae, *J. Invertebr. Pathol.* *13*:308-309.

Howland, R. B., Glancy, E. A., and Sonnenblick, B. P., 1937, Transplantation of wild-type and vermilion eye disks among four species of *Drosophila, Genetics* *22*:434-442.

Jones, J. C., 1962, Current concepts concerning insect hemocytes, *Am. Zool.* *2*:209-246.

Jones, J. C., 1964, The circulatory system of insects, in: *The Physiology of Insecta, Vol. 3,* pp. 1-106 (M. Rockstein, ed.), Academic Press, New York.

Jones, J. C., 1970, Hemocytopoiesis in insects, in: *Regulation of Hematopoiesis, Vol. 1,* pp. 7-65 (A. S. Gordon, ed.), Appleton-Century-Crofts, New York.

Judy, K. J., 1969, Cellular responses to ecdysterone *in vitro, Science* *165*:1374-1375.

Judy, K. J. and Gilbert, L. I., 1970, Histology of the alimentary canal during the metamorphosis of *Hyalophora cecropia* (L), *J. Morphol.* *131*:277-300.

Judy, K. J. and Marks, E. P., 1971, Effects of ecdysterone *in vitro* on hindgut and hemocytes of *Manduca sexta* (Lepidoptera), *Gen. Comp. Endocrinol.* *17*:351-359.

Kambysellis, M. P., 1968, Interspecific transplantation as a tool for indicating phylogenetic relationship, *Proc. Nat. Acad. Sci.* *59*:1166-1172.

Kambysellis, M. P., 1970, Compatibility in insect tissue transplantations. I. Ovarian transplantations and hybrid formation between *Drosophila* species endemic to Hawaii, *J. Exp. Zool.* *175*:169-180.

Kitano, H., 1969a, Experimental studies on the parasitism of *Apanteles glomeratus* L. with special reference to its encapsulating-inhibiting capacity, *Bull. Tokyo Gakugei Univ. Ser. Nat. Sci.* *21*:95-136.

Kitano, H., 1969b, Defensive ability of *Apanteles glomeratus* L. (Hymenoptera: Braconidae) to the hemocytic reaction of *Pieris rapae crucivora* Boisduval (Lepidoptera: Pieridae), *Appl. Entomol. Zool.* *4*:41-55.

Monod, J. and Poulson, D. F., 1937, Specific reactions of the ovary to interspecific transplantation among members of the melanogaster group of *Drosophila, Genetics* *22*:257-263.

Nappi, A. J., 1970, Defense reactions of *Drosophila euronotus* larvae against the hymenopterous parasite *Pseudeucoila bochei, J. Invertebr. Pathol.* *16*:408-418.

Nappi, A. J., 1973a, The role of melanization in the immune reaction of larvae of *Drosophila algonquin* against *Pseudeucoila bochei, Parasitology* *65*: 23-32.

Nappi, A. J., 1973b, Hemocytic changes associated with the encapsulation and melanization of some insect parasites, *Exp. Parasitol.* *33*:285-302.

Nappi, A. J. and Stoffolano, Jr., J. G., 1971, *Heterotylenchus autumnalis:* Hemocytic reactions and capsule formation in the host, *Musca domestica, Exp. Parasitol.* *29*:116-125.

Nappi, A. J. and Stoffolano, Jr., J. G., 1972a, Distribution of hemocytes in larvae of *Musca domestica* and *Musca autumnalis* and possible chemotaxis during parasitization, *J. Insect Physiol.* *18*:169-179.

Nappi, A. J. and Stoffolano, Jr., J. G., 1972b, Hemocytic changes associated with the immune reaction of nematode-infected larvae of *Orthellia caesarion, Parasitology* *65*:295-302.

Nappi, A. J. and Streams, F. A., 1969, Hemocytic reactions of *Drosophila melanogaster* to the parasites *Pseudeucoila mellipes* and *P. bochei, J. Insect Physiol.* *15*:1551-1566.

Novák, V. J. A., 1966, *Insect Hormones,* p. 478, Methuen and Co. Ltd., London.

Pflugefelder, O., 1948, Atypische Gewebsdifferenzierung bein Stabheuschrecken nach experimenteller Stoerung der inneren Sekretion, *Z. Krebsforsch.* 56:107-120.

Pipa, R. L. and Woolever, P. S., 1965, Insect neurometamorphosis. II. The fine structure of perineural connective tissue, adipohemocytes, and the shortening ventral nerve cord of a moth, *Galleria mellonella* (L.), *Z. Zellforsch.* 68:80-101.

Poinar, Jr., G. O., 1969, Arthropod immunity to worms, in: *Immunity to Parasitic Animals, Vol. 1*, pp. 173-210 (G. J. Jackson, R. Herman, and I. Singer, eds.), Appleton-Century-Crofts, New York.

Rizki, M. T., 1957a, Alterations in the hemocyte population of *Drosophila melanogaster, J. Morphol.* 100:437-458.

Rizki, M. T., 1957b, Tumor formation in relation to metamorphosis in *Drosophila melanogaster, J. Morphol.* 100:459-472.

Rizki, M. T., 1960, Melanotic tumor formation in *Drosophila, J. Morphol.* 106:147-157.

Rizki, M. T., 1962, Experimental analysis of hemocyte morphology in insects, *Am. Zool.* 2:247-255.

Rizki, M. T. and Rizki, R. M., 1959, Functional significance of the crystal cells in the larva of *Drosophila melanogaster, J. Biophys. Cytol.* 5:235-240.

Salt, G., 1956, Experimental studies in insect parasitism. IX. The reactions of a stock insect to an alien parasite, *Proc. Roy. Soc. (London) B* 146:93-108.

Salt, G., 1960, Experimental studies in insect parasitism. XI. The hemocytic reaction of a caterpillar under varied conditions, *Proc. Roy. Soc. (London) B* 151:446-467.

Salt, G., 1963, The defense reactions of insects to metazoan parasites, *Parasitology* 53:527-642.

Salt, G., 1965, Experimental studies in insect parasitism. XIII. The hemocytic reaction of a caterpillar to eggs of its habitual parasite, *Proc. Roy. Soc. (London) B* 162:303-318.

Salt, G., 1966, Experimental studies in insect parasitism. XIV. The hemocytic reaction of a caterpillar to larvae of its habitual parasite, *Proc. Roy. Soc. (London) B* 165:155-178.

Sang, J. H., 1969, Biochemical basis of hereditary melanotic tumors in *Drosophila, Nat. Cancer Inst. Monograph 31*:291-301.

Sang, J. H. and Burnet, B., 1963, Physiological genetics of melanotic tumor in *Drosophila melanogaster*. I. The effects of nutrient balance on tumor penetrance in the tu^k strain. *Genetics 48*:235-253.

Saunders, G. C., 1970, Development of the immune response, in: *Biology of the Immune Response*, pp. 93-135 (P. Abramoff and M. La Via, eds.), McGraw-Hill, New York.

Schneider, F., 1950, Die Abwehrreaktion des Insektenblutes und ihre Beeinflussung durch die Parasiten, *Vierteljahresschr. Naturforsch. Ges. Zuerich 95*:22-44.

Schrivastava, S. C. and Richards, A. G., 1965, An autoradiographic study of the relation between hemocytes and connective tissue in the wax moth, *Galleria mellonella* L., *Biol. Bull. 128*:337-345.

Shapiro, M., 1969, Immunity of insect hosts to insect parasites, in: *Immunity to Parasitic Animals, Vol. 1*, pp. 211-228 (G. J. Jackson, R. Herman, and I. Singer, eds.), Appleton-Century-Crofts, New York.

Stephens, J. M., 1959, Immune responses of some insects to some bacterial antigens, *Can. J. Microbiol.* 5:203-228.

Stephens, J. M., 1962a, Bactericidal activity of the blood of actively immunized wax moth larvae, *Can J. Microbiol.* 8:491-499.

Stephens, J. M., 1962b, Influence of active immunization on melanization of the blood of wax moth larvae, *Can. J. Microbiol.* 8:597-602.

Stephens, J. M., 1963a, Immunity in insects, in: *Insect Pathology, Vol. 1*, pp. 232-297 (E. A. Steinhous, ed.) Academic Press, New York.

Stephens, J. M., 1963b, Bactericidal activity of hemolymph of some normal insects, *J. Insect Pathol.* 5:61-65.

Stephens, J. M., 1963c, Effect of active immunization on total hemocyte counts of larvae of *Galleria mellonella* (Linnaeus), *J. Insect Pathol.* 5:152-156.

Stephens, J. M., 1963d, Protective effects of several immunizing preparations that produce active immunity in *Galleria mellonella* (Linnaeus), *J. Insect Pathol.* 5:129-130.

Stephens, J. M. and Marshall, J. H., 1962, Some properties of an immune factor isolated from the blood of actively immunized wax moth larvae, *Can. J. Microbiol.* 8:719-725.

Streams, F. A. and Greenberg, L., 1969, Inhibition of the defense reaction of *Drosophila melanogaster* parasitized simultaneously by the wasps *Pseudeucoila bochei* and *Pseudeucoila mellipes, J. Invertebr. Pathol.* 13:371-377.

Vogt, M., 1940, Zur Ursache der unterschiedlichen gonodotropen Wirkung der Ringdruse von *Drosophila funebris* und *Drosophila melanogaster, Arch. Entwicklungsmech. Organ.* 141:424.

Walker, I., 1959, Die Abwehrreaktion des Wirtes *Drosophila melanogaster* gegen die zoophage Cynipidae *Pseudeucoila bochei* Weld, *Rev. Suisse Zool.* 68:569-632.

Whitten, J. M., 1964, Hemocytes and the metamorphosing tissues in *Sarcophaga bullata, Drosophila melanogaster,* and other cyclorrhaphous Diptera, *J. Insect Physiol.* 10:409-528.

Whitten, J. M., 1968, Metamorphic changes in insects, in: *Metamorphosis: A Problem in Developmental Biology,* pp. 43-105 (W. Etkin and L. I. Gilbert, eds.), Appleton-Century-Crofts, New York.

Whitten, J. M., 1969, Hemocyte activity in relation to epidermal cell growth, cuticle secretion and cell death in a metamorphosing cyclorrhaphan pupa, *J. Insect Physiol.* 15:763-778.

Wigglesworth, V. B., 1959, Insect blood cells, *Ann. Rev. Ent.* 4:1-16.

Wigglesworth, V. B., 1970, *Insect Hormones,* p. 159, Cambridge University Press, London.

Wyatt, G. R. and Linzen, B., 1965, The metabolism of ribonucleic acid in *Cecropia* silkmoth pupae in diapause, during development and after injury, *Biochim. Biophys. Acta* 103:588-600.

Chapter 19

Lysozymelike Activities in the Hemolymph of Crassostrea virginica*

S. Y. Feng

*Marine Research Laboratory
and
Biological Sciences Group
University of Connecticut
Noank, Connecticut*

INTRODUCTION

In recent years the presence of lysozymelike activities in the hemolymph of invertebrates has been documented with increasing frequency. Mohrig and Messner (1968) report the occurrence of lysozyme at a level of 25–500 μg/ml in the hemolymph of normal *Gallaria mellonella*. This level can, however, be elevated nonspecifically up to a maximum of 9000 μg/ml of hemolymph within 24 hr by injections of sterile Ringer solution, India ink, and Gram-positive bacteria. Jolles and Zuili (1960) discovered a bacterial lytic factor in the marine polychaete worm, *Nephthys hombergi,* which Perin and Jolles (1972) characterize as lysozome. Schubert and Messner (1971) have also observed lysozymelike activities in nine species of marine, fresh-water, and terrestrial annelids: *Arenicola marina, Nereis diversicolor, Tubifex* sp., *Enchytraeus* sp., *Allolobophora caliginosa, Hirudo medicinalis, Haemopis sanguisuga, Herpobdella octoculata,* and *Glossiphonia complanta.* However, they do not observe heightened levels of lysozyme in these annelids after injection of various bacteria.

*Contribution No. 89 from Marine Research Laboratory of the Marine Sciences Institute, University of Connecticut.

The author wishes to dedicate this paper to the memory of the late Professor Leslie Alfred Stauber of Rutgers University.

In molluscs, lysozyme was first found in the hemolymph and mantle mucus of *Crassostrea virginica* By McDade and Tripp (1967a,b) and in that of *Anodonta anatina* by Messner and Mohrig (1969). Feng and Canzonier (1970) showed seasonal variations in lysozymelike activities in oyster hemolymph. Certain parasitic infections also have an effect on the lysozomelike activity which suggests the functional significance of lysozyme as an indicator of the oyster's humoral response to infections. In the study of both the immune response of *Crassostrea virginica* and the evolution of immune mechanisms in general, lysozyme appears to be a valuable tool. Lysozyme is one of the macromolecules that transcends both animal and plant kingdoms, although plant lysozyme differs chemically from the egg white lysozyme (Meyer *et al.*, 1946). It is widely distributed in animal tissues, tears, vertebrate milk and mucus (Jolles, 1960), and in plant ficus and papaya latex.

LYSOZYME CHARACTERISTICS

The designation of bacterial lytic factors as lysozyme in invertebrates is largely based upon the following three criteria: (1) reduction in the turbidity of a suspension of isolated cell-wall preparation or whole cell of *Micrococcus lysodeikticus*, (2) release of reducing groups, and (3) liberation of acetylamino-sugar complex of glucosamine and the acidic hexosamine. Although the lysozymelike material in oyster hemolymph is characterized by the three criteria (McDade and Tripp, 1967a), it differs basically from egg white lysozyme in electrophoretic mobility and probably in both molecular weight and isoelectric point (pI). In fact, the present study shows that lysozomelike activities in oyster hemolymph appear to be largely associated with acidic proteins.

ANALYTICAL DISC ELECTROPHORESIS

Since disc electrophoresis in an acidic buffer system provides a quick screening procedure for the detection of basic proteins in biological materials, oyster hemolymph containing lysozymelike activities was subjected to this precedure to determine whether a hemolymph component similar to the mobility of egg white lysozyme was, indeed, present. Specifically the disc electrophoresis system of Reisfeld *et al.* (1962) for the isolation of basic proteins was employed; it consists of a 7.5% and 15% small pore running gel (pH 4.2) with a 2.5% large pore upper gel (pH 6.8) in a β-alanine buffer (pH 4.4).

In the 15% gel, oyster hemolymph is characterized by the three prominent anodal bands exhibited in Fig. 1. A relatively diffused band (fraction a) remains in the large pore gel, while a distinct band (fraction b) and a broadly diffused band (fraction c) appear in the upper portion of the running gel. Egg white

Oyster Hemolymph
15 % gel, pH 4.2

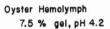

a
b

c

Fig. 1. Disc electrophoresis of oyster
hemolymph and egg white lysozyme
in 15% polyacrylamide gel (pH 4.2).
The direction of protein migration
is from anode (top) toward cathode
(bottom). Note the absence of lysozyme band in oyster hemolymph.

Oyster   Lysozyme
Hemolymph

Oyster Hemolymph
7.5 % gel, pH 4.2

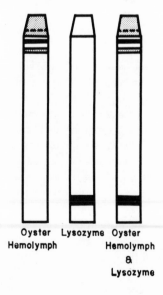

Fig. 2. Disc electrophoresis of oyster hemolymph, egg white lysozyme and a mixture of oyster hemolymph and egg white lysozyme
in 7.5% polyacrylamide gel (*p*H
4.2). The direction of protein migration is from anode (top) toward
cathode (bottom). Note again the
absence of lysozyme band in oyster
hemolymph and complete separation of oyster hemolymph proteins
from lysozyme in the gel where a
mixture of oyster hemolymph and
lysozyme was applied.

Oyster   Lysozyme   Oyster
Hemolymph   Hemolymph
                        &
                     Lysozyme

lysozyme, on the other hand, manifests itself as a clearly defined, single, cathodal fraction indicating that it is a basic protein. Thus, although oyster hemolymph seems to contain lysozymelike activities, it apparently does not contain a
band comparable to that of the egg white lysozyme.

Results of coelectrophoresis of oyster hemolymph, egg white lysozyme, and
a mixture of oyster hemolymph and egg white lysozome on three separate 7.5%
gel preparations are shown in Fig. 2. As can be seen, a considerable amount of
oyster hemolymph proteins appears to be trapped in the large pore gel. In
addition, oyster hemolymph contains two anodal bands, but it lacks, as in the
15% gel, the basic protein band that corresponds with the egg white lysozyme
band at the cathode. In the electrophoresed mixture of oyster hemolymph and
egg white lysozyme, three bands of oyster hemolymph origin appear in the
anodal region, while a faster moving band of egg white lysozyme is found at the
cathode.

PREPARATIVE DISC ELECTROPHORESIS

In order to determine which oyster hemolymph protein fraction(s)contain
lysozymelike activities, enough materials were obtained from each fraction using
the preparative disc electrophoresis technique. Fractions a, b, and c contain
0.56, 1.72, and 4.16 mg protein/ml respectively; the corresponding specific lysozymelike activity is 57, 10, and 2 units/mg of protein, 83% of which remains in
the large pore gel. Apparently little or no activity was associated with basic
proteins.

ION EXCHANGE CHROMATOGRAPHY

Oyster hemolymph was subjected to a modified cation exchange chromatography (Amberlite CG-50) described by Bonavida *et al.* (1967) and Parry *et al.*
(1969). As Fig. 3 illustrates, 14 UV absorption peaks are discernible. Lysozymelike activities are, however, only detected in peaks 4, 9, and 10, when each
peak is tested for lysozymelike activities using a standard suspension of *Micrococcus lysodeikticus.* Peaks 9 and 10 exhibit 33 units/ml of activities, while peak 4
has only 1 unit/ml. Of particular interest are the results summarized in Fig. 4.
The pooled material of peaks 9 and 10 was desalted and concentrated and then
subjected to disc and polyacrylamide gel electrophoresis (15% gel, pH 4.2; 15%
gel, *p*H 8.4). In each run, egg white lysozyme was incorporated as a control. As
is clear, the protein concentrate of peaks 9 and 10 barely enters the large pore
gel of the acidic gel, while the egg white lysozyme migrates to the cathodal
region of the gel. The isolated oyster hemolymph protein exhibits three cathodal
components in the basic gel (pH 8.4), while the egg white lysozyme, a basic
protein, does not enter the gel at all.

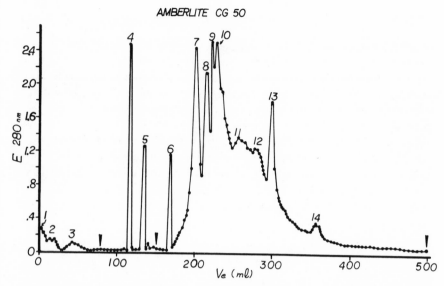

Fig. 3. Ion exchange chromatography on Amberlite CG-50 (2.5 × 11.6 cm) of oyster native hemolymph. The resin was previously equilibrated with 0.2 M sodium phosphate buffer, pH 6.5 and 3.5 ml fractions were collected. Protein concentration of each fraction was determined by UV absorption at 280 nm. Lysozymelike activity was screened for each UV absorption peak as well as valleys indicated by solid arrow heads.

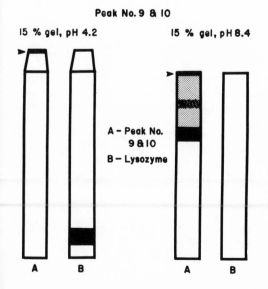

Fig. 4. Electrophoresis of materials recovered from peaks 9 and 10 in 15% polyacrylamide gel at pH 4.2 and 8.4. In the acidic gel, the oyster protein barely entered the large pore gel at the anode while the egg white lysozyme band (B) was found at its usual location near the cathode. In the basic gel, three cathodal bands of oyster hemolymph origin were found at the upper part of the gel (A) while egg white lysozyme, a basic protein, did not enter the gel (B) as expected. The direction of protein migration in the basic gel system was from the cathode (top) toward anode (bottom).

FINAL COMMENT

It is concluded that the lysozymelike activity of oyster hemolymph is associated with acidic proteins of different electrophoretic mobilities. The data illustrate the danger in relating the humoral principles of invertebrates with seemingly comparable immunological parameters or biochemical constituents of vertebrate origin. Such immunological equivalents may, indeed, exist and contribute to our understanding of the evolution of the immune mechanism. However, as there is such a tremendous diversity between the morphological structure and function of vertebrates and invertebrates, it is highly probable that invertebrates possess humoral defense mechanisms not found in vertebrates at all. Hence, the lysozymelike activity found in the oyster hemolymph may represent a case of functional convergence during the course of biochemical evolution.

REFERENCES

Bonavida, B., Sapse, A. T., and Sercarz, E. E., 1967, Human tear lysozyme. I. Purification, physicochemical, and immunochemical characterization, *J. Lab. Clin. Med. 70*:951-962.

Feng, S. Y. and Canzonier, W. J., 1970, Humoral responses in the American oyster (*Crassostrea virginica*) infected with *Bucephalus* sp. and *Minchinia nelsoni*, in: *A Symposium on Diseases of Fishes and Shellfishes, Special Pub. No. 5, pp. 497-510 (S. F. Snieszko, ed.), American Fisheries Society.*

Jolles, P., 1960, Lysozyme, in: *The Enzymes, Vol. 4*, 2nd ed., pp. 432-445 (P. D. Boyer, H. Lardy, and K. Myrback, eds.), Academic Press, New York.

Jolles, P. and Zuili, S., 1960, Purification et étude comparée de nouveaux lysozymes: extraits du poumon de poule et de *Nephthys hombergi, Biochim. Biophys. Acta 39*:212-217.

McDade, J. E. and Tripp, M. R., 1967*a*, Lysozyme in the hemolymph of the oyster, *Crassostrea virginica, J. Invertebr. Pathol. 9*:531-535.

McDade, J. E. and Tripp, M. R., 1967*b*, Lysozyme in oyster mantle mucus, *J. Invertebr. Pathol. 9*:581-582.

Messner, B. and Mohrig, W., 1969, Zum Lysozym-Vorkommen bei Muscheln, *Anodonta anatina* (L.), *Zool. Jahrb. Physiol. 74*:427-435.

Meyer, K., Hohnel, E., and Steinberg, A., 1946, Lysozyme of plant origin, *J. Biol. Chem. 163*:733-740.

Mohrig, W. and Messner, B., 1968, Immunreaktionen bei Insekten I. Lysozym als grundlegender antibakterieller Faktor im humoralen Abwehrmechanismus der Insekten. *Biol. Zb., L'vivs'k. Derzh. Univ. 87*:439-470.

Parry, Jr., R. M., Chandan, R. C., and Shahani, K. M., 1969, Isolation and characterization of human milk lysozyme, *Arch. Biochem. Biophys. 103*:59-65.

Perin, J.-P. and Jolles, P., 1972, The lysozyme from *Nephthys hombergi* (Annelid), Biochim. Biophys. Acta 263:683-689.

Reisfeld, R. A., Lewis, U. J., and Williams, D. E., 1962, Disk electrophoresis of basic proteins and peptides on polyacrylamide gels, *Nature 195*:(4838): 281-283.

Schubert, V. I. and Messner, B., 1971, Untersuchungen über das Vorkommen von Lysozym bei Anneliden, *Zool. Jahrb. Physiol.* 76:36-50.

Chapter 20

Induction of Internal Defense Mechanisms in the Lobster, Homarus americanus

James E. Stewart and B. M. Zwicker

Fisheries Research Board of Canada
Halifax Laboratory, P.O. Box 429
Halifax, Nova Scotia, Canada

INTRODUCTION

Invertebrates in general have the following nonspecific, hemolymph defense mechanisms: (1) bactericidal activity, (2) agglutinin activity, and (3) phagocytic activity which were recently reviewed in depth by Sindermann (1971) for the crustaceans. The overall effectiveness of these mechanisms in nature, together with mechanical barriers to transmission and possibly other intrinsic defenses can be judged only by the limited data available on epizootics occurring among natural stocks. Apparently, the effectiveness is high since more or less constant exposure to relatively large numbers of different microorganisms does not appear to result in epizootics until the exposure includes an infectious agent uniquely suited to overcome the invertebrate's defenses. In this, the invertebrates compare favorably with other animals.

DISEASE AND IMMUNITY IN CRUSTACEANS

Gaffkya homari, the microorganism causing the fatal infection, gaffkemia, in the American lobster, is one infective agent particularly able to overcome the lobster's defenses. A recent review of this disease (Stewart and Rabin, 1970) illustrates the inability of the lobster's phagocytic, bactericidal, and agglutinating capacities to reduce the severity of this infection. *In vitro* tests performed with lobster hemolymph agglutinin have shown that, although a wide variety of

microorganisms (*Achromobacter thalassius, Bacillus subtilis, Brevibacterium* sp.,
*Flavobacterium marinus, Gaffkya tetragena, Micrococcus conglomeratus, Micro-
coccus sedentarius,* and *Pseudomonas perfectomarinus*) were agglutinated, none
of four strains of *G. homari* were affected (Cornick and Stewart, 1968). In
addition, although *G. homari* was phagocytosed *in vivo,* this action did not clear
the pathogen from the host. The pathogen, after causing a massive decline in
circulating hemocyte numbers, flourished in the hemolymph, reaching numbers
of 1×10^8 to 1×10^9/ml considerably in advance of the death of the lobster.
The bactericidin of the lobster's hemolymph (Cornick and Stewart, 1968), as in
the case of the agglutinin, was effective against the microorganisms listed above,
but did not interfere with the growth of *G. homari.* In fact, as would be expected, the lobster hemolymph serum was an excellent growth medium for the
pathogen (Rabin, 1965; Cornick and Stewart, 1968). These data illustrated reasons for the lobster's inability to cope with *G. homari* infections initiated by
infective agent numbers ranging from very few (1×10^1/kg host body wt) to
very high (1×10^9/kg host body wt). The times to death at $15°C$ were virtually
the same, i.e., approximately 2 weeks, regardless of inoculum size.

The possibility of inducing some form of resistance to this disease has been
encouraged by the demonstration of humoral responses to the injection of foreign materials by a number of aquatic invertebrates. Recent work (Bang, 1967)
revealed that a lysin could be induced almost immediately and spontaneously in
Sipunculus by the injection of crab blood or the marine ciliate, *Anophrys.* The
immediacy of the response along with the lack of specificity led Bang to conclude that the lysin was not comparable to vertebrate antibody.

Similar findings have been reported in the extensive study of the induction
of bactericidin in invertebrates initiated by Evans *et al.* (1968) using as the
inducing agent a Gram-negative bacterium isolated from the intestine of *Panulirus argus.* The injection of formalin killed suspensions of this bacterium induced
bactericidins in the spiny lobsters, *P. argus* (Evans *et al.,* 1968 and 1969*a,* and
Weinheimer *et al.,* 1969), *P. interruptus* (Evans *et al.,* 1969*b*), the American
lobster (Acton *et al.,* 1969), the abalones, *Haliotis rufescens, H. corrugata,* and
H. cracherodii (Cushing *et al.,* 1971), and sipunculid worms (Evans *et al.,*
1969*c*). Several noteworthy general characteristics were: (1) the period required
for the induction was brief, usually around 48 hr, (2) the duration of the
enhanced bactericidal activity was relatively short (several weeks), (3) a background bactericidal level was observed in hemolymph drawn prior to injection of
the inducing agent, and (4) the induced bactericidins appeared to lack the specificity of vertebrate antibody.

Stewart and Zwicker (1972), following the lead of Evans *et al.* (1968) and
Acton *et al.* (1969), produced an enhancement of bactericidal activity of hemo-
lymph of American lobsters by injection of vaccines prepared from a strain of
Pseudomonas perolens isolated from the intestine of the lobster, *H. americanus.*

Table I. Source of Bactericidin(s)^a

I

No. of lobsters	Mean bactericidal values before and after induction^b							
	Mean hemocyte number per mm³ hemolymph		Serum		Hemocyte-free plasma		Pooled hemocyte extracts	
	A	B	A	B	A	B	A	B
10	19,400	11,300	76	608	80	264	60	43

*A represents preinduction and B represents postinduction.

II

Mean bactericidal values

Postinduction^b values

No. of lobsters	Control lobsters (noninduced)			Experimental lobsters (induced)			Combination of postinduction^b components^c mixed in equal volumes			
	Serum	Plasma	Hemocyte extracts	Serum	Plasma	Hemocyte extracts	EHE + CP	CHE + CP	CHE + EP	EHE + EP
6	93	17	<10	533	127	<10	68	50	480	352

^{a}Summarized from Stewart and Zwicker (1972).
^{b}Vaccine – *P. perolens* (all live animal work at 15° C).
^{c}E = Experimental (induced); HE = hemocyte extract; C = control (noninduced); P = plasma.

The extent of enhancement *in vivo* was roughly proportional to the concentration of the vaccine with peak activity recorded at approximately 48 hr, and the duration of the enhancement compared favorably with that observed by Evans and his co-workers; the enhancement *in vivo* was temperature-dependent. Heat stability trials suggested that more than one bactericidin was present and that the induced bactericidin(s) possibly was different from the low titer, background bactericidal activity present prior to injection of the vaccine. The bactericidal activity could be enhanced considerably, *in vitro*, by small reductions in the pH of the assay medium, e.g., by reducing normal hemolymph pH of 7.6 to pH 7.0. This *in vitro* enhancement was to a certain extent reversible. The most interesting finding, reproduced in abbreviated form in Table I, was the observation that the bactericidal principle(s) exists in the hemolymph in an inactive form until activated by material contained within the hemocytes and released upon their rupture.

Bactericidins were not induced in the American lobster within 48 hr by vaccines prepared from *G. homari* or *P. perolens* ATCC 10575 (Stewart and Zwicker, 1972). However, vaccines from several Gram-negative organisms (several pseudomonads and an *Achromobacter*), isolated from the intestine of the lobster, did induce an enhanced bactericidal titer, and, in addition, one Gram-positive intestinal isolate, *Sarcina lutea*, produced an increased titer active against the intestinal isolate, *P. perolens*, but not against itself. Attempts to demonstrate resistance among lobsters to *G. homari* upon enhancement of the bactericidal activity were uniformly negative when the lobsters were challenged with the pathogen within 4 days of injection with vaccines prepared from *P. perolens* (intestinal isolate), *G. homari*, and *S. lutea* (intestinal isolate).

Subsequent experiments in which lobsters were injected with vaccines prepared from avirulent strains of *G. homari* showed that a degree of resistance to virulent strains of *G. homari* could be induced (Table II). The degree of resistance is apparent in the increased times to death for those lobsters injected with the vaccines of the avirulent strain of *G. homari* 9 days prior to challenge. No relationship appears to exist between the bactericidal levels and the degree of resistance; repeated injections did not produce higher degrees of resistance. Further evidence of the differences exists in the shorter time necessary, 48 hr, for the induction of maximal bactericidal levels in contrast to the time required for a degree of resistance to become apparent, e.g., not evident at 4 days but observed for the lobsters injected with vaccines 9 days prior to challenge. Again, as with the bactericidins, the induced resistance appears to be short lived. Experiments are in progress to determine whether the resistance observed can be completely effective when smaller challenge doses are used.

The development in the American lobster of a degree of resistance to *G. homari*, which is apparently unrelated to bactericidal activity in the hemolymph, is comparable to the findings of McKay and Jenkin (1969). These authors, working with the fresh-water crayfish, *Parachaeraps bicarinatus*, have shown an

Table II. Relation between Bactericidin(s) and Protection[a]

Lobsters	Mean time to death days ± S.E.	Bactericidal titer P. perolens as test organism
A – Single injection of vaccine[c]		
Noninduced controls (infected)	14.6 ± 1.1	40
4 days after vaccination	15.3	160
9 days	26.0 ± 0.7	160
20 days	17.5 ± 2.58	160
30 days	17.3 ± 2.9	80
B – Multiple injections of vaccines		
Noninduced controls (infected)	14.4	40
Vaccines[b]		
P. perolens (4×)	14.8	640
G. homari ATCC 10400 (5×)	22.5	640
Formalized saline (5×)	13.6	80

[a]Methodology given in Stewart and Zwicker (1972).
[b]Given once/week
Lobsters challenged with virulent strain G. homari (approximately 2 × 10⁶ cells/kg host body wt) 2 days after last vaccination (10 lobsters/group held at 15°C).
[c]All lobsters, except for the controls, received a single injection of a vaccine of G. homari ATCC 10400, an avirulent strain. All lobsters challenged with avirulent strain of G. homari (approximately 2 × 10⁶ bacterial cells/kg host body wt). Each group contained 10 lobsters held at 15°C.

induced or adaptive resistance to a pseudomonad moderately pathogenic before immunization of the host with vaccines prepared from the pathogen as well as from two other microorganisms, *Pseudomonas fluorescens* and *Salmonella typhimurium*. They concluded that neither lytic nor cytocidal principles were involved; the induced resistance constituted a different kind of crustacean response from any previously reported.

FINAL REMARKS

McKay and Jenkin (1969) proposed, as a useful device for studies and discussions of defense mechanisms in invertebrates, the criterion of functionality. *In vitro,* the heat labile bactericidal principle of the American lobster's hemolymph did partially inhibit the growth of a number of microorganisms nonpathogenic to the lobster (Cornick and Stewart, 1968). When the bactericidin was inactivated by heat, two of the microorganisms, *A. thalassius* and *P.*

perfectomarinus, were no longer inhibited, but instead grew as well in the serum as does *G. homari*. The functionality of the bactericidin(s) may rest in its ability to eliminate microorganisms which, in its absence, would be just as pathogenic as *G. homari*.

Among the interesting, unanswered questions concerning the bactericidin(s) of invertebrates, in general, are those relating to the nature of the bactericidin, the question as to whether its enhancement is a result of *de novo* synthesis or merely the release of preformed material, the sites of synthesis and/or storage, the exact nature of the signals provoking the enhancement and controlling the circulating concentration levels, the major site of action *in vivo*, i.e., inside or outside the hemocyte, and the nature of the limited but real specificity required of the inducing agent. The other aspect of the work reviewed cursorily and briefly in this article concerns the precise nature of the induced resistance reported by McKay and Jenkin (1969) for the fresh-water crayfish and confirmed in preliminary experiments by ourselves for the American lobster.

McKay and Jenkin (1970*a*,*b*) and Sindermann (1971) suggest a central role for phagocytes in invertebrate resistance and suggest that induced resistance is a function of altered phagocytic abilities (McKay and Jenkin, 1970*a*,*b*) or, in a slightly different form, an augmentation of phagocytosis by relatively nonspecific innate or acquired humoral factors (Sindermann, 1971). With the increased effort now being applied generally to studying natural or acquired humoral factors and resistance in invertebrates, precise descriptions and understandings of these mechanisms hopefully should follow soon.

REFERENCES

Acton, R. T., Weinheimer, P. F., and Evans, E. E., 1969, A bactericidal system in the lobster *Homarus americanus*, *J. Invertebr. Pathol. 13*:463-464.

Bang, F. B., 1967, Serological responses among invertebrates other than insects, *Federation Proc. 26*:1680-1684.

Cornick, J. W. and Stewart, J. E., 1968, Interaction of the pathogen *Gaffkya homari* with natural defense mechanisms of *Homarus americanus, J. Fisheries Res. Board Can. 25*:695-709.

Cushing, J. E., Evans, E. E., and Evans, M. L., 1971, Induced bactericidal responses of abalones, *J. Invertebr. Pathol. 17*:446-448.

Evans, E. E., Painter, B., Evans, M. L., Weinheimer, P., and Acton, R. T., 1968, An induced bactericidin in the spiny lobster, *Panulirus argus, Proc. Soc. Exp. Biol. Med. 128*:394-398.

Evans, E. E., Weinheimer, P. F., Painter, B., Acton, R. T., and Evans, M. L., 1969*a*, Secondary and tertiary responses of the induced bactericidin from West Indian spiny lobster, *Panulirus argus, J. Bacteriol. 98*:943-946.

Evans, E. E., Cushing, J. E., Sawyer, S., Weinheimer, P. F., Acton, R. T., and McNeely, J. L., 1969*b*, Induced bactericidal response in the California spiny lobster, *Panulirus interruptus* (34160), *Proc. Soc. Exp. Biol. Med. 132*:111-114.

Evans, E. E., Weinheimer, P. F., and Acton, R. T., 1969c, Induced bactericidal response in a sipunculid worm, *Nature (London)* 222:695.

McKay, D. and Jenkin, C. R., 1969, Immunity in the invertebrates. II. Adaptive immunity in the crayfish (*Parachaeraps bicarinatus*), *Immunology 17*:127-137.

McKay, D. and Jenkin, C. R., 1970a, Immunity in the invertebrates. The role of serum factors in phagocytosis of erythrocytes by hemocytes of the fresh-water crayfish (*Parachaeraps bicarinatus*), *Australian J. Exp. Biol. Med. Sci. 48*:139-150.

McKay, D. and Jenkin, C. R., 1970b, Immunity in the invertebrates. Correlation of the phagocytic activity of hemocytes with resistance to infection in the crayfish (*Parachaeraps bicarinatus*), *Australian J. Exp. Biol. Med. Sci. 48*:609-617.

Rabin, H., 1965, Studies on gaffkemia, a bacterial disease of the American lobster, *Homarus americanus* (Milne Edwards), *J. Invertebr. Pathol. 7*:391-397.

Sindermann, C. J., 1971, Internal defenses of crustacea: a review, *Nat. Marine Fisheries Serv. Fisheries Bull., 69*:455-489.

Stewart, J. E. and Rabin, H., 1970, Gaffkemia, a bacterial disease of lobsters (Genus *Homarus*), in: *A Symposium on Diseases of Fishes and Shellfishes,* Spec. Publ. 5, pp. 431-439 (S. F. Snieszko, ed.), American Fisheries Society.

Stewart, J. E. and Zwicker, B. M., 1972, Natural and induced bactericidal activities in the hemolymph of the lobster, *Homarus americanus:* products of hemocyte–plasma interaction, *Can J. Microbiol. 18*:1499-1509.

Weinheimer, P. F., Acton, R. T., Sawyer, S., and Evans, E. E., 1969, Specificity of the induced bactericidin of the West Indian spiny lobster, *Panulirus argus, J. Bacteriol. 98*:947-948.

Chapter 21

Comparison of a Natural Agglutinin
in the Hemolymph of
the Blue Crab, Callinectes sapidus,
with Agglutinins of Other Invertebrates

Gilbert B. Pauley*

*National Marine Fisheries Service
Middle Atlantic Coastal Fisheries Center
Pathobiology Investigations
Oxford, Maryland*

INTRODUCTION

Cultivation of many invertebrates is of commercial value and an understanding of their immune mechanisms is important for combating the pernicious diseases that often debilitate them. Invertebrates possess a variety of humoral substances involved in internal defense that differ considerably from classical vertebrate antibodies (Bang, 1967; Carton, 1969; Feng, 1967; Sindermann, 1971; Tripp, 1970). Many of these hemolymph factors agglutinate a variety of foreign materials. Cantacuzéne (1923) summarized his findings on invertebrate humoral substances including those capable of agglutination. Although his articles contain elaborate claims of results without adequate experimental data presented in protocol form, subsequent investigators are confirming many of these claims.

Spider crab (*Maia squinado*) sera agglutinate the protozoan, *Anophrys sarcophaga* (Bang, 1962, 1967). However, it may be more common that hemolymph substances lyse Protozoa rather than agglutinate them (Bang, 1962, 1966, 1967; Feng and Stauber, 1968). Bacteria are agglutinated by sera from the sipunculid worm, *Phascolosoma agassizzi* (Blitz, 1966) and by the hemolymph

*Present address: Washington Cooperative Fishery Unit, University of Washington, Seattle, Washington.

from the lobster, *Homarus americanus,* and the crab *Cancer irroratus* (Cornick and Stewart, 1968a,b). Pauley (1971) found natural agglutinins against several marine bacteria in the sea hare, *Aplysia californica.* According to Tyler and Metz (1945), the California spiny lobster, *Panulirus interruptus,* contains tissue heteroagglutinins in the serum that act on the cells of all species belonging to the same group (Class). By exhaustive cross-adsorption tests, any single species will remove agglutinins for all species tested that belong to the same Class. Natural agglutinins against invertebrate spermatozoa are known in several invertebrate Classes (Tyler, 1946; Smith and Goldstein, 1971).

The agglutinins most commonly observed and studied among invertebrates are those which agglutinate vertebrate red blood cells (RBC). Several of these have been studied in some detail and these include RBC agglutinins of the California sea hare, *Aplysia californica* (Pauley *et al.,* 1971a); the hermit crab, *Paguristes ulreyi* (Cushing, 1967); the crayfish, *Procambarus clarkii* (Miller *et al.,* 1972); the snail, *Viviparus malleatus* (Cheng and Sanders, 1962); the coconut crab, *Birgus latro* (Cohen, 1968); the starfish, *Asterias forbesi* (Finstad *et al.,* 1972); the Murray mussel, *Velesunio ambiguus* (Jenkin and Rowley, 1970); the crayfish, *Parachaeraps bicarinatus* (McKay *et al.,* 1969); and the cockroaches, *Periplaneta americana* (Scott, 1972) and *Blabarus craniifer* (Anderson *et al.,* 1972). An agglutinating protein from the albumin gland of the snail, *Helix pomatia* (Hammarström and Kabat, 1969) is the subject of extensive study, along with similar substances from other snails of the same genus. The two most thoroughly studied invertebrate hemolymph RBC agglutinins are those in the oyster, *Crassostrea virginica* (Tripp, 1966; McDade and Tripp, 1967; Li and Flemming, 1967; Acton *et al.,* 1969) and the horseshoe crab, *Limulus polyphemus* (Cohen *et al.,* 1965; Cohen, 1968, 1970, 1971; Marchalonis and Edelman, 1968; Finstad *et al.,* 1972).

Much of the information available on invertebrate agglutinins has been reviewed recently (Cohen, 1973; Finstad, 1973; Pauley, 1973b; Tripp, 1973; Acton, this volume). Due to the extensive work on invertebrate agglutinins, it is well known that these molecules have diverse structures and functions and differ significantly from vertebrate antibodies. Continued research on invertebrate immune mechanisms will provide further insight into the evolution of immune responses in both invertebrates and vertebrates. Recently, Pauley (1973a) found that serum from the blue crab, *Callinectes sapidus,* will agglutinate RBC. This paper deals in detail with the physicochemical properties and function of this blue crab agglutinin which are compared to RBC agglutinins of other invertebrates.

DISCUSSION

General

I collected the crabs, *C. sapidus,* or obtained them from a commercial supplier at Oxford, Maryland. They were housed in tanks supplied with aerated running water from the Tred Avon River, a tributary of Chesapeake Bay. The water was maintained at ambient summer temperatures. Crabs were fed raw chicken or fish *ad libitum,* but cannibalistic tendencies tended to select survival for the stronger crabs. Unless cannibalized, crabs survive several weeks under the above conditions.

All crabs were bled only once using a sterile 5.0 or 10.0 ml syringe and 20-gauge 1½" needle. The posterior portion of the carapace was swabbed with 70% ethanol before withdrawing hemolymph from the pericardial cavity. Hemolymph from a minimum of five male and five female crabs with a carapace width of five inches or more was collected for each test to be performed and was allowed to clot around an applicator stick. The clot was then easily removed. The resultant serum was pooled and passed through a Swinnex-25 millipore filter (0.45 μ pore size) into sterile tubes and utilized immediately or dated and frozen at $-25°C$.

Agglutinin Titers

A 0.05 ml suspension of 2.0% (by volume) rabbit RBC in saline was added to Kahn tubes containing serial twofold dilutions of 1.0 ml crab serum in 0.15 M NaCl. Just prior to use, RBC were washed three times in 0.15 M saline and centrifuged at 2500 RPM/10 min at 4°C. Each agglutination test was conducted in triplicate, and the degree of agglutination was determined after 24 hr incubation at 27°C. The degree of agglutination was judged from a very strong (++++) to a very weak (+) reaction with a dissecting microscope (30X) and the titer was expressed as the reciprocal of the dilution. Control tubes contained 0.5 ml of either untreated serum or 0.15 M saline inoculated with RBC. All agglutination experiments were repeated at least once with rabbit RBC preserved in modified Alsevers solution.

Normal serum agglutination titers of *Callinectes sapidus* against vertebrate RBC varied between individuals, although never more than twofold (Table I). Rabbit RBC gave the highest titer, 64. These results corroborate earlier work by several investigators who found that titers of invertebrate hemolymph agglutinins are in general very low, usually < 1:500 (Tripp, 1966; McKay *et al.,* 1969; Pauley *et al.,* 1971; Miller *et al.,* 1972). An exception to this condition is the agglutinin in the snail, *Helix lactea,* which has a titer of > 1:8,000 (Boyd and Brown, 1965; Boyd *et al.,* 1966). Moreover, these titers cannot be increased substantially by prior injections of either bacteria (Pauley, 1971) or RBC (Tripp, 1966; Pauley, 1973a). Blue crab agglutinin can be increased slightly for a short period of time, but the reaction is nonspecific, since both chicken RBC and sterile saline evoke a slight increase in titer comparable to that caused by rabbit RBC (Pauley, 1973a). Studies of other invertebrates show that humoral immune responses, in general, are ephemeral and nonspecific (Bang, 1966; Chadwick, 1967; Sindermann, 1971; Stewart and Zwicker, 1972). Exceptions to these generalities

Table I. Range of Serum Agglutination Titers
from Five Male and Five Female Blue Crabs
(Callinectes sapidus)[a]

Test cells	Titer range
Human RBC (type O)	8–32
Rabbit RBC	16–64
Chicken RBC	8–32
Saline control	0

[a] Serum was not pooled for this test.

apparently exist, such as a complete lack of any type of immune response (Teague and Friou, 1964), or a prolonged period before any response is noticed (Evans *et al.*, 1969).

The titer of blue crab agglutinin is sex related (Table II) and is significantly higher in males (P = 0.01). Cushing (1967) noted that the hemagglutinin in the hermit crab varies among individuals but is not correlated with the animal's sex. Kothbauer and Brunner (1971) found no sexual relationship to agglutinins in several species of snails. The hemagglutinin in the serum of the coconut crab is apparently related to weight and possibly sexual development; agglutinins are completely absent in the sera of the very young (Cohen, 1968). According to Bang (1967), spider crab agglutinin spontaneously disappears during the molting cycle. The findings of Kothbauer *et al.*, (1972) indicate a close relationship between the agglutinin and the development of the reproductive apparatus in snails *(Helix pomatia)*; the agglutinin is found only in fully developed animals. Agglutinin titers are directly proportional to the total protein content of hemolymph in snails (Cheng and Saunders, 1962) and in oysters (Tripp, 1966). However, Pauley *et al.* (1971a) did not find the same relationship between hemolymph proteins and titers in the California sea hare.

Table II. Relationship of Blue Crab (*Callinectes
sapidus*) Serum Agglutinin against Rabbit
RBC to Sex of the Crab

Sex	Number of test animals	Mean agglutination titer	Range of agglutination titer
Male	9	48	16–64
Female	12	28	16–64

Physical and Chemical Properties

The effect of temperature on agglutinin activity was studied by assaying crab serum with rabbit RBC after the following treatments: (1) repeated freezing and thawing in a dry ice–ethanol bath, (2) freezing for 2 weeks to 6 months at −25°C, and (3) heating at various temperatures from 40°C to 80°C for 30 min followed by rapid cooling in an ice bath. To test the effect of dialysis on agglutinin activity, sera were dialyzed in 8 × 100 Visking tubing (Union Carbide Corporation) for 24 hr at 4°C against 0.15 M NaCl, 0.01 M hydroxymethyl aminomethane (TRIS) buffer ("TB") adjusted to a pH of 7.5, the mean physiological pH of crab serum. TB baths were changed three times during each dialysis. To test the effect of pH on the agglutinin, sera were separated into 2.5 ml portions and the pH was adjusted to various levels by adding appropriate amounts of 1.0 M and 10.0 M HCl or NaOH. After 4 hr incubation at room temperature, any precipitate formed was centrifuged at 5000 RPM/15 min at 4°C and the supernatant dialyzed for 24 hr against three changes of TB. The dialyzed serum was subsequently tested for agglutinating activity.

The naturally occurring agglutinin in *C. sapidus* serum was stable at low temperatures (−25°C) and after repeated freezing and thawing (Table III). The

Table III. Tests Performed to Determine the Stability and Nature of the Natural Agglutinin in the Serum of *Callinectes sapidus*

Experimental procedure	No inactivation	Partial inactivation	Total inactivation
Physical treatments			
Prolonged freezing (6 months)	+		
Repeated freezing and thawing	+		
Heat (50°C)	+		
Heat (60°C)			+
Alkaline pH extremes			+
Acidic pH extremes			+
Dialysis		+	
Chemical treatments			
Trichloroacetic acid extraction			+
Phenol extraction			+
Diethyl ether extraction	+		
Na citrate chelation	+		
Urea incubation		+	
Enzyme treatments			
Trypsin	+		
Pepsin	+		

agglutinin was stable after incubation at 50°C/30 min but was completely inactivated after incubation at 60°C/30 min (Table III). It was active at pH values
between 6 and 11 and was completely inactivated at acidic and alkaline pH
beyond these values (Fig. 1). Dialysis for 24 hr partially inactivated the agglutinin.

Crab sera were subjected to the following chemical tests: (1) dialysis against
0.4 *M* sodium citrate for 24 hr at 4°C (Acton *et al.*, 1969); (2) phenol extraction, according to the method of Kolb and Granger (1970), using diethyl ether
extraction as one type of control (Pauley *et al.*, 1971*a*); (3) 8.0 *M* urea (pH 7.0)
incubation (1 part urea:1 part serum incubated for 24 hr at 27'C); (4) 10%
trichloroacetic acid (TCA) extraction (1 part 20% TCA:1 part serum for 2 hr at
4°C). Formed precipitates were removed and all test sera were dialyzed at 4°C
for 24 hr, and then were subjected to agglutination assay with rabbit RBC.
Undialyzed and dialyzed sera served as controls.

Trypsin and pepsin (Worthington Laboratories) were incubated at 37°C
with pooled crab sera (1.0 μg or 10.0 μg enzyme/ml of serum) at pH 8.0 and 6.0,
respectively. After 24 hr the enzyme-treated sera were assayed for agglutinating
activity against rabbit RBC. A number of procedures were employed to determine the stability and nature of the agglutinating substance present in the serum

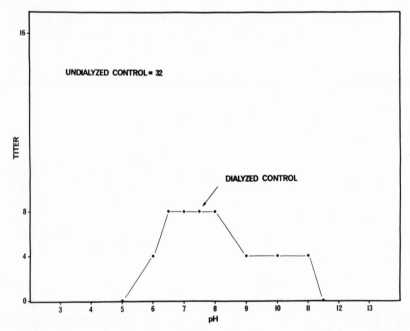

Fig. 1. Range of pH stability of blue crab agglutinin. Normal, undialyzed, control
serum exhibited a titer of 32. Note that dialysis reduces the agglutination titer.

of the blue crab. The results of these tests are presented in Table III. Only phenol and TCA were capable of completely inactivating the agglutinin, while urea partially inactivated the agglutinin.

The sensitivity of *Callinectes sapidus* agglutinin to phenol and TCA extraction suggests that its biological activity is not dependent upon nucleic acids or polysaccharides but may be due to a protein or lipoprotein. Although lipoproteins are dissolved in phenol (Nowotny, 1969), a lipid component in the agglutinin was ruled out on the basis of its stability to diethyl ether (Scanu, 1965), to prolonged freezing, and to three repeated freezings and thawings (Hatch and Lees, 1968). Cohen (1968) found that ten repeated freezings and thawings were needed to inhibit the agglutinin of *Limulus polyphemus*. At present it is assumed that the blue crab agglutinin is protein or contains a major protein component. This assumption is based on the agglutinin's susceptibility to heat, pH extremes, and to extractions with phenol, TCA, and urea. The inactivation of *C. sapidus* agglutinin by heat and pH extremes is characteristic of proteins (Fox and Foster, 1957; Florkin and Stotz, 1963). Proteins may be precipitated by phenol (Nowotny, 1969) and TCA (MacInnis and Voge, 1970). Urea will cause dissociation of hydrogen bonds in proteins and will often separate a protein into component subunits, as it does in horseshoe crab hemagglutinin (Marchalonis and Edelman, 1968). Enzymes indicate that either the blue crab agglutinin is not a protein or that the enzymes did not affect the active site of the molecule. Since trypsin causes hydrolysis of peptide bonds between the carboxyl group of only arginine or lysine, these amino acids may not be present in the active site of the agglutinin molecule, or, if they are, they may be protected from enzymatic action by the configuration of the agglutinin. Kolb and Granger (1968, 1970) observed that although both human and mouse lymphotoxin were protein as determined by their buoyant densities, they were resistant to trypsin digestion. The inability of pepsin to affect the agglutinin may have been due to the inactivity of the enzyme at pH 6.0, since its pH optimum is 2.0. Antibacterial factors in sipunculid worms are insensitive to pepsin for possibly the same reason (Krassner and Flory, 1970). Molluscan hemagglutinins are resistant to proteases (Pauley *et al.*, 1971a; Uhlenbruck *et al.*, 1971), and this may be a specific and peculiar property of invertebrate agglutinins. Uhlenbruck *et al.* (1971) suggested the use of protein digesting enzymes as a method of purifying molluscan hemagglutinins. Crayfish agglutinin is also resistant to proteolytic enzymes (Miller *et al.*, 1972).

Only a few invertebrate agglutinins are characterized in any great detail, and all exhibit certain common properties. However, when compared with vertebrate immunoglobulin, agglutinins show some obvious differences. *C. virginica* hemagglutinin is unaffected by dialysis, although aging renders it dialyzable, and it is heat labile (Tripp, 1966; Li and Flemming, 1967; Acton *et al.*, 1969). Oyster hemagglutinin is stable from pH 6–9 and breaks down into subunits beyond pH 7–8 (Li and Fleming, 1967; Acton *et al.*, 1969). It is therefore very similar to *A*.

californica agglutinin, and the reduced titer of sea hare agglutinin at pH extremes may indeed indicate dissociation of the molecule into subunits (Pauley *et al.*, 1971a).

Horseshoe crab (*L. polyphemus*) hemagglutinin has been studied extensively by Marchalonis and Edelman (1968), who found that, like oyster hemagglutinin, it could be separated into subunits by exposure to pH 3.0 or 9.6 followed by treatment with 8.0 M urea. They also showed that horseshoe crab hemagglutinin was stabilized by calcium ions and had no covalent linkages, such as disulfide bonds, between the subunits. In addition to hydrogen bonds, some invertebrate agglutinins are stabilized by covalent disulfide bonds because of their susceptibility to 2-mercaptoethanol (Sprenger and Uhlenbruck, 1971; Pauley *et al.*, 1971a). Sodium citrate had no effect on blue crab agglutinin, indicating a lack of 1968). Sodium citrate had no effect on blue crab agglutinin, indicating a lack of dependence on bivalent cations for stabilization as are those of the oyster, *C. virginica,* the horseshoe crab, *L. polyphemus,* the starfish, *A. forbesi* (Acton, *et al.,* 1969; Finstad, *et al.,* 1972). The sea hare agglutinin was not dependent upon divalent cations for stabilization (Pauley *et al.,* 1971a). However, the susceptibility of blue crab agglutinin to dialysis may indicate a need for calcium, which, if removed by dialysis, would not be replaced by the calcium-free dialysis fluid. Crayfish (*P. clarkii*) shares many of the same properties of blue crab agglutinin (Miller *et al.,* 1972). Crayfish activity was normal between pH 6.4 and 10.4, but was inactivated at both pH extremes. It was almost completely inactivated at 60°C and was inactivated with phenol and TCA.

Antisera were produced in rabbits. Freund's complete adjuvent (Difco) was mixed with an equal amount of antigen, either human gamma globulin (Hyland), crab serum, or crab agglutinin. These mixtures were administered weekly for 5 weeks as 1.0 ml subcutaneous and 2.0 ml intramuscular injections in the rabbits. Two weeks after the last injection, antiserum was collected by cardiac puncture, filter sterilized, and frozen at −25°C. Crab agglutinin was prepared by adsorbing crab serum with rabbit RBC for 24 hr. These RBC were then washed three times in 0.15 M NaCl, resuspended in saline, and mixed with adjuvent.

Immunoelectrophoresis was carried out with Gelman immunoelectrophoresis apparatus. Noble Agar (Difco) was washed for 72 hr in distilled water and made up as a 1.0% mixture in 0.05 ionic strength barbitol buffer at pH 8.2. Both the crab serum and rabbit antiserum were used undiluted. Electrophoretic separation of the crab serum was for 1 hr at 200 V. Precipitation was allowed to proceed at room temperature for 24 hr. Nonprecipitated protein was removed by rinsing in 0.15 M NaCl for 3 days followed by distilled water rinse for 2 hr. Slides were stained while wet by fixing in 2.0% acetic acid for 30–40 min and staining in 3.0% amido Schwartz (Buffalo black) for 1–5 seconds. Differentiation was accomplished in a solution of 225 ml methanol, 50 ml glacial acetic acid, and 500 ml distilled water.

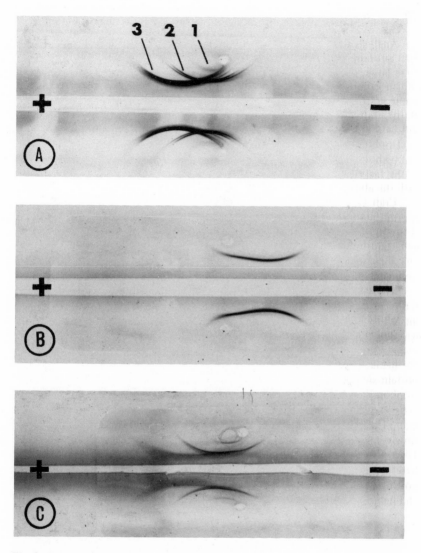

Fig. 2. Immunoelectrophoresis. (*a*). Normal crab serum showing two very small bands near the origin in region I and three large arcs in both regions II and III. (*b*). Purified human gamma globulin. Note lack of gamma globulin in normal crab serum. (*c*). Crab agglutinin appears to involve molecules in regions I and II and, to a lesser degree, those in region III.

Analysis of whole crab serum by immunoelectrophoresis showed eight distinct protein arcs (Fig. 2a): two very small arcs near the origin in region I and three large, distinct ones in both regions II and III. By comparison with purified human gamma globulin (Fig. 2b), clearly no gamma globulin fraction occurs in whole crab serum, since all of the crab proteins migrated toward the anode. All of the crab serum proteins showed a migratory pattern similar to human alpha and beta globulins. The crab agglutinin could not be isolated as a single immunoelectrophoretic band by adsorption with rabbit RBC. A strong arc was isolated from whole serum in both groups I and II, as well as a lighter more indistinct arc of the fastest moving group III (Fig. 2c), indicating that more than one molecule with the ability to agglutinate RBC is present in blue crab hemolymph.

Crab serum, human gamma globulin, and rabbit antiserum were placed in appropriate wells of immunodiffusion plates (Hyland) and allowed to precipitate at room temperature for 24 hr. Ouchterlony analysis showed that the crab hemagglutinin, although not in purified form, was apparently concentrated in one slow migrating protein band (Fig. 3a). No crab protein resembled human gamma globulin, as indicated by a lack of cross-reactivity (Figs. 3a,b).

The lack of any protein migrating in the gamma globulin region agreed with serum protein analysis of other invertebrate fluids (Woods et al., 1958). Adsorbing whole crab hemolymph with rabbit RBC indicates that agglutinating activity was possibly due to more than one protein, which was corroborated by Sephadex column chromatography of blue crab serum. Scott (1972) found that the hemagglutinin of the cockroach, Periplaneta americana, is a slowly migrating protein similar to an alpha globulin. Starch-gel electrophoresis and immunoelectrophoresis revealed that horseshoe crab (L. polyphemus) hemagglutinin is associated with an electrophoretically slowly moving protein (Marchalonis and Edelman, 1968; Finstad et al., 1972). Starfish (Asterias forbesi) agglutinin is also a slowly moving protein demonstrable by immunoelectrophoresis (Finstad et al., 1972). According to Tyler and Scheer (1945), spiny lobster (P. interruptus) heteroagglutinins were found in a single, slowly migrating electrophoretic component that was not hemocyanin. However, antisera indicated that agglutinins and hemocyanin are serologically equivalent.

Molecular Weight Studies

The partial stability of the agglutinin to dialysis indicates that a macromolecule is involved in addition to a small dialyzable factor. The approximate molecular weight of the blue crab agglutinin was estimated by molecular-sieve column chromatography. Sephadex G-50 or G-100 gel was poured in a 2.3 cm diameter Siliclad (Clay-Adams) coated glass column to a final height of 36.5 cm, and the column was equilibrated 24 hr with TB at pH 7.5. The column was loaded with 5 ml of pooled crab serum and eluted with TB at 4°C, and the flow

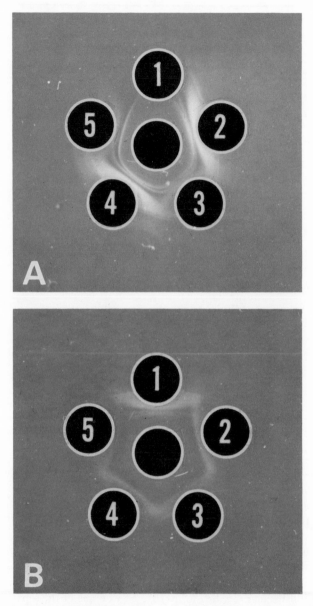

Fig. 3. Ouchterlony immunodiffusion analysis. (*a*). Center well contains normal blue crab serum. Crab hemagglutinin (well 5) appears to be concentrated primarily in one slow, migrating, protein and shows obvious identity reaction with normal crab hemolymph (wells 2–4). As expected, there is no response with antiserum to human gamma globulin (well 1). (*b*). Center well contains antiserum to normal crab serum and to human gamma globulin. Note nonidentity between crab serum (well 1) and gamma globulin (wells 2–5).

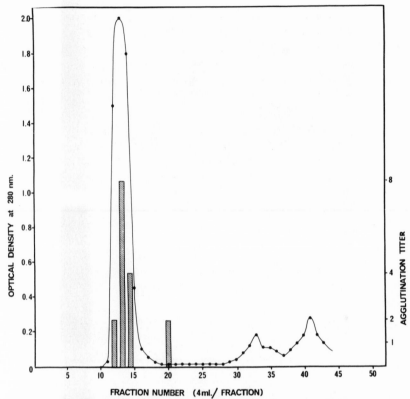

Fig. 4. Sephadex column chromatography separation of *C. sapidus* serum. Note majority of the agglutinating activity occurs with the single, major, protein peak, while a smaller, secondary localization of activity follows by several fractions. Blue dextran was located in fractions 12–14 and phenol red was in tubes 39–43.

rate was adjusted to 4.0 ml/8 min. Four-milliliter fractions were collected and assayed for protein concentration by measuring their absorption at 280 nm in a Beckman DU-2 Spectrophotometer and then were tested for agglutinating activity using rabbit RBC. A control titer was run on the pooled crab serum. Molecular-sieve column chromotography on Sephadex beads indicated that two separate agglutinins may exist. The weight of the larger molecule is at least 150,000, assuming that it is a globular protein (Fig. 4). The elution pattern of the large molecule on Sephadex G-50 and G-100 columns was the same as blue dextran, which has a molecular weight of 2×10^6. An example of the separation pattern in a G-50 column is shown in Fig. 4. Most of the agglutinating activity appeared in the single, major protein fraction which was eluted with the blue dextran. A smaller peak of activity could always be retrieved from the column a few tubes behind the blue dextran. Although no loss in agglutinin titer could be detected following freezing at $-25°C$, crab serum frozen for six months and then passed through a Sephadex G-50 column apparently lost most of the large molecular weight activity, but the smaller activity peak was usually unaffected by this process (Pauley, 1973b). Freezing may alter the blue crab agglutinin enough so that it is fixed to the Sephadex beads, as occurs at specific pH with anti-A agglutinin of *Helix pomatia* (Ishiyama and Uhlenbruck, 1972). Li and Flemming (1967) found oyster hemagglutinin activity associated with two distinct protein peaks after separation by Sephadex G-75 columns, indicating a molecular weight less than 75,000. This is in fair agreement with McDade and Tripp (1967), who estimated a molecular weight above 65,000. These authors were probably working with the subunits rather than the intact molecule because Acton *et al.* (1969) have since shown that oyster hemagglutinin is composed of noncovalently linked subunits with a molecular weight of 20,000, and that the entire molecule with all its subunits intact has a very high sedimentation coefficient of 33.4 S. This is farily close to the minor 31 S activity peak of sea hare agglutinin (Pauley *et al.*, 1971a). Two studies have shown that oyster hemagglutinin subunits were stabilized by calcium ions (McDade and Tripp, 1967; Acton *et al.*, 1969), but this was not true for *A. californica* agglutinin since it was not inactivated by sodium citrate (Pauley *et al.*, 1971a).

A hemagglutinin present in the mussel *V. ambiguus* has recently been purified and characterized (Jenkin and Rowley, 1970). The material was precipitated by 50% saturated ammonium sulfate, and subsequently purified by sucrose density-gradient centrifugation. Its sedimentation coefficient 28 S is similar to the minor 31 S activity peak of sea hare serum. Marchalonis and Edelman (1968) estimated a molecular weight of about 400,000 for horseshoe crab agglutinin, and it could be separated into subunits by pH extremes and urea. These observations have been corroborated by Cohen (1968) and Finstad *et al.* (1972).

Specificity and Function

In an attempt to immunize blue crabs with RBC (Pauley, 1973a), the agglutinin was found to be nonspecific. Both a heterologous antigen (chicken RBC) and sterile saline evoked a slight increase in titer, comparable to that of homologous antigen (Rabbit RBC). This response was thought to represent a simple variation of the normal titer range due to any nonspecific stress. The titer of *A. californica* agglutinin cannot be increased by prior bacterial challenge (Pauley, 1971) as would occur with vertebrate agglutinating antibodies.

Boyd and Brown (1965) indicated that *Helix lactea* agglutinin is highly specific. Subsequent studies by Boyd *et al.* (1966) revealed that this agglutinin is not present in the hemolymph but is confined to the snail's albumin gland. Kothbauer *et al.* (1972) found a close relationship between this agglutinin and sexual development, and assigned it some important role in reproduction. Boyd *et al.* (1966) did not find this high degree of specificity among other mollusks. The *Helix* sp. agglutinin is specific for human-A RBC. Uhlenbruck and Prokop (1966) accounted for this by the fact that human-A cells contain the sugar *N*-acetyl-D-galactosamine, which in a nonreducing terminal position will inhibit hemagglutination. Hammerström and Kabat (1969) provided an excellent analysis of the *H. pomatia* combining site. Specific agglutination of human RBC occurs in the butter clam, *Saxidomus giganteus* (Johnson, 1964), and the sugars, *N*-acetyl-galactosamine and *N*-acetyl-D-glucosamine, inhibit *S. giganteus* agglutinin. Sprenger and Uhlenbruck (1971) showed that the snail (*Caucasotachea atrolabiata*) agglutinins are capable of reacting with both terminal and nonterminal *N*-acetyl-D-galactosamine. The hemolymph agglutinins found in many other invertebrates do not appear to have the high degree of specificity of snail (*Helix* sp.) agglutinins. This is not surprising in view of the hypothesis that albumin gland agglutinins from snails probably have a reproductive function; thus it would be advantageous to possess a highly specific molecule. However, the hemolymph agglutinins, although capable of multiple functions, apparently act as components only of the internal defense machinery or immune system to help eliminate foreign substances and potential pathogenic organisms. It is obvious that with regard to immunity, it would be a distinct advantage to possess a molecule or group of molecules with the ability to agglutinate a variety of receptor sites.

The spiny lobster, *P. interruptus,* apparently has a group of molecules in the hemolymph capable of reacting with certain cell surface combining sites (Tyler and Metz, 1945). Adsorption of lobster serum with cells of any single species removed agglutinins for all animal species that belonged to the same group (Class) but left agglutinins against cells of all other groups. Although some cross-reactions occurred, Tyler and Metz (1945) concluded that at least 10 class-specific agglutinins existed in lobster serum. The serum of American lobsters (*Homarus americanus*) contained strong and specific natural agglutinins for an antigen present on the red blood cells of the sea herring, *Clupea harengus* (Sindermann and Mairs, 1959). Cornick and Stewart (1968*a*) found that the bacterial agglutinin in *H. americanus* could be adsorbed from the serum by preincubation with various bacteria. Finstad *et al.* (1972) indicated a high degree of RBC specificity in the horseshoe crab, *L. polyphemus.*

Tripp (1966) demonstrated that oyster (*C. virginica*) agglutinin is relatively nonspecific, since the component responsible for agglutination of chicken, guinea pig, and bovine RBC was completely removed by treatment with RBC from any species. However, agglutinins for sheep, rabbit, and horse cells were not completely removed by adsorption with heterologous RBC. Other studies revealed that a variety of sugars inhibited oyster agglutinin (McDade and Tripp, 1967). Sea hare agglutinin was apparently nonspecific. Cross-agglutination tests showed that any of four marine bacteria completely adsorbed, out of normal *A.*

californica serum, the agglutinin against itself, the other marine bacteria, and two types of RBC (Pauley *et al.*, 1971*a*). However, *Serratia marcescens* was incapable of adsorbing sea hare agglutinin, which is not surprising since it was not agglutinated. Partial inactivation of the agglutinin by *Escherichia coli* "O" antigen indicated that the attachment site of the agglutinin was, at least in part, a polysaccharide similar in structure to "O" antigen (Pauley *et al.*, 1971*a*). Crayfish (*P. clarkii*) serum did not agglutinate *S. marcescens* and cross-adsorption tests showed that chicken RBC and *Micrococcus aquivivus* were both capable of completely adsorbing crayfish agglutinin activity against each other (Miller *et al.*, 1972). Rabbit RBC were also capable of adsorbing activity against *M. aquivivus*, but complete cross-adsorption was not found between any of the other bacteria and RBC combinations tested. For example, chicken RBC were not capable of eliminating activity against rabbit RBC. McKay *et al.* (1969) indicated some specificity by cross-adsorption tests in the clam, *Tridacna fossor;* the Murray mussel, *Velesunio ambiguus;* and the crayfish, *Parachaeraps bicarinatus*. However, their results are very similar to those obtained in the oyster (Tripp, 1966) and the crayfish (Miller *et al.*, 1972).

Agglutinins of several invertebrates appear to play an important role in defense mechanisms against potential pathogens. Spider crabs lacking an agglutinin against a marine ciliate (*Anorphrys sarcophaga*) were killed by this protozoan, whereas those possessing the agglutinin survived injections of the parasite (Bang, 1962; 1967). Cornick and Stewart (1968*a*) found that a single bacterium of *Gaffkya homari* was sufficient to produce a fatal infection in the American lobster, *H. americanus*, while other bacteria including *Gaffkya tetragena* did not produce serious infections. They attributed this phenomenon to the ability of lobster serum to agglutinate all bacteria tested except *G. homari*. They also found that *G. homari* was only moderately pathogenic in the crab, *Cancer irroratus* (Cornick and Stewart, 1968*b*). The milder effect of this pathogen on *C. irroratus* was possibly due to the agglutinin in this crab against *G. homari*. Pauley *et al.* (1971*b*) found that marine bacteria, which were agglutinated by sea hare hemolymph, were cleared very rapidly from these animals, while *S. marcescens*, which was not agglutinated, was not cleared from this mollusk. Feng (1966) noted a very slow removal of bacteria from oysters; this is interesting because this mollusk apparently lacks any bacterial agglutinins (Tripp, 1966). Bayne (1973) found that *S. marcescens* was rapidly cleared from the octopus, *Octopus dofleini*, apparently by agglutinins in the hemolymph. Stuart (1968) did demonstrate agglutinins in another species of octopus (*Eledon cirrosa*). Tubiash and Krantz (1970) found the blue crab, *C. sapidus*, highly susceptible to some bacteria, but relatively refractory to other bacteria. This may be due to either the presence or lack of agglutinins against these various bacteria, since several RBC are agglutinated in the serum (Pauley, 1973*a*). Agglutinin titers in the sea hare were greatly depressed following bacterial injections but returned to normal as the bacteria were cleared from the hemolymph (Pauley *et al.*, 1971*b*). Although secondary bacterial injections were cleared more rapidly than primary injections in several invertebrates, this secondary clearance did not appear to be related to any increase in agglutinin titer (McKay and Jenkin, 1970*a*; 1970*c*; Pauley *et al.*, 1971*b*; Pauley, 1971; Bayne, 1973).

Although Scott (1971) was not able to find any opsonic activity in cockroach hemolymph, the majority of recent evidence indicates that invertebrates possess serum opsonins, which are probably the same molecules that cause agglutination. Tripp (1966) was the first to find an opsonic effect in an invertebrate. He observed the number of oyster hemocytes phagocytizing rabbit RBC in 30 min, which nearly doubled when the RBC were pretreated with oyster hemagglutinin. The number of ingested RBC per phagocyte was also greatly increased by pretreatment with hemagglutinin. These results were subsequently corroborated (Tripp and Kent, 1967). The snail, *Helix aspersa,* possessed opsonic factors capable of increasing the phagocytosis of both yeast and sheep RBC (Prowse and Tait, 1969). They observed that phagocytosis of each of these particles occurred in normal serum and in serum adsorbed with the heterologous materials. They also observed that these serum factors not only influenced the rate of phagocytosis but were necessary for any pahgocytosis at all to occur in *H. aspersa.* Stuart (1968) also found opsonic factors in octopus serum that were necessary for phagocytosis of RBC. McKay and Jenkin (1970*a,c*) found that crayfish serum contains opsonins that enhance greatly phagocytosis of RBC. Serum from the reef crab, *Ozius truncatus,* can opsonize RBC for subsequent phagocytosis by crayfish hemocytes (McKay and Jenkin, 1970*a*). These investigators indicated, as did Tripp (1966), that the naturally occurring hemagglutinins are the same molecules responsible for the opsonic activity. Pauley *et al.* (1971*b*) observed that chicken RBC are phagocytosed more quickly if pretreated with sea hare serum containing hemagglutinin; the opsonic factor and the agglutinin are presumed to be the same molecule.

In analyzing any aspect of invertebrate immunity, it should be kept in mind that all aspects of the immune mechanisms in these animals is profoundly influenced by the ambient temperature. The lack of a lytic effect in the serum of an invertebrate combined with the presence of an agglutinin, which probably functions as an opsonin, leads to the following proposed mechanism of pathogen or antigen clearance from these animals. After entering the invertebrate, foreign material is quickly agglutinated, after which a dramatic drop in agglutinin titer occurs. At this time, the antigen also is opsonized or prepared for phagocytosis. With the antigen properly prepared, active phagocytosis ensues, accompanied by a reduction in the number of circulating hemocytes. If possible, intracellular digestion of the foreign material occurs at this point most likely by lysosomal enzymes similar to those in vertebrates. If intracellular digestion is not possible, then the material is either sequestered *in situ* or removed by phagocytic migration across epithelial borders, which leads to elimination of these cells. As the foreign substance is removed from the hemolymph, the agglutinin titer returns to normal, ready to aid the animal to eliminate any future inimical substances. These agglutinins function in the nonspecific anamnestic responses observed in invertebrates exactly as they do in primary reactions but they may not be responsible for these specific secondary responses which are attributed to cellular memory mechanisms (Cooper, 1969).

SUMMARY

A natural agglutinin to vertebrate red blood cells occurs in blue crab (*C. sapidus*) hemolymph. The agglutinin appears to be protein because of sensitivity to heat, pH extremes, TCA, phenol, and urea. It does not resemble immunoglobulins in that it can be enhanced only slightly and nonspecifically by prior injection. Immunoelectrophoresis and Ouchterlony immunodiffusion further support its lack of similarity to vertebrate gamma globulin. There are possibly two distinct agglutinins demonstrable by immunoelectrophoresis and Sephadex column chromatography. Most of the agglutinin possesses a molecular weight of over 100,000 and is unique among invertebrate agglutinins. It is partially inactivated by dialysis, probably due to a dependence on divalent cations. These results suggest a large molecular-weight protein component containing subunits. The blue crab agglutinin, like other invertebrate agglutinins, plays an important role in defense against potential pathogens by acting as an opsonin. This agglutinin is undoubtedly responsible for crab resistance to infection.

REFERENCES

Acton, R. T., Bennett, J. C., Evans, E. E., and Schrohenloher, R. E., 1969, Physical and chemical characterization of an oyster hemagglutinin, *J. Biol. Chem.* 244:4128-4135.

Anderson, R. S., Day, N. K. B., and Good, R. A., 1972, Specific hemagglutinin and a modulator of complement in cockroach hemolymph, *Infect. Immunol.* 5:55-59.

Bang, F. B., 1962, Serological aspects of immunity in invertebrates, *Nature (London)* 196:88-89.

Bang, F. B., 1966, Serologic response in a marine worm, *Sipunculus nudus, J. Immunol.* 96:960-972.

Bang, F. B., 1967, Serological responses among invertebrates other than insects, *Federation Proc.* 26:1680-1684.

Bayne, C. J., 1973, Internal defense mechanisms of *Octopus dofleini, Malacological Rev.* 6:13-17.

Blitz, R. R., 1966, The clearance of foreign material from the coelom of *Phascolosoma agassizii, Dissertation Abstr.* 26:3584.

Boyd, W. C. and Brown, R., 1965, A specific agglutinin in the snail *Otala (Helix) lactea, Nature* 208:593-594.

Boyd, W. C., Brown, R., and Boyd, L. G., 1966, Agglutinins to human erythrocytes in mollusks, *J. Immunol.* 96:301-303.

Brown, R., Almodovar, L. R., Bhatia, H. M., and Boyd, W. C., 1968, Blood group specific agglutinins in invertebrates, *J. Immunol.* 100:214-216.

Cantacuzéne, J., 1923, Le problème de l'immunité chez les Invertébrés, *Comp. Rend. Soc. Biol.* Celeb. du 75 Anniversaire: 48-119.

Carton, Y., 1969, Données récentes sur les phénomènes d' immunité humorale acquise chez les invertébrés, *Ann. Biol.* 8:657-682.

Chadwick, J. S., 1967, Serological responses of insects, *Federation Proc.* 26:1675-1679.

Cheng, T. C. and Sanders, B. G., 1962, Internal defense mechanisms in Molluscs and an electrophoretic analysis of a naturally occurring serum hemagglutinin in *Viviparus malleatus* Reeve, *Proc. Penn. Acad. Sci.* 36:72-83.

Cohen, E., 1968, Immunologic observations of the agglutinins of the hemolymph of *Limulus polyphemus* and *Birgus latro, Trans. N.Y. Acad. Sci.* 30:427-443.

Cohen, E., 1970, A review of the nature and significance of hemagglutinins of selected invertebrates, in: *Protein Metabolism and Biological Function,* pp. 87-93, (C. P. Bianchi and R. Half, eds.), Rutgers University Press, New Brunswick, N.J.

Cohen, E., 1971, A biomedical perspective of agglutinins of *Limulus polyphemus* (Horseshoe crab), *The Serological Museum, Bull.* 45:3-4.

Cohen, E., 1973, Agglutinins of selected marine invertebrates, *Ann. N.Y. Acad. Sci.* (in press).

Cohen, E., Rose, A. W., and Wissler, F. C., 1965, Heteroagglutinins of the horseshoe crab *Limulus polyphemus, Life Sci.* 4:2009-2016.

Cooper, E. L., 1969, Specific tissue graft rejection in earthworms, *Science* 166:1414-1415.

Cornick, J. W. and Stewart, J. E., 1968a, Interaction of the pathogen *Gaffkya homari* with natural defense mechanisms of *Homarus americanus, J. Fisheries Res. Board. Can.* 25:695-709.

Cornick, J. W. and Stewart, J. E., 1968b, Pathogenicity of *Gaffyka homari* for the crab *Cancer irroratus, J. Fisheries Res. Board Can.* 25:795-799.

Cushing, J. E., 1967, Invertebrates, immunology, and evolution, *Federation Proc.* 26:1666-1670.

Evans, E. E., Cushing, J. E., Sawyer, S., Weinheimer, P. F., Acton, R. T., and McNeely, J. L., 1969, An induced bactericidal response in a sipunculid worm, *Nature (London)* 222:695.

Feng, S. Y., 1966, Experimental bacterial infections in the oyster *Crassostrea virginica, J. Invertebr. Pathol.* 8:505-511.

Feng, S. Y., 1967, Responses of molluscs to foreign bodies, with special reference to the oyster, *Federation Proc.* 26:1685-1692.

Feng, S. Y. and Stauber, L. A., 1968, Experimental hexamitiasis in the oyster *Crassostrea virginica, J. Invertebr. Pathol.* 10:94-110.

Finstad, C., 1973, The erythrocyte agglutinin in *Limulus polyphemus* serum: molecular structure and biological function, *Ann. N.Y. Acad. Sci.* (in press).

Finstad, C. L., Litman, G. W., Finstad, J., and Good, R. A., 1972, The evolution of the immune response. XIII. The characterization of purified erythrocyte agglutinins from two invertebrate species, *J. Immunol.* 108:1704-1711.

Florkin, M. and Stotz, E. H., 1963, *Comprehensive Biochemistry, Proteins,* Part 1, p. 280, Elsevier, Amsterdam.

Fox, S. W. and Foster, J. F., 1957, *Introduction to Protein Chemistry,* pp. 459, Wiley, New York.

Hammarström, S. and Kabat, E. A., 1969, Purification and characterization of a bloodgroup A reactive hemagglutinin from the snail *Helix pomatia* and a study of its combining site, *Biochemistry* 8:2696-2705.

Hatch, F. T. and Lees, R. S., 1968, Practical methods for plasma lipoprotein analysis, *Adv. Lipid Res.* 6:1-68.

Ishiyama, I. and Uhlenbruck, G., 1972, Further studies on the specificity of the anti-A agglutinin from *Helix pomatia, Comp. Biochem. Physiol.* 42A:269-276.

Jenkin, C. R. and Rowley, D., 1970, Immunity in invertebrates. The purification of a hemagglutinin to rat and rabbit erythrocytes from the hemolymph of the Murray mussel (*Velesunio ambiguus*), *Australian J. Exp. Biol. Med. Sci.* 48:129-137.

Johnson, H. M., 1964, Human blood group A, specific agglutinins of the butter clam *Saxidomus giganteus, Science* 146:548-549.

Kolb, W. P. and Granger, G. A., 1968, Lymphocyte *in vitro* cytotoxicity: characterization of human lymphotoxin, *Proc. Nat. Acad. Sci. U.S.* 61:1250-1255.

Kolb, W. P. and Granger, G. A., 1970, Lymphocyte *in vitro* cytotoxicity: characterization of mouse lymphotoxin, *Cellular Immunol. 1*:122-132.

Kothbauer, H. and Brunner, H. S., 1971, Haemagglutinine aus Schnecken: zur Frage ihrer biologischen Funktion, *Z. Naturforschung 26*:1082-1084.

Kothbauer, H., Nopp, H., and Brunner, H. S., 1972, Haemagglutinine aus Schnecken: Auswirkung der Amputation der Augententakel; Einfluss des Entwicklungszustandes des Genitaltraktes, *Immunol-Information 6*:2-4.

Krassner, S. M. and Flory, B., 1970, Antibacterial factors in the sipunculid worms *Goldfingia gouldii* and *Dendrostomum pyroides, J. Invertebr. Path. 16*:331-338.

Li, M. F. and Flemming, C., 1967, Hemagglutinins from oyster hemolymph, *Can. J. Zool. 45*:1225-1234.

MacInnis, A. J. and Voge, M., 1970, *Experiments and Techniques in Parasitology*, pp. 232, Freeman, San Francisco.

McDade, J. E. and Tripp, M. R., 1967, Mechanism of agglutination of red blood cells by oyster hemolymph, *J. Invertebr. Pathol. 9*:523-530.

McKay, D. and Jenkin, C. R., 1970*a*, Immunity in the invertebrates. The role of serum factors in phagocytosis of erythrocytes by hemocytes of the fresh-water crayfish (*Parachaeraps bicarinatus*), *Australian J. Exp. Biol. Med. Sci. 48*:139-150.

McKay, D. and Jenkin, C. R., 1970*b*, Immunity in the invertebrates. The fate and distribution of bacteria in normal and immunized crayfish (*Parachaeraps bicarinatus*), *Australian J. Exp. Biol. Med. Sci. 48*:599-607.

McKay, D. and Jenkin, C. R., 1970*c*, Immunity in the invertebrates. Correlation of the phagocytic activity of hemocytes with resistance to infection in the crayfish (*Parachaeraps bicarinatus*), *Australian J. Exp. Biol. Med. Sci. 48*:609-617.

McKay, D., Jenkin, C. R., and Rowley, D., 1969, Immunity in the invertebrates. I. Studies on the naturally occurring hemagglutinins in the fluid from invertebrates, *Australian J. Exp. Biol. Med. Sci. 47*:125-134.

Marchalonis, J. J. and Edelman, G. M., 1968, Isolation and characterization of a hemagglutinin from *Limulus polyphemus, J. Mol. Biol. 32*:453-465.

Miller, V. H., Ballback, R. S., Pauley, G. B., and Krassner, S. M., 1972, A preliminary physicochemical characterization of an agglutinin found in the hemolymph of the crayfish *Procambarus clarkii, J. Invertebr. Pathol. 19*:83-93.

Nowotny, A., 1969, *Basic Exercises in Immunochemistry*, pp. 197, Springer-Verlag, New York.

Pauley, G. B., 1971, Bacterial clearance in the marine gastropod mollusk *Aplysia californica* (Cooper), *Proc. Nat. Shellfisheries Assoc. 61*:11-12.

Pauley, G. B., 1973*a*, An attempt to immunize the blue crab, *Callinectes sapidus*, with vertebrate red blood cells, *Experientia 29*:210-211.

Pauley, G. B., 1973*b*, Physicochemical properties of the natural agglutinins of some mollusks and crustaceans, *Ann. N. Y. Acad. Sci.* (in press).

Pauley, G. B., Granger, G. A., and Krassner, S. M., 1971*a*, Characterization of a natural agglutinin in the hemolymph of the California sea hare, *Aplysia californica, J. Invertebr. Pathol. 18*:207-218.

Pauley, G. B., Krassner, S. M., and Chapman, F. A., 1971*b*, Bacterial clearance in the California sea hare, *Aplysia californica, J. Invertebr. Pathol. 18*:227-239.

Prowse, R. H. and Tait, N. N., 1969, *In vitro* phagocytosis by amoebocytes from the hemolymph of *Helix aspera* (Müller). I. Evidence for opsonic factor(s) in serum. *Immunology 17*:437-443.

Scanu, A. M., 1965, Factors affecting lipoprotein metabolism, *Adv. ·Lipid Res. 3*:63-138.

Scott, M. T., 1971, Recognition of foreignness in invertebrates. II. *In vitro* studies of cockroach phagocytic hemocytes, *Immunology 21*:817-828.

Scott, M. T., 1972, Partial characterization of the hemagglutinating activity in the hemolymph of the American cockroach (*Periplaneta americana*), *J. Invertebr. Pathol. 19*:66-71.

Sindermann, C. J., 1971, Internal defenses of crustacea: a review, *Fisheries Bull. 69*:455-489.

Sindermann, C. G. and Mairs, D. F., 1959, A major blood group system in Atlantic sea herring, *Copeia 1959*:228-232.

Smith, A. C. and Goldstein, R. A., 1971, "Natural" agglutinins against sea urchin sperm in the hemolymph of the crab, *Cardisoma guanhumi, Marine Biol. 8*:6.

Sprenger, I. and Uhlenbruck, G., 1971, On the specificity of broad spectrum agglutinins XI. The reaction of the agglutinin from the snail *Caucasotachea atrolabiata, Z. Immunol.-Forsch. 142*:254-259.

Stewart, J. E. and Zwicker, B. M., 1972, Natural and induced bactericidal activities in the hemolymph ot the lobster, *Homarus americanus:* products of hemocyte–plasma interaction, *Can. J. Microbiol. 18*:1499-1509.

Stuart, A. E., 1968, The reticulo-endothelial apparatus of the lesser octopus, *Eledone cirrosa, J. Pathol. Bacteriol. 96*:401-412.

Teague, P. O. and Friou, G. J., 1964, Lack of immunological responses by an invertebrate, *Comp. Biochem. Physiol. 12*:471-478.

Tripp, M. R., 1966, Hemagglutinin in the blood of the oyster *Crassostrea virginica, J. Invertebr. Pathol. 8*:478-484.

Tripp, M. R., 1970, Defense mechanisms of mollusks, *J. Reticuloendothelial Soc. 7*:173-182.

Tripp, M. R., 1973, Agglutinins and opsonins of oyster hemolymph, *Ann. N. Y. Acad. Sci.* (in press).

Tripp, M. R. and Kent, V. E., 1967, Studies on oyster cellular immunity, *In Vitro 3*:129-135.

Tubiash, H. S. and Krantz, G. E., 1970, Experimental bacterial infection of the blue crab, *Callinectes sapidus. Bacteriol. Proc. 1970*:G80.

Tyler, A., 1946, Natural hemagglutinins in the body fluids and seminal fluids of various invertebrates, *Biol. Bull. 90*:213-219.

Tyler, A. and Metz, C. B., 1945, Natural heteroagglutinins in the serum of the spiny lobster, *Panulirus interruptus.* I. Taxonomic range of activity, electrophoretic and immunizing properties, *J. Exp. Zool. 100*:387-406.

Tyler, A. and Scheer, B. T., 1945, Natural heteroagglutins in the serum of the spiny lobster, *Panulirus interruptus.* II. Chemical and antigenic relation to blood proteins, *Biol. Bull. 89*:193-200.

Uhlenbruck, G. and Prokop, O., 1966, An agglutinin from *Helix pomatia,* which reacts with terminal N-acetyl-D-galactosamine, *Vox Sanguinis 11*:519-520.

Uhlenbruck, G., Reifenberg, U., and Prokop, O., 1971, Resistance to proteases of *Helix pomatia* anti-A: consequences for tumor cell A-like antigen, *Acta Biol. Med. Ger. 27*:455-457.

Woods, K. R., Paulsen, E. C., Engle, Jr., R. L., and Pert, J. H., 1958, Starch gel electrophoresis of some invertebrate sera, *Science 127*:519-520.

Chapter 22

Characteristics of the Agglutinin in
the Scorpion, Androctonus australis*

Zacharie Brahmi

Institut Pasteur d'Algerie
Algiers, Algeria

and

Edwin L. Cooper

Department of Anatomy, School of Medicine
University of California
Los Angeles, California

Entre Balance et Sagittaire
Jadis il fut machine de guerre.
Redoutable adversaire,
Son nom, il vaut mieux taire.

Anonymous, n.d.

INTRODUCTION

The hemolymph of most invertebrates contains naturally occurring hemagglutinins with specificities comparable to the isohemagglutinins present in vertebrate sera (Tyler, 1946; Cushing *et al.*, 1963; Tripp, 1966; Marchalonis and Edelman, 1968; McKay *et al.*, 1969). Similarly, the hemolymph of some invertebrates, such as the oyster (Tripp, 1966), the horseshoe crab (Marchalonis and Edelman, 1968), and the crayfish (McKay and Jenkin, 1969) contains elements analogous to vertebrate antibodies, for both increase the rate of phagocytosis of erythrocytes. Several investigators have tried to characterize the factors involved in invertebrate phagocytosis. Acton *et al.* (1969), for example, observed that an

*Supported in part by NSF Grant GB17767; two grants from The California Institute for Cancer Research and a grant from the Brown-Hazen Corporation to Edwin L. Cooper.

261

oyster agglutinin has a sedimentation coefficient of 33 S and that it can be dissociated into polypeptide chains having a molecular weight of 20,000. Likewise, Marchalonis and Edelman (1968) isolated an agglutinin from the horseshoe crab and determined that it has a sedimentation coefficient of 13.5 S and that it too can be dissociated to yield polypeptide chains of a molecular weight of 22,500. Miller *et al.* (1971) found an agglutinin in the serum of the crayfish which is of particular interest, as it has a molecular weight greater than 150,000 and is, thus, probably a protein. This agglutinin resembles the agglutinin Pauley *et al.* (1971) found in the sea hare and the one Jenkin and Rowley (1970) observed in the mussel. Whether or not these factors in invertebrate hemolymph are, in fact, related structurally to immunoglobulins requires further physicochemical analyses.

Our recent attempt revealed that the hemolymph of the Algerian scorpion, *Androctonus australis,* contains a naturally occurring hemagglutinin for vertebrate erythrocytes. Its properties are reminiscent of the agglutinins which occur naturally in the variety of invertebrates noted by Scott (1971). It is, briefly, nondialyzable, heat labile, and precipitates in distilled water.

ELIMINATION OF SRBC BY SCORPIONS AND INCREASE IN HEMOCYTES

To study its elimination of foreign particles, we injected seven scorpions with SRBC and at 10 min intervals determined both the number of recognizable SRBC and the number of hemocytes. As Table I and Fig. 1 illustrate, the number of SRBC decreases in 50 min from, for example, 42 to 4 in scorpion 1 and from 190 to 6 in scorpion 7. On the other hand, the number of hemocytes at first decreases and then increases. As can be seen, the number is 44 in scorpion 1 before immunization; it decreases to 14, 30 min after immunization, but reaches 140, 3 hr later. Similarly, in scorpion 7 the number of hemocytes decreases after immunization from 58 to 22, but increases to 138 after 3 hr.

INCREASE IN HEMAGGLUTININS AFTER IMMUNIZATION

The hemagglutinin titers of 10 of the 47 scorpions immunized with SRBC exhibit a two to fourfold increase in titers. Thus, as Table II indicates, there is some degree of increase in titer, especially on day 1 following immunization in 21% of injected scorpions. This increase, however, does not persist, and begins to decline on day 2. As peak titers usually occur 24 hr after immunization, the scorpion's response differs from the classic vertebrate response. Of particular interest, too, is the fact that the increase in titer usually occurs in scorpions with a low initial agglutinating titer.

Table I. Rate of SRBC Elimination and Simultaneous Increase in Hemocytes in Scorpions Injected with 0.02 ml (Scorpions 1–5) and 0.04 ml (Scorpions 6–7) of a Suspension of 5% SRBC

Time after injection, min	Scorpion 1		Scorpion 2		Scorpion 3		Scorpion 4		Scorpion 5		Scorpion 6		Scorpion 7	
	SRBC	Hemo.[a]	SRBC	Hemo.	SRBC	Hemo.	SRBC	Hemo.	SRBC	Hemo.	SRBC	Hemo.	SRBC	Hemo.
0	—	*44*	—	*48*	—	*58*	48	*36*	—	—	—	—	—	—
10	42	24	42	44	24	28	22	24	28	84	320	104	190	58
20	28	16	28	36	12	18	10	16	16	136	107	111	34	46
30	22	14	20	12	8	30	12	16	14	85	38	87	9	41
40	14	40	10	22	12	26	2	26	14	56	8	32	5	20
50	4	48	2	32	0	40	0	34	2	9	12	12	6	22
180	0	140	0	162	0	150	0	88	0	170	6	104	1	138
72 hr	0	52	0	186	0	170	—	—	—	—	—	—	—	—

[a] The number of SRBC and of hemocytes represents the total number of cells in 10 squares in a hemocytometer. The numbers in italics represent the number of hemocytes before injection of SRBC.

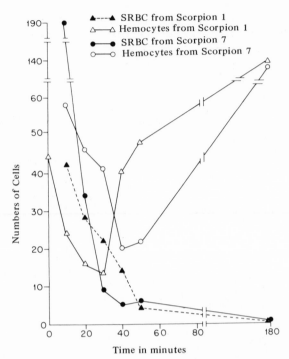

Fig. 1. Rate of elimination of SRBC and simultaneous increase in circulating hemocytes in two scorpions injected with 0.02 ml (scorpion 1) and 0.04 ml (scorpion 7) of 5% SRBC. Number of cells represent the total number of SRBC and of hemocytes in 10 squares of a Malassaz hemocytometer.

SPECIFICITY OF NATURALLY OCCURRING AGGLUTININS

The hemolymph of freshly captured scorpions is, evidentally, capable of agglutinating human, horse, and sheep erythrocytes (Hu, Ho and SRBC). To determine the specificity of the scorpion's response to these hemagglutinins, we absorbed normal hemolymph with one type of erythrocyte and examined the titers for all three. As can be seen in Table III, absorption of hemolymph with HuRBC, for example, lowers the titers for HuRBC from 1:512 to 1:2. The titers against HoRBC drop only slightly from 1:256 to 1:128, and the titers against SRBC drop from 1:64 to 1:4. On the other hand, absorption of the same hemolymph with HoRBC completely eliminates all the hemagglutinins against HoRBC. The titers against HuRBC decrease significantly from 1:512 to 1:256, and the titers against SRBC drop from 1:64 to 1:8. As absorption of the agglutinin with one type of RBC only slightly lowers the titer against the other types

Table II. Agglutinating Titers of Scorpions Which
Showed an Increase of 2 Dilutions or More Following
a Single Injection with 0.02 ml of 5% SRBC

Scorpion No.[a]	Titer before immunization[b]	Titers after immunization on day[b]			
		1	2	3	4
J-1	8	128	16	–	
J-2	8	64	16	–	
J-14	32	128	–	–	
J-18	2	16	8	4	
J-28	4	32	8	8	–
J-29	4	32	16	–	
A-4	4				32
A-5	32				128
A-10	2				32
A-11	32				128

[a]37 scorpions were also injected but showed no significant increase over initial titer.
[b]Titers represent the last dilution showing microscopic agglutination.

of RBC, the presence of different agglutinins in the hemolymph of the scorpion is clearly indicated. McKay *et al.* (1969) and Scott (1971) report similar results for the clam mussel and crayfish. Miller *et al.* (1971) suggest that there are even more specific agglutinins in the crayfish *Procambarus clarkii.*

Table III. Specificity of the Hemagglutinins
in the Scorpion *Androctonus australis*

Absorbing red cell	Red cell used in titration		
	Human	Horse	Sheep
Human	2[a]	128	4
Horse	256	0	8
None	512	256	64

[a]Titers represent the last dilution showing macroscopic agglutination.

Table IV. Effect of Temperature and Dialysis
on the Naturally Occurring Hemagglutinins
in Scorpion Hemolymph

Treatment of hemolymph	Agglutinating titers[a]
None	32
30 min at 25°C	32
30 min at 45°C	32
30 min at 56°C	64
30 min at 65°C	0
Dialyzed 15 hr[b] against distilled H_2O	8
Dialyzed 15 hr against saline	32

[a] Reciprocal of the last hemolymph dilution that agglutinated SRBC.
[b] Presence of a white precipitate in the dialysis tube.

EFFECT OF TEMPERATURE AND DIALYSIS

If small aliquots of normal hemolymph are incubated for 30 min at 25°C, 45°C, 56°C, and 65°C, the titers are similar. There is a small increase at 56°C, but, as Table IV reveals, the agglutinating activity is completely destroyed by 30 min at 65°C.

Dialysis of normal hemolymph against distilled water for 15 hr at room temperature results in the formation of a white precipitate. Moreover, the titer of the hemolymph drops form 1:32 to 1:8 after slight centrifugation. However, there is no change in titer when the same hemolymph is dialyzed against saline for 15 hr. According to our results then, the hemagglutinins are nondialyzable.

IMMUNOELECTROPHORESIS AND PAPER
ELECTROPHORESIS OF HEMOLYMPH

As illustrated by Fig. 2a, immunoelectrophoresis of a pool of freshly drawn hemolymph reveals 13 arcs of precipitation though none in the gamma region. Most of the proteins migrate toward the anode, but some migrate toward the cathode. Immunoelectrophoresis of normal human serum depicted in Fig. 2b makes it clear that scorpion hemolymph lacks any fraction in the gamma region. Similarly, when normal hemolymph is tested with normal human serum on

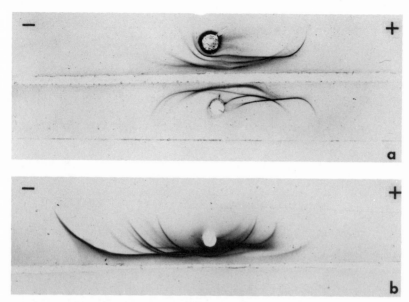

Fig. 2. (*a*) Immunoelectrophoresis patterns of freshly drawn scorpion hemolymph. Upper well undiluted hemolymph. Lower well hemolymph diluted 1:2. (*b*) Immunoelectrophoretic patterns of normal human serum obtained under the same conditions as in (*a*).

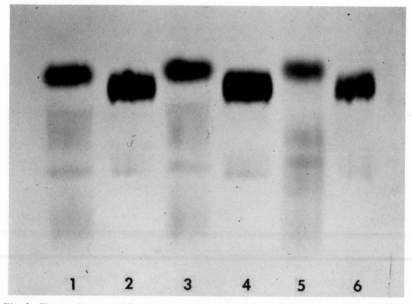

Fig. 3. Electrophoresis of freshly drawn hemolymph from 3 scorpions (strips 2, 4, 6), 2 normal human serums (strips 1 and 3), and 1 normal horse serum (strip). Notice the lack of migration of hemolymph components in the γ region.

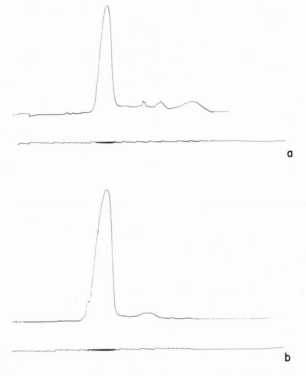

Fig. 4. (*a*) Densitometer absorption curve of freshly drawn hemolymph (Analytrol, Beckman instruments). (*b*) Densitometer absorption curve of normal human serum under the same conditions as in (*a*).

cellulose acetate paper, the main fractions of hemolymph migrate in the range of human albumin. Some fractions are detected in the alpha and beta regions, but none migrate in the gamma region, as Figs. 3, 4*a,b* reveal.

THE CELLULAR MACHINERY

Particularly at the cellular level, the scorpion is an excellent species for studying invertebrate immune phenomena. In that there appears to be a rapid increase in the total number of cells after scorpions are injected with SRBC, one might infer that there is no significant difference between scorpions that exhibit an increase in titer and those that do not.

However, we made no differential cell counts to ascertain which, if any, of the cells increased more than the others. Normal hemolymph usually contains three types of mature circulating hemocytes: a basophilic cell (60%), an acidophilic cell (25%), and a cell which resembles the mammalian granulocyte (15%) (Potier and Goyffon, 1967; Gysin, 1969). It would be worthwhile to note if there is a significant increase in any one of these over the other two. Finally, there is a lymphatic gland that some investigators believe to be involved in hemopoiesis (Blanc, 1967; Kowalewsky, 1903; Cuénot, 1897) and which may be the source of leukocytes. Whether the increase in circulating hemocytes is due to the recruitment of new cells from this gland, or to proliferation of existing peripheral hemocytes, or to a combination of both factors is not yet determined.

SUMMARY

The hemolymph of the scorpion, *Androctonus australis,* contains agglutinins capable of agglutinating vertebrate erythrocytes (RBC). Absorption of the hemolymph with one type of RBC removes the agglutinins against the absorbing RBC but lowers only slightly the titers against nonabsorbing RBC. Of the scorpions injected with sheep red blood cells (SRBC), 21% show some increase in agglutinating titers with peaks usually reached 24 hr after immunization. After injection with SRBC and bleeding every 10 min, we observed: (1) a rapid clearance of the SRBC, complete after 60 min; (2) an initial drop of circulating hemocytes in the first 40 to 50 min, after which their numbers quickly increased suggesting recruitment and/or proliferation. Heating the hemolymph at 65°C for 30 min completely destroyed all the agglutinins, but dialysis against saline had no effect. Immunoelectrophoresis of a pool of normal hemolymph gave 13 arcs of precipitation: heavier arcs migrate toward the anode, lighter ones toward the cathode. No migration occurred in the α region. These results were confirmed by cellulose acetate electrophoresis with no marked differences between the immunoelectrophoresis of male and female scorpions. Because of the presence of a lymph or organ that produces hemocytes, the scorpion is particularly advantageous for exploring further the evolution of cellular immunity.

ACKNOWLEDGMENTS

We thank Mrs. Frances Brahmi for assistance in preparation of the manuscript.

REFERENCES

Acton, R. T., Bennett, J. C., Evans, E. E., and Schrohenloher, R. E., 1969, Physical and chemical characterization of an oyster hemagglutinin, *J. Biol. Chem.* 224:4128.

Blanc, P. L., 1967, Etude des elements figures de l'hemolymphe de quelques scorpions africains, *Biol. Eco.,* Rapport particulier No. *14*:I.

Cuénot, L., 1897, Les globules sanguins et les organes lymphoides des invertebres, *Arch. Anat. Microbiol. 1*:1.

Cushing, G. E., Calaprice, N. L., and Trump, G., 1963, Blood group reactive substances in some marine invertebrates, *Biol. Bull. 125*:69.

Gysin, J., Le Corroler, Y., and Irunberry, J., 1969, Cytologie sanguine du scorpion, *Arch. Inst. Pasteur Algerie 47*:73.

Jenkin, C. R. and Rowley, D., 1970, Immunity in invertebrate. The purification of a hemagglutinin to rat and rabbit erythrocytes from the hemolymph of the murray mussel (*Velesunia ambiguus*), *Australian J. Exp. Biol. Med. Sci. 48*:129.

Kowalewsky, A., 1903, Une nouvelle glande lymphatique chez le scorpion d'Europe, *Ann. St. Petersburg I.*

Marchalonis, J. J. and Edelman, G. M., 1968, Isolation and characterization of a hemagglutinin from *Limulus polyphemus, J. Mol Biol. 32*:453.

McKay, D. and Jenkin, C. R., 1969, Immunity in invertebrates. II. Adaptive immunity in the crayfish (*Parachaeraps bicarinatus*), *Immunology 17*:127.

McKay, D., Jenkin, C. R., and Rowley, D., 1969, Immunity in the invertebrates. I. Studies on the naturally occurring hemagglutinins in the fluids from invertebrates, *Australian J. Exp. Biol. Med. Sci. 47*:125.

Miller, V. H., Ballback, R., Pauley, G. B., and Krassner, S. M., 1971, A preliminary physico-chemical characterization of an agglutinin found in the hemolymph of the crayfish, *Procambarus clarkii, J. Invertebr. Pathol. 19*:83.

Pauley, G. B., Granger, G. A., and Krassner, S. M., 1971, Characterization of a natural agglutinin in the hemolymph of the California sea hare, *Aplysia californica, J. Invertebr. Pathol. 18*:207.

Potier, H. and Goyffon, M., 1967, Numeration des hemocytes chez le scorpion *Androctonus australis, Biol. Eco.,* Rapport particulier No. *27*:I.

Scott, M. T., 1971, A naturally occurring hemagglutinin in the hemolymph of the American cockroach, *Arch. Zool. Exp. Gen. 112*:73.

Tripp, M. R., 1966, Hemagglutinin in the blood of the oyster, *Crassostrea virginica, J. Invertebr. Pathol. 8*:478.

Tyler, A., 1946, Natural heteroagglutinins in the body fluid and seminal fluids of various invertebrates, *Biol. Bull.90*:213.

Chapter 23

Hemagglutinins: Primitive Receptor Molecules Operative in Invertebrate Defense Mechanisms *

Ronald T. Acton†

Division of Biology
California Institute of Technology
Pasadena, California

and

Peter F. Weinheimer ‡

Department of Medicine
Division of Clinical Immunology and Rheumatology
University of Alabama in Birmingham
Birmingham, Alabama

INTRODUCTION

In recent years those of us who hold an interest in comparative immunology have witnessed an increased emphasis in deciphering the molecular events operative in invertebrate defense mechanisms. Our own efforts have centered mainly on the role of various hemolymph factors in invertebrate immunity, and whether these factors bear any relationship to components of vertebrate immune mechanisms. From our studies and those of others, there exists several lines of evidence that: (1) hemagglutinins (HA) represent primitive receptor molecules operative in the immune mechanism of invertebrates, and (2) the hemagglutinins of several key invertebrate species are related chemically. In addition, HA is apparently

*Supported in part by the Atomic Energy Commission Contract No. AT(04-3)767, grants from the U.S. Public Health Service (AI-02693, AI-9153, and AM-03555) and the National Science Foundation (Grant GB-5983).
†Smith Kline and French Research Fellow, California Institute of Technology. Present address: Department of Microbiology, University of Alabama in Birmingham, University Station, Birmingham, Alabama 35294.
‡Research Scholar, American Cancer Society.

related to other hemolymph factors such as inducible bactericidins, naturally occurring hemolysins, and clotting factors. Thus, in this presentation, we would like to present a unifying concept of how these molecules with seemingly diverse functions may be related, and how they may have evolved from a common ancestral gene. We will also question whether analogies exist between invertebrate hemolymph factors and the immunoglobulins, complement and clotting systems of vertebrates. Admittedly, much will be speculative. However, if one closely peruses the literature, tersely reviewed here, it may be obvious that many of our conclusions have substance.

BIOLOGICAL STUDIES

Naturally occurring HA are found in the hemolymph of almost every species of advanced invertebrate (Acton and Evans, 1968; Bernheimer, 1952; Boyd *et al.*, 1966; Brown *et al.*, 1968; Cohen *et al.*, 1962; Cushing *et al.*, 1963; McKay *et al.*, 1969; Tripp, 1966; Tyler, 1946; Weinheimer, 1970*a,b*; Weinheimer *et al.*, 1970). Investigations have been directed broadly in two directions. First, there are those studies concentrating on the usefulness of invertebrate hemagglutinins as reagents for blood group determinations (Bizot, 1971; Boyd and Brown, 1965; Brown *et al.*, 1968; Hammarström and Kabat, 1969, 1971; Ishiyama and Uhlenbruck, 1972; Kühnemund and Kohler, 1969; Prokop *et al.*, 1965, 1968; Schnitzler and Kilias, 1970; Tyler and Metz, 1945; Tyler and Scheer, 1945). In this regard, various species of land snails have been studied in great detail. Land snail albumin glands have agglutinins for human A or B erythrocytes. Prokop *et al.* (1965) found that anti-A agglutinins from *Helix pomatia* react with terminal nonreducing *N*-acetyl-D-galactosamine (GalNAc) residues. Other investigators provided confirmation, and apparently snail agglutinins react with GalNAc and *N*-acetyl-D-glucosamine (GNAc) sugar residues on erythrocyte membranes (Uhlenbruck and Prokop, 1966; Prokop *et al.*, 1968). Further studies by Hammarström and Kabat (1969, 1971) provided more evidence that the anti-A agglutinin of *Helix pomatia* has a combining site for GalNAc and GNAc in the α and β form. Ishiyama and Uhlenbruck (1972) recently showed that the combining site of the snail agglutinin is directed, in addition to *N*-acetylated aminosugars, to a wide spectrum of glucose and galactose polymers of α-anomeric-($1\rightarrow6$) structure. Studies by Bizot (1971) with other species of snails revealed that albumin extracts contain at least two agglutinins. One agglutinin has anti-A activity which probably reacts with α-*N*-acetyl-D-galactosamine residues, and another agglutinin reacts with human red cells of any ABO group. HA from invertebrate species, as widely separated in taxonomy as the oyster and horseshoe crab, are also inhibited from agglutinating erythrocytes by *N*-acetylated aminosugars (Cohen, 1968; McDade and Tripp, 1967), linking these molecules functionally and chemically.

One of the more attractive ideas on the role of invertebrate HA is that these molecules may serve as recognition factors which function in immunity against infectious agents (Boyden, 1966). Moreover, Burnet (1968) suggested that HA are the forerunners of vertebrate immunoglobulins. Before discussing these possibilities, we should like to review the pertinent literature with evidence for participation of HA molecules in an invertebrate's defense against foreign intrusion.

Perhaps Tripp (1966) was the first to provide a clue that HA are active in defense mechanisms. He demonstrated that rabbit red cells treated *in vitro* with oyster hemolymph are more readily phagocytized by oyster leukocytes than nontreated cells. HA could be absorbed by a variety of mammalian erythrocytes. Whether the HA functions *in vivo* in a like manner is open to question. Similarly, Stuart (1968) found that in the octopus, another mollusc, phagocytosis of erythrocytes depends on a hemolymph factor. In an effort to determine if oyster HA was functioning *in vivo* in an immune situation analogous to vertebrates, Acton and Evans (1968) injected different groups of oysters with varying amounts of sheep erythrocytes. A rise in HA titers, as a consequence of the injection schedule, was not observed. During the course of the experimental period, the HA titer did fluctuate but this was attributable to environmental factors.

McKay *et al.* (1969) likewise questioned the role of invertebrate HA. They found that in different invertebrates hemolymph proteins agglutinate the erythrocytes of several vertebrate species. Following absorption of hemolymph with one species of erythrocyte, molecules remain specific for erythrocytes taken from other vertebrates. These molecules may function biologically. Erythrocytes treated with crayfish hemolymph adhere more readily to crayfish phagocytic cells. It is of interest that this enhanced adhesion is not observed if mouse peritoneal macrophages are exposed to mouse erythrocytes pretreated with crayfish hemolymph. *In vivo* studies suggest that crayfish HA may have a functional role. Following injections of erythrocytes into crayfish, circulating hemocyte numbers decrease and erythrocyte agglutinin titers drop. This is parallel to a fall in the number of injected erythrocytes.

There is evidence for opsonic factors in hemolymph from the snail, *Helix aspersa* (Prowse and Tait, 1969). Yeast cells are not phagocytized by snail amoebocytes unless treated with hemolymph. Moreover, opsonic factors in the hemolymph possess some degree of specificity. Hemolymph absorbed with yeast still contains factors which increase sheep erythrocyte phagocytosis but is depleted of yeast opsonic factor.

Further studies by McKay and Jenkin (1970a) gave additional insight into the biological role of hemolymph factors in phagocytosis. Utilizing the crayfish, *Parachaeraps bicarinatus,* pretreatment of sheep erythrocytes with crayfish hemolymph is essential for efficient adherence to hemocytes. For phagocytosis to occur, it is mandatory to pretreat erythrocytes. Adherence of treated erythrocytes to crayfish hemocytes is the initial step before phagocytosis and is unaffected by low temperatures of 8°C and 0°C; phagocytosis is affected at 8°C and completely inhibited at 0°C. Since at least three species of molluscs contain hemolymph opsonic factors (Tripp, 1966; Stuart, 1968; Prowse and Tait, 1969), McKay and Jenkin investigated the possibility that mollusc HA could enhance erythrocyte phagocytosis by crayfish hemocytes. Of two species of molluscs and one crustacean tested, only hemolymph from the reef crab was effective in enhancing phagocytosis. Hemocytes from crayfish immunized with erythrocytes show far greater phagocytic activity than normal hemocytes, although increased activity could only be demonstrated in the presence of hemolymph.

In another series of experiments, McKay and Jenkin (1970b,c) found that crayfish eliminate several bacterial species from the hemolymph more effectively following immunization with the bacteria. These increased clearance rates could not, however, be correlated with hemolymph opsonins. Furthermore, hemocytes from crayfish immunized with bacteria are more active in phagocytosing opsonized erythrocytes than hemocytes from unimmunized crayfish. This suggests that hemocyte recognition of erythrocytes is mediated by hemolymph factors, the hemagglutinins. In these experiments, however, the HA titer did not increase in immunized animals, lending support to the observations of Acton and Evans (1968).

Pauley et al. (1971a) found rapid bacterial clearance in another invertebrate, the sea hare, Aplysia californica, concomitant with decreases in hemolymph bacterial agglutinin titers and hemocytes. Opsonic factors occur in the hemolymph and enhance the phagocytosis of chicken erythrocytes. This factor appears to be equally responsible for bacterial agglutination and opsonic activity.

Hemolymph from the American cockroach, Periplaneta americana, contains erythrocyte agglutinins (Scott, 1971a,b; 1972). However, contrary to the findings just reviewed, cockroach HA does not enhance phagocytosis of vertebrate erythrocytes. Thus, some species of invertebrates seem to lack HA molecules possessing opsonic activity, although the cockroach and other related species should be reevaluated to clarify this point.

PHYSICAL AND CHEMICAL STUDIES

In Table I some of the physicochemical properties of invertebrate hemagglutinins are summarized. Various species have molecules with similar properties. However, it should be stressed that several characteristics of these HA have rendered isolation and further studies difficult. First, HA molecules have a tendency to aggregate and dissociate depending on pH and Ca^{++} ion concentration. This makes molecular weight studies extremely difficult. Also, sedimentation of HA molecules is usually dependent upon concentration. In some results, sedimentation coefficients were not determined over several concentrations and extrapolated to infinite dilution (Table I). Thus, this would account for some of

Table I. Comparison of the Physicochemical Properties of Invertebrate Hemagglutinin and Fibrinogen

	Horseshoe crab HA[a]	Oyster HA[b]	Snail HA[c]	Murray mussel HA[d]	Sea hare HA[e]	Starfish HA[f]	Crayfish HA[g]	Spiny lobster HA[h]	Spiny lobster fibrinogen[i]
Molecular weight	400,000	–	100,000	–	>150,000	–	>150,000	400,000	420,000
$S^\circ_{20,w}$	13.5	33.4	5.3	28	18.5,31	6.5	–	10.3	14.5
$D^\circ_{20,w}$								2.4	2.9
Subunit molecular weight	22,500	20,000	–	–	–	30,000	–	68,500	70,000
Carbohydrate (!)	–	8.8	7	–	–	–	–	4.6	3
Amino-terminal residues	Leucine	Threonine	–	–	–	Threonine, serine, aspartic acid, glutamic acid	–	Phenylalanine	Leucine
Calcium Dependence	+	+	–	–	0	+	–	+	+

[a] Marchalonis and Edelman, 1968a.
[b] Acton et al., 1969b.
[c] Hammarström and Kabat, 1969.
[d] Jenkin and Rowley, 1970.
[e] Pauley et al., 1971b.
[f] Finstad et al., 1972.
[g] Miller et al., 1972.
[h] Weinheimer et al., 1972.
[i] Fuller and Doolittle, 1971a,b.

the differences. The isolated molecules do not readily dissociate into respective subunits and require strong denaturing solvents in order to effect dissociation. Although reduction and alkylation are not imperative to achieve dissociation, thiol-binding reagents must be a part of the dissociating solvents to inhibit disulfide interchange and subsequent aggregation (Acton, 1970). In spite of these difficulties, it appears that the molecules share many properties. A close similarity is observed between the molecules from horseshoe crabs, oysters, and spiny lobsters where amino acid compositions and peptide maps are available. Furthermore, the importance of calcium in stabilizing the molecules and their greater effectiveness in a pH range of 7–8 suggest common properties. As previously stated, many of these molecules have specificities for N-acetylated aminosugars.

Table II depicts an analysis of carbohydrate moieties found associated with the oyster and spiny lobster HA subunit (Acton, *et al.,* 1972). Fucose, mannose, galactose, glucosamine, and sialic acid are common to both subunits. On a molar basis, the spiny lobster HA contains approximately twice as much total carbohydrate as the oyster HA. The molar quantities of the mannose and galactose were approximately proportional to the molecular weights of the subunits and accounted for most of the difference in total carbohydrate content. The ratio of galactose to mannose was approximately 1:4 in both subunits. It is tempting to speculate that both HA subunits contain an oligosaccharide of similar composition. With the spiny lobster subunit containing an additional carbohydrate moiety, the carbohydrate residues, tentatively identified from the snail HA and spiny lobster fibrinogen molecule, are also similar to those from the oyster and spiny

Table II. Carbohydrate Composition
of Hemagglutinin Subunit

	Oyster		Lobster	
	%	Moles per subunit[a]	%	Moles per subunit[b]
Fucose	0.6	0.8	0.1	0.4
Mannose	3.7	4.2	2.9	10.9
Galactose	1.5	1.1	0.6	2.4
Glu $NH_2^{[c]}$	2.7	3.0	0.8	3.0
Sialic acid[d]	0.2	0.1	0.2	0.5
Total CHO[e]	8.8	9.2	4.6	17.2

[a]Molecular weight of subunit = 20,000.
[b]Molecular weight of subunit = 68,000.
[c]Glucosamine as free base.
[d]Sialic acid as N-acetylneuraminic acid.
[e]Total carbohydrate as sum of monosaccharides.

lobster HA. Perhaps what is most intriguing about the physicochemical data is the similarity of spiny lobster fibrinogen with HA molecules.

COMMENTS AND CONCLUSIONS

We will now turn to a final discussion of the significance of these similarities and attempt to present a unifying concept of their relationship to invertebrate defense mechanisms. The data just presented suggest that invertebrate hemagglutinins are functionally and structurally related. Since many invertebrate species can synthesize bactericidins, hemolysins, and other factors that rid hosts of infectious agents, we can speculate more easily about analogies between these components and those involved in vertebrate immunity (Acton et al., 1969a; Day et al., 1970; Evans et al., 1968, 1969a,b,c; Cushing et al., 1969; McKay and Jenkin, 1970b; Weinheimer et al., 1969a; Weinheimer et al., 1970). At least in the spiny lobster, the hemagglutinins, bactericidins, and erythrocyte hemolysins are apparently separate entities (Weinheimer, 1970b). Furthermore, there seems to be a progression from the primitive invertebrates toward a more complex system, as that of the spiny lobster. For example, the oyster, which possesses hemagglutinins, lacks hemolysins, bactericidins, and clotting factors (Acton et al., 1968; Weinheimer, et al., 1969b). The earthworm may lack bactericidins but not clotting factors (Cooper et al., 1969, 1973), while the sipunculid worm only lacks clotting factors (Cushing et al., 1969; Evans, et al., 1969b; Weinheimer et al., 1970). Thus, primitive creatures may not have acquired the complexity of hemolymph components operative in arthropods (Evans et al., 1969d). The similarities between the HA prompts speculation that such molecules were the primitive receptor molecules that evolved in invertebrates to assist in the protection against foreign intrusion by pathogens, the precursor gene being one which coded for a molecule of about 20,000 molecular weight. By fused and contiguous gene duplication and possible translocation, genes evolved coding for hemagglutinin molecules of about 69,000, as found in the spiny lobster. These genes underwent considerable mutation producing molecules with diverse functions such as hemolysins, bactericidins, and clotting factors. This speculation is supported by the physicochemical relationship between spiny lobster hemagglutinins and fibrinogen (Weinheimer et al., 1972; Fuller and Doolittle, 1971a). However, it should be stressed that final resolution will emerge only when detailed structural analysis of these molecules has been carried out.

Finally, we reiterate that all invertebrate hemolymph components interact to provide immune defense mechanisms. One can easily visualize how molecules which agglutinate and lyse bacteria would be essential. Additional evidence implies that invertebrate clotting mechanisms are involved in responses to disease agents (Bang, 1970; Rabin, 1970; Stewart et al., 1969). In many ways, such reactions mimic those of vertebrate immune mechanisms. In vertebrate animals, foreign antigenic material stimulates antibody synthesis which binds to antigens forming complexes. These complexes bind complement that initiates a whole array of inflammatory reactions (Gigli and Austen, 1971). Moreover, much evidence points to participation of various components of vertebrate blood coagulation system in inflammatory responses (Austen, 1971; McKay, 1972). One manner for effecting this is by activating the complement system via a pathway that bypasses the need for antigen and antibody. In other words, complement is a system of proteins which mediates a number of reactions such as cell lysis, chemotaxis, agglutination, and phagocytosis. Although antigen and antibody complexes can initiate the reaction mechanisms of complement, there exist other means of accomplishing this.

Certainly, many molecules mediating reactions of the complement system could have evolved before those requiring antigen and antibody complexes. The molecular mechanisms responsible for generating antibody diversity, whereby an array of antibody molecules are synthesized with specificities for an almost infinite number of antigens, is such a complicated one that it may have evolved quite late or to only a limited extent earlier. Thus, some resemblance of the vertebrate complement system with several effector mechanisms of sequestering infectious agents may have evolved early and still be operative in present-day invertebrates. Evidence supporting this view is derived from studies by Day et al. (1970). According to their findings, some species of invertebrates possess hemolymph activities resembling those mediated by the terminal components of the vertebrate complement system. This is an important clue and represents the most striking similarity yet between invertebrate and vertebrate components involved in immunity. Finally, the available physical and chemical data on invertebrate hemagglutinins suggest no homology with vertebrate immunoglobulins. However, detailed primary structural data must be available to settle this question unequivocally.

An alternative hypothesis holds that many genes coding for invertebrate hemolymph factors were lost with the emergence of vertebrates. A hemagglutinin molecule has, in fact, been demonstrated in the lamprey, the most primitive vertebrate, which differs from lamprey immunoglobulins (Marchalonis and Edelman, 1968b). It would be interesting to investigate this molecule further since it may be a remnant from invertebrates.

Hopefully, this review will stimulate additional work to either prove or disprove our speculations. If that is the case, then we shall be pleased, for it is our conviction that the invertebrates can serve as useful models to aid in achieving greater insight into the evolution of immunity and to the means of manipulating this mechanism.

ACKNOWLEDGMENTS

During the years that we have been involved with various aspects of invertebrate immunity, there have been several individuals who have contributed experimentally or conceptually to our approaches. Most notable are Drs. E. E. Evans, J. Claude Bennett, Ralph E. Schrohenloher, Bill Niedermeier, Edwin L. Cooper, and Ray D. Owen, to whom we express our great appreciation. We would also like to thank Robert Mathewson of the Lerner Marine Laboratory, Bimini, Bahamas, and Lt. Gordon McCall of the Florida Board of Conservation, Panama City, Florida, for providing facilities.

REFERENCES

Acton, R. T., 1970, Immunobiological and Immunochemical Studies of the Oyster, *Crassostrea virginica,* pp. 86; Doctoral Thesis, Department of Microbiology, University of Alabama in Birmingham, Birmingham, Alabama.

Acton, R. T. and Evans, E. E., 1968, Comparative immunological studies with the oyster, *Crassostrea virginica, In Vitro 3*:146-153.

Acton, R. T., Bennett, J. C., Evans, E. E., and Schrohenloher, R. E., 1969*b*, Physical and chemical characterization of an oyster hemagglutinin, *J. Biol. Chem. 244*:4128-4135.

Acton, R. T., Weinheimer, P. F., and Evans, E. E., 1969, A bactericidal system in the lobster, *Homarus americanus, J. Invertebr. Pathol. 13*:463-464.

Acton, R. T., Weinheimer, P. F., and Niedermeier, W., 1973, The carbohydrate composition of invertebrate hemagglutinin subunits isolated from the lobster *Panulirus argus* and the oyster *Crassostrea virginica, Comp. Biochem. Physiol. 44*:185-189.

Austen, K. F., 1971, Chemical mediators of the acute inflammatory response in man, in: *Progress in Immunology,* pp. 723-744, (B. Amos, ed.), Academic Press, New York.

Bang, F. B., 1970, Cellular aspects of blood clotting in the seastar and the hermit crab, *J. Reticuloendothelial Soc. 7*:161-172.

Bernheimer, A. W., 1952, Hemagglutinins in caterpillar blood, *Science 155*:150-151.

Bizot, M., 1971, Hemagglutinin from the snail *Eobania vermiculate, Vox Sanguinis 21*:465-468.

Boyd, W. C. and Brown, R., 1965, A specific agglutinin in the snail *Otala (Helix) lactea, Nature 208*:593-594.

Boyd, W. C., Brown, R., and Boyd, L. G., 1966, Agglutinins for human erythrocytes in Mollusks, *J. Immunol. 96*:301-303.

Boyden, S. V., 1966, Natural antibodies and the immune response, *Adv. Immunol. 5*:1-28.

Brown, R., Almodovar, L. R., Bhatia, H. M., and Boyd, W. C., 1968, Blood group specific agglutinins in invertebrates, *J. Immol. 100*:214-216.

Burnet, F. M., 1968, Evolution of the immune process in vertebrates, *Nature 218*:426-430.

Cohen, E., 1968, Immunological observations of the agglutinins of the hemolymph of *Limulus polyphemus* and *Birgus latro, Trans. N. Y. Acad. Sci. 30*:427-443

Cohen, E., Rose, A. W., and Wissler, F. C., 1962, Heteroagglutinins of the horseshoe crab, *Limulus polyphemus, Life Sci. 4*: 2009-2015.

Cooper, E. L., Acton, R. T., Weinheimer, P. H. and Evans, E. E., 1969, Lack of a bactericidal response in the earthworm *Lumbrious terrestris* after immunization with bacterial antigens, *J. Invertebr. Pathol. 14*:402-406.

Cooper, E. L., Lemmi, M. A., and Moore, T., 1973, Agglutinins and cellular immunity in earthworms, *Ann. N. Y. Acad. Sci. (in press).*

Cushing, J. E., Calaprice, N. L., and Trump, G., 1963, Blood group reactive substances in some marine invertebrates, *Biol. Bull. 125*:69-80.

Cushing, J. E., McNeely, J. L., and Tripp, M. R., 1969, Comparative immunology of sipunculid coelomic fluid, *J. Invertebr. Pathol. 14*:4-12.

Day, N. K. B., Gewarz, H., Johannsem, R., Finstad, J., and Good, R. A., 1970, Complement and complement-like activity in lower vertebrates and invertebrates, *J. Exp. Med.* *132*:941-950.

Evans, E. E., Painter, B., Evans, M. L., Weinheimer, P., and Acton, R. T., 1968, An induced bactericidin in the spiny lobster, *Panulirus argus, Proc. Soc. Exp. Biol. Med.* *128*:394-398.

Evans, E. E., Weinheimer, P. F., Painter, B., Acton, R. T., and Evans, M. L., 1969*a*, Secondary and tertiary responses of the induced bactericidin from the West Indian spiny lobster, *Panulirus argus, J. Bacteriol.* *98*:943-946.

Evans, E. E., Weinheimer, P. F., Acton, R. T., and Cushing, J. E., 1969*b*, Induced bactericidal response in a sipunculid worm, *Nature 223*:695.

Evans, E. E., Cushing, J. E., Sawyer, S., Weinheimer, P. F., Acton, R. T., and McNeely, J. L., 1969*c*, Induced bactericidal response in the California spiny lobster *Panulirus interruptus, Proc. Soc. Exp. Biol. Med. 132*:111-114.

Evans, E. E., Acton, R. T., Bennett, J. C., and Weinheimer, P. F., 1969*d*, Evolution of the immune response. In: *Protides of the Biological Fluids,* (H. Peeters, ed.), Pergamon Press, Oxford, pp. 29-38.

Finstad, C. L., Litman, G. W., Finstad, J., and Good, R. A., 1972, The evolution of the immune response. XIII. The characterization of purified erythrocyte agglutinins from two invertebrate species, *J. Immunol. 108*:1704-1711.

Fuller, G. M. and Doolittle, R. F., 1971*a*, Studies of invertebrate fibrinogen. I. Purification and characterization of fibrinogen from the spiny lobster, *Biochemistry 10*:1305-1311.

Fuller, G. M. and Doolittle, R. F., 1971*b*, Studies of invertebrate fibrinogen. II. Transformation of lobster fibronogen into fibrin, *Biochemistry 10*:1311-1315.

Gigli, J. and Austen, K. F., 1971, Phylogeny and function of the complement system, *Ann. Rev. Microbiol. 25*:309-332.

Hammarström, S. and Kabat, E. A., 1969, Purification and characterization of a bloodgroup. A reactive hemagglutinin from the snail *Helix pomatia* and a study of its combining site, *Biochemistry 8*:2696-2705.

Hammarström, S. and Kabat, E. A., 1971, Studies on specificity and binding properties of the blood group. A reactive hemagglutinin from *Helix pomatia, Biochemistry 10*:1684-1692.

Ishiyama, I. and Uhlenbruck, G., 1972, Further studies on the specificity of the anti-A agglutinin from *Helix pomatia, Comp. Biochem. Physiol. 42A*:269-276.

Jenkins, C. R. and Rowley, D., 1970, Immunity in invertebrates. The purification of a hemmaglutinin to rat, rabbit erythrocytes from the hemolymph of the murray mussel (*Velesunio ambiguus*), *Australian J. Exp. Biol. Med. Sci. 48*: 129-137.

Kühnemund, O. and Kohler, W., 1969, Untersuchungen uber die Reingung des Protectins Anti-Anel (Anti-A$_{HP}$) aus *Helix pomatia, Experientia 25*:1137-1138.

McDade, J. E. and Tripp, M. R., 1967, Mechanisms of agglutination of red blood cells by oyster hemolymph, *J. Invertebr. Pathol. 9*:523-530.

McKay, G. D., 1972, Participation of components of the blood coagulation system in the inflammatory response, *Am. J. Pathol. 67*:181-204.

McKay, D. and Jenkin, C. R., 1970*a*, Immunity in the invertebrates. The role of serum factors in phagocytosis of erythrocytes by hemocytes of the fresh-water crayfish (*Parachaeraps bicarinatus*), *Australian J. Exp. Biol. Med. Sci. 48*:139-150.

McKay, D. and Jenkin, C. R., 1970*b*, Immunity in the invertebrates. The fate and distribution of bacteria in normal and immunized crayfish (*Parachaeraps bicarinatus*),, *Australian J. Exp. Biol. Med. Sci. 48*:599-607.

McKay, D. and Jenkins, C. R., 1970c, Immunity in the invertebrates. Correlation of the phagocytic activity of hemocytes with resistance to infection in the crayfish (*Parachaeraps vicarinatus*), *Australian J. Exp. Biol. Med. Sci. 48*:609-617.

McKay, D., Jenkin, C. R., and Rowley, D., 1969, Immunity in the invertebrates I. Studies on the naturally occurring hemagglutinins in the fluid from invertebrates. *Australian J. Exp. Biol. Med. Sci. 47*:125-134.

Marchalonis, J. J. and Edelman, G. M., 1968a, Isolation and characterization of a hemagglutinin from *Limulus polyphemus*, *J. Mol. Biol. 32*:453-465.

Marchalonis, J. J. and Edelman, G. M., 1968b, Phylogenetic origins of antibody structure. III. Antibodies in the primary immune response of the sea lamprey, *Petromyzon marinus*, *J. Exp. Med. 127*:891-914.

Miller, V. H., Ballback, R. S., Pauley, G. B., and Krassner, S. M., 1972, A preliminary physiochemical characterization of an agglutinin found in the hemolymph of the crayfish *Procambarus clarkii*, *J. Invertebr. Pathol. 19*:83-93.

Pauley, G. B., Granger, G. A., and Krassner, S. M., 1971a, Characterization of a natural agglutinin present in the hemolymph of the California sea hare, *Aplysia californica*, *J. Invertebr. Pathol. 18*:207-218.

Pauley, G. B., Krassner, S. M., and Chapman, F. A., 1971b, Bacterial clearance in the California sea hare, *Aplysia californica*, *J. Invertebr. Pathol. 18*:227-239.

Prokop, O., Schlesinger, D., and Rackwitz, O., 1965, Uber eine thermostabile "antibody-like substance" (Anti-A$_{hel}$) bei *Helix pomatia* und derem Herkunft, *Z. Immunitaetsforsch. 129*:402-412.

Prokop, O., Uhlenbruck, G., and Kohler, W., 1968, A new source of antibody-like substance having anti-blood groups specificity, *Vox Sanguinis 14*:321-333.

Prowse, R. H. and Tait, N. N., 1969, *In vitro* phagacytosis by amoebocytes from the hemolymph of *Helix aspersa* (Muller). I. Evidence for opsonic factor(s) in serum, *Immunology 17*:437-443.

Rabin, H., 1970, Hemocytes, hemolymph and defense reactions in Crustaceans, *J. Reticuloendothelial Soc. 1*:195-207.

Schnitzler, St. and Kilias, R., 1970, Uber das Vorkommen von Hamagglutinin bei Landlungenschnecken, *Blut. 20*:221.

Scott, M. T., 1971a, A naturally occurring hemagglutinin in the hemolymph of the American cockroach, *Arch. Zool. Exp. Gen.* 112:73-80.

Scott, M. T., 1971b, Recognition of foreignness in invertebrates. II. *In vitro* studies of cockroach phagocytic hemocytes, *Immunology 21*:817-828.

Scott, M. T., 1972, Partial characterization of the hemagglutinating activity in hemolymph of the American cockroach (*Periplaneta americana*), *J. Invertebr. Pathol. 19*:66-71.

Stewart, J. E., Arie, B., Zwicker, B. U., and Dingle, J. R., 1969, Gaffkemia, a bacterial disease of the lobster, *Homarus americanus:* Effects of the pathogen, *Gaffkya homari*, on the physiology of the host, *Can. J. Microbiol. 15*:925-932.

Stuart, A. E., 1958, The reticuloendothelial apparatus of the lesser octopus, *Eledone cirrosa*, *J. Pathol. Bacteriol. 96*:401.

Tripp, M. R., 1966, Hemagglutinin in the blood of the oyster, *Crassostrea virginica*, *J. Invertebr. Pathol. 8*:478-484.

Tyler, A., 1946, Natural heteroagglutinins in the body fluids and seminal fluids of various invertebrates, *Biol. Bull. 90*:213-219.

Tyler, A. and Metz, C. B., 1945, Natural heteroagglutinins in the serum of the spiny lobster, *Panulirus interruptus*. I. Taxonomic range of activity of electrophoretic and immunizing properties, *J. Exp. Zool. 100*:377-406.

Tyler, A. and Scheer, B. T., 1945, Natural heteroagglutinins in the serum of the spiny lobster, *Panulirus interruptis.* II. Chemical and antigenic relation to blood proteins, *Biol. Bull. 89*:193-200.

Uhlenbruck, G. and Prokop, O., 1966, An agglutinin from *Helix pomatia* which reacts with terminal *N*-acetyl-D-galactosamine, *Vox Sanguinis 11*:519-520.

Weinheimer, P. F., 1970*b*, "Characterization of erythrocyte-reactive factors of *Panulirus argus:* A contribution to immunophylogeny," Doctoral Thesis, Department of Microbiology, University of Alabama in Birmingham, Birmingham, Alabama.

Weinheimer, Peter F., 1970*a*, Immunophylogeny. A review of immune-like mechanisms of invertebrate species, *Alabama J. of Med. Sci. 7*:451-460.

Weinheimer, P. F., Evans, E. E., Stroud, R. M., Acton, R. T., and Painter, B., 1969*a*, Comparative Immunology: Natural hemolytic system of the spiny lobster, *Panulirus argus, Proc. Soc. Exp. Biol. Med. 130*:322-326.

Weinheimer, P. F., Acton, R. T., and Evans, E. E., 1969*b*, An attempt to induce a bactericidal response in the oyster, *J. Bacteriol. 97*:462-463.

Weinheimer, P. F., Acton, R. T., Cushing, J. E., and Evans, E. E., 1970, Reactions of sipunculid coelomic fluid with erythrocytes, *Life Sci. 9*:145-152.

Weinheimer, P. F., Acton, R. T., Evans, E. E., and Bennett, J. C., 1974, Characterization of the natural hemagglutinin from the spiny lobster, *Panulirus argus, Biochemistry* (submitted for publication).

Chapter 24

Tumors in Drosophila
and Antibacterial Immunity

Walter J. Burdette

The University of Texas
Medical School at Houston
Houston, Texas

TUMORS IN *DROSOPHILA*

Melanotic tumors in *Drosophila* have been the subject of much interest and some controversy since the first strain bearing these hereditary tumors was reported by Bridges in 1916. The tumors consist of aggregates of polygonal and fusiform cells that appear early in life, do not divide, but gradually undergo dissolution and pigmentation as metamorphosis proceeds. They are usually scored by determining the residual melanin in larval, pupal, and imaginal stages (Fig. 1). We collected a large number of strains and studied their behavior in response to various treatments (Burdette, 1951, 1959a; Burdette and Carver, 1970). All those which we examined were benign, and susceptibility was found to be related to multiple genes. Usually there are modifying genes that enhance or suppress respectively the main gene(s). Some of the main genes have been located precisely, and more of the genes for susceptibility are located on the second chromosome than elsewhere. However, one, two, three, or all chromosomes carry these genes in some strains. In a series of interstrain crosses, we found that very few of the genes are alleles (Burdette and Olivier, 1951). Penetrance varies from less than 1 to more than 99%, depending on the strain, temperature, nutrition, and other conditions of culture (Burdette, 1952a 1959a; Herskowitz and Burdette, 1951). Chromosomal aberrations are not obligate for tumors to appear, and we were able to obtain back mutation with x-irradiation in one strain, thus eliminating the possibility that the effect resulted from a small deletion (Burdette, 1959a). No consistent increment or decrement in inci-

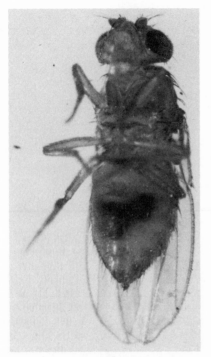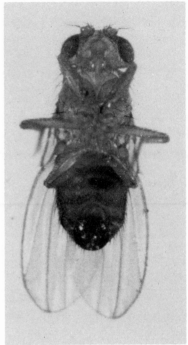

Fig. 1. *Drosophila* with melanotic tumors.

dence was obtained when heterochromatin in the form of hyperploid or hypo-
ploid Y chromosomes were varied in tumor strains of *Drosophila* (Burdette,
1959*b*).

Nitrogen mustard (Burdette, 1952*b*), 20-methylcholanthrene (Burdette,
1952*c*), irradiation, and other agents increase the numbers of tumors that appear
in the population of these strains (Burdette, 1959*a*). Introduction of the genoid
for CO_2 sensitivity seemed to lower the incidence of the turmors (Burdette,
1958). When tumor genes were introduced into Florida stocks that exhibited
high spontaneous rates of mutation, no consistent alteration in incidence of
tumors was obtained (Burdette, 1954*a*). The introduction of both oncogenic
RNA and DNA virus by feeding and inoculation increased the incidence of these
tumors (Burdette, 1968; Burdette and Yoon, 1967).

We (Burdette, 1954*b,c* 1964) found that genetic damage to ring gland and
ligation of larvae at appropriate stages to impede the flow of hormone from the
gland resulted in more tumors. Recently, Madhavan (1972) has been able to
increase the number of tumors appearing by administering juvenile hormone.
Thus the cells constituting the tumors still respond to the stimulus of molting
and juvenile hormones.

In addition to these hereditary melanotic tumors, flies with tumorous head appearing when the tu^h gene is homozygous (Newby, 1948), transplantable imaginal discs that do not metamorphose autotypically (Gateff and Schneiderman, 1968), and the ovarian tumors that appear when *fes* and *fu* genes (King, 1968; Ghelelovitch, 1959) act, represent aggregations of cells similar to those occurring normally at their point of origin. Also, Gateff and Schneiderman (1968) found they could transplant a malignant neuroblastoma, derived from the brain of flies with the *l(2)gl*^{4} gene homozygones as serial transfers, to the abdomens of adults. However, the probable aggregation of hemocytes along with a stroma of fusiform cells that constitutes the hereditary melanotic tumors in many of the strains (King, 1968; Ghelelovitch, 1959) identifies this group as most suitable for use in scrutinizing immune mechanisms.

BACTERIAL IMMUNITY IN STRAINS OF *DROSOPHILA* WITH AND WITHOUT HEREDITARY MELANOTIC TUMORS

Since hemocytes have been looked upon as constituting the principal component in aggregates of cells that are called hereditary melanotic tumors in some strains of *Drosophila*, the antibacterial immunity in a strain of *Drosophila* with known major genes for susceptibility to these tumors has been compared to one without. Bowman *et al.* (1972) have reported that inducible bacterial defenses can be demonstrated in *Drosophila* by using strains of bacteria resistant to antibiotics and determining number of bacteria present after a single injection of organisms subsequent to vaccination with organisms frozen and thawed.

Parallel studies were carried out with the *Oregon R* and $tu^{48a}vg\,bw$ strains of *Drosophila*. Males up to 4 days of age were inoculated with 1×10^2 to 1×10^5 streptomycin-sensitive *Aerobacter cloacae* that had been attenuated or killed by rapid freezing and thawing in 0.025 µl of *Drosophila* Ringer's solution. Then, injections were repeated later with a similar dose of streptomycin-resistant organisms of the same strain as follows. Flies used as controls received an initial injection of 0.025 µl of saline without the organisms, and in 48 hr one group received another similar injection of saline and another group was inoculated with the same titer of streptomycin-resistant *Aerobacter cloacae* in 0.025 µl of *Drosophila* Ringer's solution. Groups of ten flies were homogenized after the intervals given in the tables and plated in appropriate dilution for tabulating the number of colonies growing out in 24 hr on medium containing streptomycin. Two hundred males were inoculated at each interval, and numerous experiments were done to obtain individuals not affected by the procedure of injection itself. The results are presented in four tables in order to group them by strain of *Drosophila* tested and numbers of bacteria in the inoculum.

Table I. Mean Number of *Aerobacter cloacae* Growing after
Vaccination and Administration of the Organisms by
Abdominal Injection to the *Oregon R* Strain of *Drosophila*

Interval	Bacteria × 10^2/Fly	
	Controls	Vaccinated
Dosage	6.0	6.0
10 min	2.2	1.4
20 min	2.1	1.4
40 min	1.2	0.67
20 hr	1.3	0.05

Table II. Mean Number of *Aerobacter cloacae* Growing after
Vaccination and Administration of the Organisms by
Abdominal Injection to the *Oregon R* Strain of *Drosophila*

Interval	Bacteria × 10^2/Fly	
	Controls	Vaccinated
Dosage	130.0	130.0
10 min	13.6	6.6
30 min	10.0	3.0
2 hr	10.0	0.66
4 hr	3.0	0.10
20 hr	2.6	0.15

Table III. Mean Number of *Aerobacter cloacae* Growing after
Vaccination and Administration of the Organisms by Abdominal
Injection to the $tu^{48a}vg\ bw$ Strain of *Drosophila*

Interval	Bacteria × 10^2/Fly	
	Controls	Vaccinated
Dosage	65	65
10 min	5.3	9.5
30 min	3.0	2.9
2 hr	2.6	2.4
20 hr	3.6	6.0

Table IV. Mean Number of *Aerobacter cloacae* Growing
after Vaccination and Administration of the Organisms by Abdominal
Injection to the $tu^{48a}vg\ bw$ Strain of *Drosophila*

Interval	Bacteria $\times 10^2$/Fly	
	Controls	Vaccinated
Dosage	700	700
10 min	1.2	5
2 hr	2.5	5.7

The cultures grew only the resistant organisms, and no problems were encountered in identifying the numbers evolved from the original inoculum of resistant organisms. Exactly the same inoculum of resistant bacteria was not used in each group of experiments, but a high and low dosage was used in both strains of *Drosophila* tested.

The information in Tables I and II clearly suggests that the vaccination procedure was associated consistently with lower numbers of surviving bacteria in the *Oregon R* strain at all intervals of time tested from 10 min to 20 hr with both the high and low titers. On the other hand, lower numbers of bacteria were found after vaccination in only two intervals with the lower initial titer in the $tu^{48a}vg\ bw$ strain, and these differences were only slight (Table III). For all other tests, the counts were higher after vaccination (Tables III and IV). Therefore, the tumor strain was more susceptible to the organisms after vaccination than the *Oregon R* strain in these preliminary experiments. In the tumor strain, which exhibits a very high incidence of spontaneous melanotic tumors, the antibacterial-defense system apparently is impaired. Since the tumors probably represent altered behavior of hemocytes, it is possible that the immune-defense mechanism detected by such experiments is, at least in part, cellular.

ACKNOWLEDGMENTS

This study was aided by a grant, CA 10037, from the National Cancer Institute, U.S. Public Health Service. The technical assistance of Claudia Chen, Matilda Olive, and Karen Robertson is gratefully acknowledged.

REFERENCES

Boman, H. G., Nilsson, Ingrid, and Rasmuson, Bertil, 1972, Inducible antibacterial defence system in *Drosophila. Nature 237*:232-235.
Bridges, C. B., 1916, Non-disjunction as proof of the chromosome theory of heredity, *Genetics 1*:107-163.

Burdette, W. J., 1951, Incidence of Tumors in Different Strains of *Drosophila, D.I.S.* 25:101-102.

Burdette, W. J., 1952*a*, Incidence of tumors in isogenic strains, *J. Nat. Cancer Inst.* 12:709-714.

Burdette, W. J., 1952*b*, Effect of nitrogen mustard on tumor incidence and lethal mutation rate in *Drosophila, Cancer Res.* 12:366-368.

Burdette, W. J., 1952*c*, Tumor incidence and lethal mutation rate in *Drosophila* treated with 20-methylcholanthrene, *Cancer Res.* 12:201-205.

Burdette, W. J., 1954*a*, Effect of mutator, *HIGH*, on tumor incidence in *Drosophila, Cancer Res.* 14:149-153.

Burdette, W. J., 1954*b*, Effect of ligation of *Drosophila* larvae on tumor incidence, *Cancer Res.* 14:780-782.

Burdette, W. J., 1954*c*, Effect of defective ring gland in incidence of tumors in *Drosophila, J. Nat. Cancer Inst.* 15:367-376.

Burdette, W. J., 1958, The effect of the genoid for CO_2 sensitivity on tumor incidence, *Proc. Am. Assoc. Cancer Res.* 2:285.

Burdette, W. J., 1959*a*, Tumors in *Drosophila*, Biological Contributions, *Texas Univ. Publ.* No. 5914:57-68.

Burdette, W. J., 1959*b*, Mutagenesis and carcinogenesis, in: *Radiation Biology and Cancer*, pp. 349-358, University of Texas Press, Austin.

Burdette, W. J., 1964, The significance of invertebrate hormones in relation to differentiation, *Cancer Res.* 24:520-536.

Burdette, W. J., 1968, Visible alterations in gene activation caused by hormone and oncogenic viruses, in: *Exploitable Molecular Mechanisms and Neoplasia* (A Collection of Papers Presented at the Twenty-second Annual Symposium on Fundamental Cancer Research), pp. 507-520, Williams and Wilkins Co., Baltimore.

Burdette, W. J. and Carver, J. E., 1970, Frequency of tumors in several laboratory stocks of *D. melanogaster, D.I.S.* 45:151.

Burdette, W. J. and Olivier, H. R., 1951, Tumor incidence and lethal mutation rate in a tumor strain of *Drosophila* treated with formaldehyde, *Cancer Res* 11:555-558.

Burdette, W. J. and Yoon, J. S., 1967, Mutations, chromosomal aberrations, and tumors in insects treated with oncogenic virus. *Science* 155:340-341.

Gateff, E. and Schneiderman, H. A., 1968, Neoplasms in mutant and cultured wild-type tissues of *Drosophila*, in: *Smithsonian Institution Symposium on Neoplasia of Invertebrate Animals*, pp. 365-397, U.S. Government Printing Office, Washington, D.C.

Ghelelovitch, S., 1959, Une Tumeur Héréditaire de la Drosophile (*Drosophila melanogaster Meig.*), in: *Etude Génétique, Physiologique, et Histologique*, pp. 153, Maurice Declum, Paris.

Herskowitz, I. H. and Burdette, W. J., 1951, Some genetic and environmental influences on the incidence of a melanotic tumor in *Drosophila, J. Exp. Zool.* 117:499-522.

King, R. C., 1968, Hereditary ovarian tumors of *Drosophila melanogaster*, in: *Smithsonian Institution Symposium on Neoplasia of Invertebrate Animals*, pp. 323-345, U.S. Government Printing Office, Washington, D.C.

Madhaven, K., 1972, Induction of melanotic pseudotumors in *Drosophila melanogaster* by juvenile hormone, *Arch. Entwicklungsmech. Organ.* 169:345-349.

Newby, W. W., 1948, Abnormal growths on the head of *Drosophila melanogaster, J. Morphol.* 85:177-195.

Chapter 25

A Final Comment on Invertebrate Immunity

M. R. Tripp

Department of Biology
University of Delaware
Newark, Delaware

It is often assumed that we know enough about the immune mechanisms of animals to arrange them in linear sequence from the first eukaryote cell through to man. There is no compelling reason to believe that this is true. The underlying assumption made is that protective devices found in one group are elaborated in the next, more complex group. This is not true for other homeostatic devices, and the evidence available now does not support the notion that there has been straight-line evolution of immune mechanisms. Invertebrates have been around longer than vertebrates and have found a variety of solutions to common problems in the course of their evolutionary histories. The findings reported in this volume support this contention.

Consider first the principles of vertebrate immune responses. The general pattern involves endocytosis of antigen, intracellular "processing" of antigen, passing information to other cells (B + T cells in mammals), and in many cases the elaboration of immunoglobulins by immunocytes. The complex cellular machinery needed for this immune response is housed in an organism of some size with physiological stability guaranteed by a series of homeostatic devices. The complex immunoglobulin molecules represent a significant part (approximately 0.02% according to Hood and Prahl, 1971) of the genetic coding in the system and require a relatively large energy investment also. These organisms typically have long generation times and few progeny compared to invertebrates. Thus, the individual vertebrate has a complex specific response to immunogens that tend to protect the individual and ensure survival for reproduction.

The invertebrates, on the other hand, present a different situation. Foreign substances in their tissues also elicit phagocytosis (or encapsulation) and intracellular destruction of some materials, but immunoglobulins are not produced.

Protective humoral substances are elaborated, but they are nonspecific, of short duration, and are not protein. The evidence available to date suggests that the combination of cellular and humoral factors in invertebrates confers only minimal protection for the individual. Other characteristics of invertebrates are small size, more direct effects of the environment on individuals, shorter generation times, and large numbers of progeny. This suggests a very different evolutionary strategy for invertebrates, namely, minimal protection for the individual with heavy reliance on high reproductive potential to replace diseased individuals. If this is the strategy used, there is no need to assume any appreciable correspondence between defense mechanisms of invertebrates and vertebrates. Yet, these reports, when taken together, represent an impressive start on a reexamination and elaboration of our concepts about the basis of invertebrate immunologic responses.

REFERENCES

Hood, L. and Prahl, J., 1971, The immune system: a model for differentiation in higher organisms, *Adv. Immunol. 14*:291-351.

Index